Handbook of Health Geography

Editor: Caleb Coleman

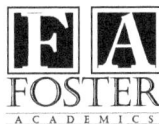

FA FOSTER
ACADEMICS

www.fosteracademics.com

www.fosteracademics.com

FA
FOSTER
ACADEMICS

Cataloging-in-Publication Data

Handbook of health geography / edited by Caleb Coleman.
     p. cm.
Includes bibliographical references and index.
ISBN 978-1-63242-950-6
1. Medical geography. 2. Medical climatology. 3. Health. 4. Medical care. I. Coleman, Caleb.
RA792 .H36 2020
614.42--dc23

Foster Academics,
118-35 Queens Blvd., Suite 400,
Forest Hills, NY 11375, USA

ISBN 978-1-63242-950-6 (Hardback)

Contents

Preface

Health geography is the field concerned with the analysis of spatial patterns of disease and healthcare provision. Geography encompasses the study of human-environment interaction and influences of the biophysical, social and built environment. Health geography is a holistic field, which draws on the principles and concepts of geography, and the social and biophysical sciences. Various quantitative and qualitative methodologies are incorporated for guiding such studies. The geography of health services involves the study of the access to healthcare services, their planning and delivery. Medical geographic studies of diseases are placed in the context of disease ecology, while spatial or geographic epidemiology studies focus on the spatial aspects of healthcare. This book discusses the fundamentals as well as modern approaches of health geography. It elucidates the concepts and innovative models around prospective developments with respect to health geography. This book, with its detailed analyses and data, will prove immensely beneficial to professionals and students involved in this area at various levels.

The information shared in this book is based on empirical researches made by veterans in this field of study. The elaborative information provided in this book will help the readers further their scope of knowledge leading to advancements in this field.

Finally, I would like to thank my fellow researchers who gave constructive feedback and my family members who supported me at every step of my research.

Editor

Effects of health intervention programs and arsenic exposure on child mortality from acute lower respiratory infections in rural Bangladesh

Warren C. Jochem[1*], Abdur Razzaque[2] and Elisabeth Dowling Root[3]

Abstract

Background: Respiratory infections continue to be a public health threat, particularly to young children in developing countries. Understanding the geographic patterns of diseases and the role of potential risk factors can help improve future mitigation efforts. Toward this goal, this paper applies a spatial scan statistic combined with a zero-inflated negative-binomial regression to re-examine the impacts of a community-based treatment program on the geographic patterns of acute lower respiratory infection (ALRI) mortality in an area of rural Bangladesh. Exposure to arsenic-contaminated drinking water is also a serious threat to the health of children in this area, and the variation in exposure to arsenic must be considered when evaluating the health interventions.

Methods: ALRI mortality data were obtained for children under 2 years old from 1989 to 1996 in the Matlab Health and Demographic Surveillance System. This study period covers the years immediately following the implementation of an ALRI control program. A zero-inflated negative binomial (ZINB) regression model was first used to simultaneously estimate mortality rates and the likelihood of no deaths in groups of related households while controlling for socioeconomic status, potential arsenic exposure, and access to care. Next a spatial scan statistic was used to assess the location and magnitude of clusters of ALRI mortality. The ZINB model was used to adjust the scan statistic for multiple social and environmental risk factors.

Results: The results of the ZINB models and spatial scan statistic suggest that the ALRI control program was successful in reducing child mortality in the study area. Exposure to arsenic-contaminated drinking water was not associated with increased mortality. Higher socioeconomic status also significantly reduced mortality rates, even among households who were in the treatment program area.

Conclusion: Community-based ALRI interventions can be effective at reducing child mortality, though socioeconomic factors may continue to influence mortality patterns. The combination of spatial and non-spatial methods used in this paper has not been applied previously in the literature, and this study demonstrates the importance of such approaches for evaluating and improving public health intervention programs.

Keywords: Acute lower respiratory infection, Arsenic, Child mortality, Spatial scan statistic, Zero-inflated negative binomial, Bangladesh

*Correspondence: w.c.jochem@soton.ac.uk
[1] Department of Geography and Environment, University of Southampton, University Road, Southampton SO17 1BJ, UK
Full list of author information is available at the end of the article

Background

Acute lower respiratory infections (ALRI) are the leading cause of childhood morbidity and mortality globally and are responsible for 18 % of all deaths in children under 5 years [1, 2]. Children in less-developed countries bear the majority of the burden of disease, experiencing 97 % of the estimated 156 million new cases of pneumonia each year [3–6]. Regionally, South and Southeast Asia have some of the highest rates of respiratory infection-related mortality, with approximately 21 % of all deaths in children under 5 years old attributed to pneumonia [1]. In Bangladesh ALRI are a leading cause of morbidity and mortality among children [4, 7, 8]. Children on average experience between 0.23 and 0.47 events per year [5, 6] and over 25,000 die from pneumonia alone each year [1]. Prior studies have found that childhood ALRI is associated with poverty, malnutrition, indoor air pollution, crowded living conditions, as well as access to medical care [2, 3, 7, 9], all factors which affect immune status or increase exposure to pathogens or lung irritants [3, 10].

ALRI continues to be a serious health concern, though it is largely treatable and preventable. Vaccines designed to target two of the major causes of ALRI, pneumococcus (*Streptococcus pneumonia*) and Hib (*Haemophilus influenzae* type b), are currently available and have been found to be effective against invasive disease; however, there are significant political, economic, and logistical challenges to distributing vaccines, particularly in developing countries [11]. Additionally, since a wide variety of pathogens can cause ALRI, vaccines can only prevent a small proportion of disease and a significant number of new cases are still likely to develop [5, 10]. In the absence of these prevention strategies, community-based intervention programs designed for early ALRI case detection and treatment with antibiotics can be successful in reducing child mortality from ALRI [12].

In Matlab, Bangladesh an ALRI intervention program implemented in 1988 was successful in quickly reducing child mortality by over 50 % [13]. An evaluation of the program by Ali and colleagues [7] identified considerable geographic variation in the ALRI mortality rates experienced by groups of households (known as *baris*) in that community; however, their work was largely a descriptive visualization of smoothed rates to accompany a non-spatial regression analysis. They stopped short of testing whether those geographic patterns of mortality events occurred due to chance and exploring which contextual and environmental factors contributed to the observed differences over space. ALRI remains a persistent problem in Matlab [6, 13, 14] and there are local clusters of elevated all-cause child mortality that remain unexplained [15], necessitating this spatial study of ALRI mortality patterns.

In addition to ALRI, the widespread contamination of drinking water by inorganic arsenic in Bangladesh (see [16]) is a health threat which must be considered when examining the effects of the health intervention programs in Matlab. The arsenic contamination is an unintended consequence of successful programs begun in the 1970s that installed wells, also called *tubewells*, across the region in order to provide clean drinking water and prevent diarrheal diseases [17, 18]. Arsenic-contaminated water has no distinguishing color, smell, or taste, and it was not routinely tested for in well installations, so the contamination was not detected until health problems were identified in the mid-1990s.

Inorganic arsenic is a potent toxin that causes wide-ranging health problems as a result of its damaging effects on the immune system [19, 20]. Despite being ingested rather than inhaled, lung cells seem particularly sensitive to arsenic-contaminated drinking water as the arsenic disrupts the inflammatory response and innate immune system signaling, increasing the risk of a lower respiratory infection [21, 22]. Previous epidemiological studies have found that people exposed to arsenic are more likely to report symptoms such as frequent coughs and to show decreased lung function [23–28]. Exposure to arsenic is also associated with increasing mortality from lung cancer [29], bronchiectasis [30], and tuberculosis [31], as well as decreasing lung function [32], and increasing susceptibility to lower respiratory infections [33, 34].

The objectives of this study are twofold. The first objective is to further develop spatial statistical methods to identify local spatial clusters while testing for known and hypothesized risk factors. This work makes use of zero-inflated negative binomial regression models (ZINB) [35] and the spatial scan statistic [36], and it demonstrates the potential for using non-spatial regression techniques to adjust spatial cluster detection tests for known risk factors. The second objective is to apply these methods to re-examine an ALRI control program that was introduced in Matlab, Bangladesh and to evaluate its effects on local child mortality patterns. While the ALRI intervention program was discussed by Ali et al. [7], the methodological approach developed here provides a more appropriate test of the geographic patterns of ALRI mortality in young children. Studying spatial disease patterns is vital for understanding the role of known risk factors in order to provide more targeted and appropriate public health interventions. Spatial analysis also can be hypothesis generating and exploratory of additional factors that could generate disparities in mortality. Arsenic exposure was not considered in any earlier study evaluating the impact of the ALRI program in Matlab and the possible link between child mortality from ALRI and arsenic exposure has not been well studied. Therefore this paper reports on the population-level relationship between arsenic in drinking water and child mortality from ALRI.

Methods

Study area

This study was conducted in Matlab, a rural group of 142 villages located approximately 50 km southeast of the capital city Dhaka in central Bangladesh (Fig. 1). Since the 1960s, Matlab has been the site of a comprehensive health and demographic surveillance system (HDSS) organized by icddr,b (formerly known as the International Center for Diarrheal Disease Research, Bangladesh) which has recorded all births, deaths, and migrations as well as conducted periodic censuses in the region. The population of Matlab lives primarily in patrilineally-related groups of housing units known as *baris*, which are the unit of analysis for this study.

Starting in 1977 icddr,b initiated a series of community-based projects in Matlab providing family planning services, immunizations, and perinatal care [37]. A key feature of the project was the use of local,

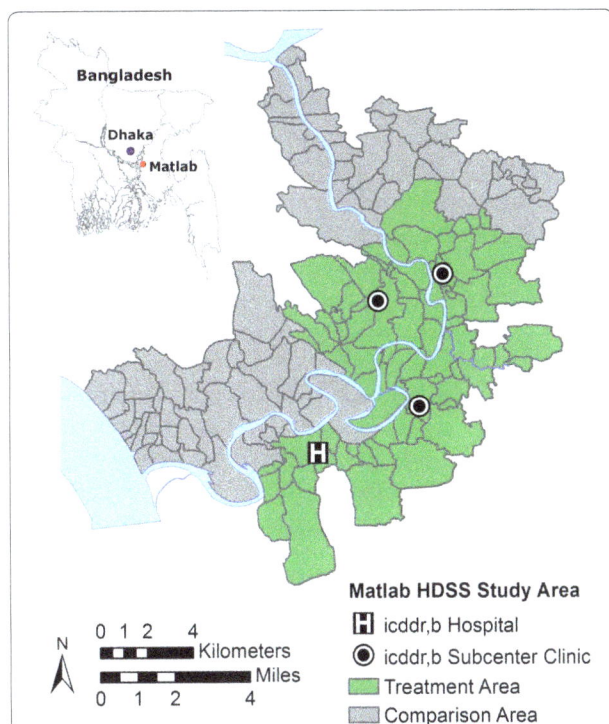

Fig. 1 The study area of Matlab, Bangladesh. The Health and Demographic Surveillance System (HDSS) area of Matlab is located in central Bangladesh. Villages were divided into two groups, one group had access to specialized medical facilities operated by icddr,b and treatment for acute lower respiratory infections and the other group (referred to as the comparison group) received standard government care. Data source: icddr,b CPUCC/GIS Unit

specially-trained, female community health workers (CHW) for service delivery and demographic surveillance. Referred to collectively as the maternal and child health and family planning program (MCH/FP), the interventions in Matlab were successful in reducing fertility and mortality by increasing the prevalence of contraceptives and vaccine use [37–39]. The MCH/FP interventions were implemented only in half of the villages in Matlab, called the "treatment area" (Fig. 1). The other villages in Matlab form two "comparison areas" adjacent to the treatment area, one in the north and the other in the southwest (Fig. 1). These areas received standard government services, but both the treatment and comparison area populations are recorded in the HDSS. Prior to the start of the MCH/FP the treatment and comparison areas had similar health and demographic measures.

ALRI control program

Beginning in 1988 the MCH/FP project expanded to include an ALRI control program [13, 40]. This community-based program was designed to reduce mortality in children under 5 years old from ALRI through a combination of health education activities for caregivers, early case detection, and management of cases using antibiotic treatment. Three outpatient, subcenter clinics as well as hospital facilities were used to treat ALRI (locations shown in Fig. 1). The ALRI program was managed by the CHWs who regularly visited households to give caretakers information on symptoms and treatment of ALRI and to identify new ALRI cases using a modified WHO case definition based on respiratory rates and other visible symptoms such as chest retractions [40, 41]. ALRI was classified as mild, moderate, or severe. Mild cases were monitored by CHW and mothers were given additional health information for supportive care. A moderate case, diagnosed as respiratory rates greater than 50 breathes per minute but without other symptoms, was treated with antibiotics. Severe pneumonia cases, defined by the presence of chest retractions and other symptoms along with respiratory rates above 50 breathes per minute or any lung infection in children under 1 month old regardless of symptoms, were referred to the icddr,b hospital in Matlab where oxygen, intravenous fluids and antibiotics were available.

Arsenic exposure

While contamination of drinking water by arsenic occurs throughout Bangladesh, the area of Matlab experiences some of the highest rates as a result of local geologic conditions [42]. The first arsenic survey of wells within Matlab conducted in 2002–2003 found 62 % of over 13,000 wells had arsenic levels above the Bangladeshi-government recommended level of 50 µg/L [43]. Studies using the HDSS data from Matlab have found that exposure to arsenic-contaminated drinking water increases risks of skin lesions, hypertension, diabetes mellitus, lung disease, and is resulting in excess adult and infant mortality [44]. Even within Matlab, arsenic contamination exhibits local-scale spatial variation due to differences in geologic conditions as well as the depth of the well [45]. Wells that tap shallower, younger aquifers are more likely to be contaminated with arsenic, while deeper wells beyond 150 m are almost entirely free of arsenic [42]. Therefore, even closely neighboring households can have different levels of arsenic exposure, and this variation in arsenic could contribute to spatial variation in disease risk.

Study data

Data for this study come from the Matlab HDSS records and include all deaths reported from pneumonia or other ALRI. Similar to Ali et al. [7], this study focuses on the population with the highest rates of ALRI, children under 2 years old, and during the years immediately following the full implementation of the ALRI control program (1989–1996) to evaluate the program's effects. This period also covers the years before knowledge of arsenic contamination was widespread and the use of wells for drinking water was common, resulting in high levels of exposure [46, 47]. HDSS data for each individual in Matlab can be linked across study years to incorporate additional census and survey data as well as linked spatially to the *bari* locations in the Matlab Geographic Information System (MGIS) [48]. Person-years for children under age 2 years in each *bari* define the population at risk. To calculate person years, each child is linked to their *baris* using a unique identification number and then followed through the HDSS records until one of three outcomes occurs: permanently out-migrate, die, or turn 2 years old. HDSS events are aggregated by *bari* across the study period to calculate the total ALRI deaths and person-years of children under 2 years (the population at risk). *Baris* are represented as point locations in the MGIS and become the unit of analysis for all analyses. A total of 7846 unique *baris* were identified during the 1989–1996 study period; though 1157 did not contain any children and were excluded from the analyses because they have no population at risk, leaving 6693 *baris*.

A *bari*-level estimate of arsenic exposure was created using data from the Matlab arsenic survey conducted in 2002–2003 which measured arsenic by lab-based hydride generation atomic absorption spectrometry (HG-AAS) and mapped wells using global position system receivers [49]. A retrospective estimate of potential exposure was created in two steps. First the 1996 census was used to find households drinking from tubewells versus surface

water sources (i.e. ponds, rivers, canals). Surface water is largely free of arsenic, but *baris* with households using tubewells are potentially exposed. *Baris* were assumed to experience the average concentration of arsenic in all wells owned by the *bari*. Following a similar procedure to Carrel et al. [50], well ownership was based on HDSS identification numbers linking wells to *baris*. If a *bari* did not have a tubewell defined by the identification number, but still reported drinking from a well, the arsenic concentration of the nearest well (based on straight line distance) identified in the MGIS was used. Arsenic levels are generally stable over time [42, 51, 52], lending support for this approach; however, the differences in study years and arsenic measures presents certain limitations to our study which we discuss later.

Additional covariates used when adjusting the models include whether the *bari* was located in the treatment area, *bari*-level socioeconomic status, and cost distance to an ALRI treatment center. Area-level socioeconomic status (SES) has been shown to influence lower respiratory infections in other contexts [53, 54], and, within Matlab, SES is linked with nutritional status which has implications for a child's immune system health [40]. It can be difficult to estimate household wealth or status in contexts without well-defined income. Therefore, similar to previous studies [15, 55–57], SES was estimated using a principal component analysis (PCA) of 1996 census data indicating the ownership of household assets (blanket/quilt, bed, lamp, watch, bicycle) as well as the material of the house walls. The *bari*-level SES score is the average of the first principal component score for all households in the *bari*. The *bari* SES was then divided into quintiles, and dichotomized with the top two quintiles considered high socioeconomic status.

Cost distance is a measure of accessibility or effort to reach a treatment center that considers both distance and physical barriers. A similar measure was found to be significant in the earlier study of ALRI mortality in Matlab [7] and the same procedure is used here. The accessibility from each *bari* point location was measured as the minimum number of cells on a raster surface (30 m resolution) needed to reach the nearest ALRI treatment center. Crossing one cell on land is assigned a value of 1, while travelling across water incurs a cost value of 5 per cell, reflecting a greater travel effort needed. Roads were not taken into consideration for accessibility because they were not well-developed during the study period. Calculations were performed in ArcGIS 10.2.1 (ESRI, Redlands, CA USA). Cost distance is included in the models for all *baris* even though all clinics are located in the treatment area in order to be consistent with the previous study [7]. An additional consideration and justification for including the measure is the possibility of spatial spillover effects—households in the comparison area who are closer to treatment area clinics, could have their health seeking behavior influenced by their neighbors.

Higher densities of people can increase the transmission of pathogens that cause ALRI [58]. The population density of the area surrounding each *bari* was calculated using a circular neighborhood with a radius of 200 meters centered on each *bari*. This distance was selected to replicate the measure used by [7]. The total population of each *bari* in the 1993 census was used for the density calculation.

Statistical methods

The analyses proceeded in two stages. First, zero-inflated negative binomial (ZINB) regression was used to model *bari*-level mortality rates. ZINB models are two-part mixture models that adjust for overdispersion (when the variance exceeds the mean) in the outcome and excess zeros produced by rare events [35, 59]. The results tables show both components of the model separately, though they are estimated at the same time. The first component is the count model using the negative binomial distribution and log-link function used to describe the number of ALRI mortality events at a *bari*. The parameter estimates for this component describe the associations with counts of mortality events after accounting for excess zeros. The negative binomial distribution includes zero as a valid event, but for rare events, the inflated number of zeroes can bias the model. The second component explicitly models the likelihood of zero mortality events (relative to 1 or more) at a *bari* using a binary model. For our models, both components used the same covariate adjustments. The log of the person-years of children under 2 years was included as an offset population to account for differences in the population at risk across *baris*. Covariates were added iteratively and goodness of fit was assessed with deviance and Akaike Information Criterion (AIC) scores. All analyses were conducted using R 2.12.1 [60]. ZINB regression was carried out with the *zeroinfl* procedure in the *pscl* package [61, 62]. Only the results of the final models are presented here.

Following the regression models, spatial cluster detection tests were performed using the spatial scan statistic implemented in the SaTScan software package [36, 63]. The spatial scan statistic is a technique for detecting local clusters which operates by placing a large number of circles of varying radii at each location, and calculating the ratio of observed events to expected events in the population within each scanning window. A likelihood ratio test is calculated for each circle to test whether the observed to expected ratio within a scanning window is different from the risk in the total population outside of the scanning window. The maximum likelihood ratio identifies the most likely cluster at a location and statistical significance is determined using Monte Carlo simulations of the locations of observed cases under the null hypothesis that events are distributed over the study area proportionally to the population. We scanned for high or low clusters of ALRI. The number of deaths to children under 2 years in each *bari* is assumed to be Poisson distributed. The maximum scanning window was limited to up to 50 % of the population at risk. Additional tests were performed with this setting limited to $\leq$10 % of the population at risk in order to assess whether smaller clusters or alternative patterns were being hidden. In all tests, clusters were considered to be significantly different from the null hypothesis of complete spatial randomness at the $\alpha = 0.1$ level as determined by 999 Monte Carlo simulations. Only clusters with no geographic overlap are presented.

Three separate cluster analyses were performed in this study—one unadjusted and two adjusted models. The unadjusted model used observed counts of ALRI and the person-years at risk to scan for clusters. The adjusted models first incorporated only the treatment area as a covariate. Next the fitted values from the ZINB models, which estimated ALRI mortality counts after adjusting for known risk factors (including the treatment area), were used. In the adjusted models, the observed number of deaths in a *bari* remains the same in each analysis and is derived from the HDSS records. The expected number of deaths at a location, used as the denominator in the spatial scan calculation, varies as covariate adjustments are made. These changes in the expected cases and subsequent changes in the risk within a scanning window are the basis for interpreting the relationships between risk factors and disease patterns. If a covariate is related to an increase in mortality rate, the expected number of deaths will be increased following adjustment and the observed to expected ratio will be reduced compared with a non-adjusted analysis. Thus, if a significant high cluster found in a given location in an unadjusted analysis is no longer significant after introduction of a covariate adjustment, we can say that the observed cluster was due to the uneven spatial distribution of that risk factor. Clusters which persist or appear after adjustment are not fully explained by a given model. Therefore cluster detection can be useful for generating research questions and hypotheses regarding additional risk factors for a given disease process.

This study differs from most previous applications of the spatial scan statistic by using regression models to calculate expected mortality counts. This approach is more flexible than entering covariate information into the SaTScan software, which is limited to a small number of categorical covariates. The regression preprocessing step allows the spatial scan statistic to effectively use continuous covariates as well as take advantage of more sophisticated, non-spatial modeling that could include non-linear relationships or more sophisticated model forms such as multilevel models [64].

The first cluster analysis is unadjusted to provide a baseline for comparison. Without adjustment, the expected number of deaths in a *bari* is proportional to the population of children under 2 years old at risk. As the ALRI control program was implemented in a geographically defined area of Matlab and did reduce mortality, we can be confident that it will also affect spatial mortality patterns. The second analysis introduces an adjustment for whether a *bari* is located within the treatment area. In this analysis the expected mortality events are calculated using the treatment/comparison area-specific rates. The third analysis uses expected counts calculated from the previously constructed ZINB model that adjusts for treatment area effects, as well as *bari*-level socioeconomic status, cost distance to a medical facility, and exposure to inorganic arsenic from contaminated drinking water. This model incorporates continuous measures of the cost surface and arsenic exposure, as well as the categorical variables for treatment area and high socioeconomic status. Results from all three analyses are presented graphically after importing the results from SaTScan into ArcGIS, to identify the locations of significant clusters as well as in tabular format to compare changes in likelihood and relative risk among clusters. This study (protocol number 12-0183) was reviewed by the Institutional Review Board of the University of Colorado Boulder and granted exempt status. All data were anonymized by icddr,b before being released to the investigators.

Results

Between 1989 and 1996, 816 deaths from ALRI were reported in children under 2 years old (276 in the treatment area, 540 in the comparison area), and the mortality rates were almost 50 % lower within the treatment area (6.18 per 1000 person-years vs. 10.74 per 1000 person-years). These deaths are 84 % of ALRI deaths across all ages in Matlab during that period. Out of 6693 *baris*, only 691 (10.3 %) reported at least 1 death, producing a larger proportion (89.7 %) of *baris* without any deaths (Fig. 2). The distribution of mortality events in the *baris* was also slightly overdispersed (variance divided by the mean = 1.278), prompting our decision to use the more flexible negative binomial rather than Poisson distribution.

Table 1 presents characteristics of the *baris* stratified by treatment and comparison area villages. Relative to the comparison area, the treatment area had slightly smaller populations at risk in each *bari*, lower average arsenic

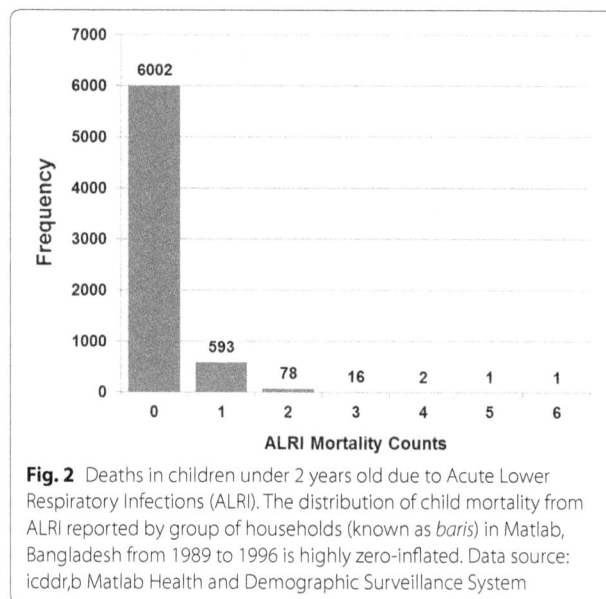

Fig. 2 Deaths in children under 2 years old due to Acute Lower Respiratory Infections (ALRI). The distribution of child mortality from ALRI reported by group of households (known as *baris*) in Matlab, Bangladesh from 1989 to 1996 is highly zero-inflated. Data source: icddr,b Matlab Health and Demographic Surveillance System

exposure levels, a larger proportion (62.9 %) of higher socioeconomic status *baris*, and a lower average population density. As all clinics are located within the treatment area, these *baris* also had lower average travel cost distances to reach a clinic. Use of tubewells and exposure to arsenic is widespread: only 179 *baris* (2.7 %) reported using a surface water source in 1996. These *baris* were assigned an arsenic exposure of 0. For the remaining *baris*, 29.4 % (n = 1912) were linked by identification number to one or more wells and assigned the average arsenic levels. The final 4781 *baris* were assumed to use the nearest tubewell, which was an average of 78 meters away from the *bari*. Overall, 69.3 % of all *baris* (n = 4636) have estimated arsenic levels above the Government of Bangladesh-recommended level of 50 µg/L.

Table 2 shows the results of the final model from the ZINB analysis. The upper panel of the table presents coefficients and standard errors from a negative binomial component while the lower panel shows coefficients and standard errors from the logit model component predicting that a *bari* reports no deaths. In preliminary tests population density was found not to be significantly related to the outcome and omitted from results shown here. While none of the covariates were significantly associated with reporting zero events, being located within the ALRI treatment area and living in a high socioeconomic status significantly reduced mortality rates. Potential arsenic exposure and the cost distance to the nearest clinic were not significantly associated with ALRI mortality in children <2 years.

The results of the ZINB model can be expressed as the expected mean counts for each *bari*. Figure 3 shows

Table 1 Sample characteristics

	Treatment	Comparison	p value
Bari person-years (children <2 years)			
Mean (SD)	13.7 (13.3)	14.6 (16.6)	0.018
Arsenic (μg/L)			
Mean (SD)	186.9 (183.0)	253.1 (225.3)	0.001
Higher socioeconomic status			
N (%)	2046 (62.9)	1937 (56.3)	0.001
Cost distance to clinic			
Mean (SD)	2225.4 (1161.8)	5864.8 (2224.4)	0.001
Population density (population in 1993 per sq. km)			
Mean (SD)	2500.0 (2143.9)	2812.5 (1633.9)	0.001
N	3251	3442	

Descriptive comparisons of *bari* characteristics of the treatment and comparison areas within Matlab, Bangladesh. Tests of differences based on two sample t-tests or Chi squared, as appropriate. Data source: icddr,b, Matlab Health and Demographic Surveillance System

Table 2 Regression results

	β	SE	p
Negative binomial model			
Treatment area	−0.580	0.108	0.000
Arsenic (100 μg/L)	0.009	0.020	0.644
High socioeconomic status	−0.302	0.076	0.000
Cost distance to clinic[a]	−0.092	0.052	0.077
(Intercept)	−4.359	0.073	0.000
Log (theta)	1.704	0.595	0.004
Zero-inflated model			
Treatment area	11.985	76.145	0.875
Arsenic (100 μg/L)	−2.633	2.769	0.342
High socioeconomic status	1.007	1.334	0.450
Cost distance to clinic[a]	1.206	1.339	0.368
(Intercept)	−15.708	76.162	0.837
N	6693		

Zero-inflated negative binomial regression analysis of *bari*-level acute lower respiratory infection (ALRI) mortality rates in children under 2 years of age in Matlab, Bangladesh, 1989–1996. Data source: icddr,b, Matlab Health and Demographic Surveillance System

[a] Centered to the mean and scaled by the standard deviation

these counts predicted for varying levels of arsenic for a *bari* in the treatment and control areas while holding constant SES at low, and cost distance and person-years at their means. The expected count of ALRI deaths only slightly increases with increasing arsenic, but, at all levels of exposure, *baris* in the treatment area, on average, experience lower numbers of ALRI deaths than the comparison area. Table 3 shows the results of the ZINB models stratified by treatment and comparison areas in the upper and lower panels of the table, respectively. When analyzed separately, the patterns of associations remain largely consistent with the combined model.

Higher socioeconomic status *baris* in both the treatment and comparison areas have lower ALRI mortality risk in young children. In the comparison area, one difference that emerges is that increasing cost distances are associated with lower counts of ALRI mortality.

Figure 4 and related Table 4 show the results of the unadjusted scan statistic which identified two statistically significant clusters. The most likely cluster is a large area of lower mortality risk (relative risk, RR = 0.53, p = 0.000) centered over the treatment area. The second most likely cluster is an area of elevated risk (RR = 1.45, p = 0.051) in the southwest area of Matlab in the comparison area. The results of sensitivity testing of the unadjusted model, limiting the maximum population size to ≤10 % of the total, are shown in Fig. 5 and Table 4. While three statistically significant clusters are found, they all follow the already reported pattern of an area of low risk in the treatment area and an area of higher risk in the southern comparison area. Therefore, further spatial scan tests proceeded with the 50 % population limit. Figure 6 and Table 4 show the results after adjusting for the location of the treatment area. The most likely cluster is now an area of lower risk (RR = 0.41, p = 0.046) in the southwestern edge of the study area, part of the comparison area. There are no longer any areas of significantly elevated risk and the two clusters initially identified in the unadjusted analysis are no longer significant. The final spatial scan statistic test included adjustments using the combined ZINB model (e.g., treatment area, socioeconomic status, cost distance, arsenic exposure). After this adjustment the previously identified cluster of lower than expected ALRI mortality risk is no longer significant at the α = 0.1 level and no significant clusters are found in the study area (no map shown).

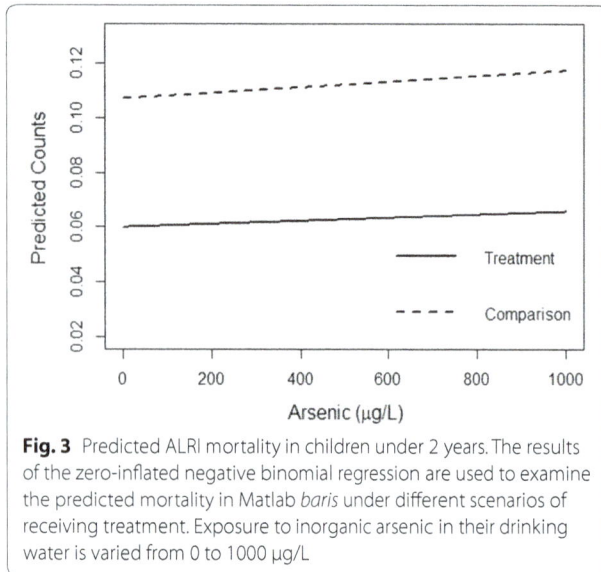

Fig. 3 Predicted ALRI mortality in children under 2 years. The results of the zero-inflated negative binomial regression are used to examine the predicted mortality in Matlab *baris* under different scenarios of receiving treatment. Exposure to inorganic arsenic in their drinking water is varied from 0 to 1000 μg/L

Table 3 Regression results of stratified models

	β	SE	p
Treatment area			
Negative binomial model			
Arsenic (100 μg/L)	0.010	0.042	0.807
High socioeconomic status	−0.348	0.140	0.013
Cost distance to clinic[a]	0.125	0.147	0.396
(Intercept)	−4.777	0.195	0.000
Log(theta)	0.674	0.559	0.228
Zero-inflated model			
Arsenic (100 μg/L)	−2.921	2.742	0.287
High socioeconomic status	0.502	1.677	0.765
Cost distance to Clinic[1]	1.945	1.488	0.191
(Intercept)	−3.214	1.405	0.022
N	3251		
Comparison area			
Negative binomial model			
Arsenic (100 μg/L)	0.008	0.022	0.702
High socioeconomic status	−0.302	0.090	0.001
Cost distance to clinic[a]	−0.151	0.058	0.010
(Intercept)	−4.306	0.084	0.000
Log (theta)	2.807	1.815	0.122
Zero-inflated model			
Arsenic (100 μg/L)	−1.686	3.006	0.575
High Socioeconomic Status	−1.310	1.712	0.444
Cost Distance to Clinic[a]	−5.137	3.003	0.087
(Intercept)	−8.242	2.693	0.002
N	3442		

Zero-inflated negative binomial regression analysis of *bari*-level acute lower respiratory infection (ALRI) mortality rates in children under 2 years of age in Matlab, Bangladesh, 1989–1996 by treatment versus comparison area. Data source: icddr,b Matlab Health and Demographic Surveillance System

[a] Centered to the mean and scaled by the standard deviation

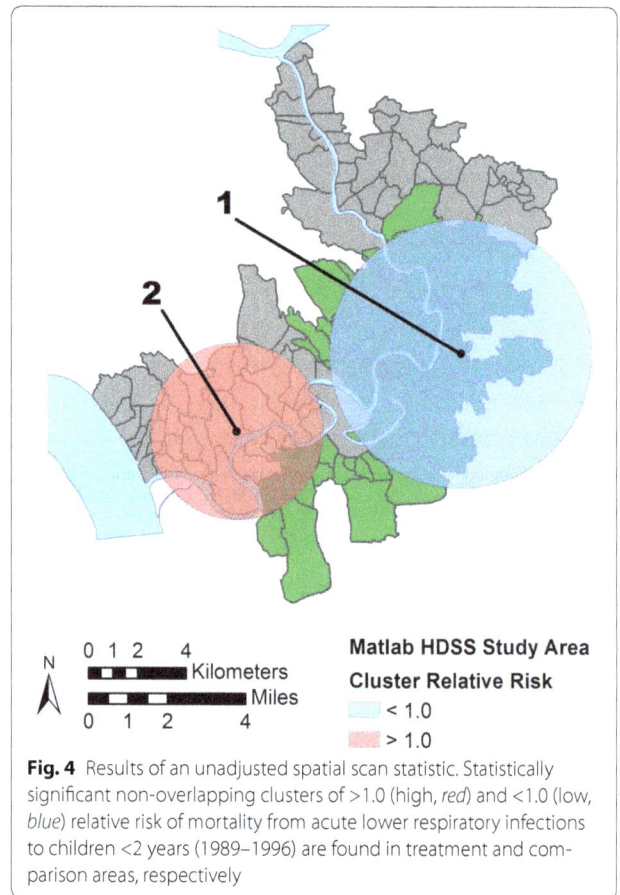

Fig. 4 Results of an unadjusted spatial scan statistic. Statistically significant non-overlapping clusters of >1.0 (high, *red*) and <1.0 (low, *blue*) relative risk of mortality from acute lower respiratory infections to children <2 years (1989–1996) are found in treatment and comparison areas, respectively

Discussion

While previous studies of acute lower respiratory infections have primarily focused on individual-level risk factors [4, 6, 9], this research sought to highlight the broader contextual and environmental characteristics that can influence mortality rates. Part of the objectives of this study were to evaluate these risk factors for childhood ALRI mortality in the contexts of a community-based control program and exposure to inorganic arsenic from contaminated drinking water in Matlab, Bangladesh. This study found that living within the area served by the ALRI control program was strongly associated with reduced mortality rates measured at the *bari* level. This finding is consistent with previous studies [7, 13, 40] that found that the control program in Matlab was successful at reducing ALRI mortality in young children by up to 50 % during the period from 1989 to 1993. The study of ALRI mortality by Ali et al. [7] used a spatial filtering technique to map smoothed rates and qualitatively observed fewer areas of elevated rates in the Matlab MCH/FP treatment area. The present study also detected that pattern and the spatial scan statistic allows for statistical inferences which show that the spatial clustering is

Effects of health intervention programs and arsenic exposure on child mortality from acute lower respiratory...

9

Table 4 Results of cluster analyses

	Observed deaths	Expected deaths	Radius (km)	Relative risk	Likelihood ratio	p value
Unadjusted (Fig. 4)						
Cluster 1	141	229.9	5.4	0.53	26.4	0.000
Cluster 2	259	197.8	3.5	1.45	11.8	0.051
Unadjusted, max size ≤10 % of population at risk (Fig. 5)						
Cluster 1	36	77.8	2.8	0.44	15.2	0.002
Cluster 2	0	14.3	0.9	0.00	14.4	0.003
Cluster 3	96	58.0	1.5	1.74	11.3	0.061
Treatment area adjusted (Fig. 6)						
Cluster 1	22	52.0	1.3	0.41	11.6	0.046
Model adjusted (*no figure*)						
	No statistically significant clusters found					

Spatial cluster analysis of childhood deaths from acute lower respiratory infections (ALRI) in Matlab, Bangladesh, 1989–1996. Results are from the spatial scan statistic implemented in SaTScan and include only statistically significant clusters at the α = 0.1 level

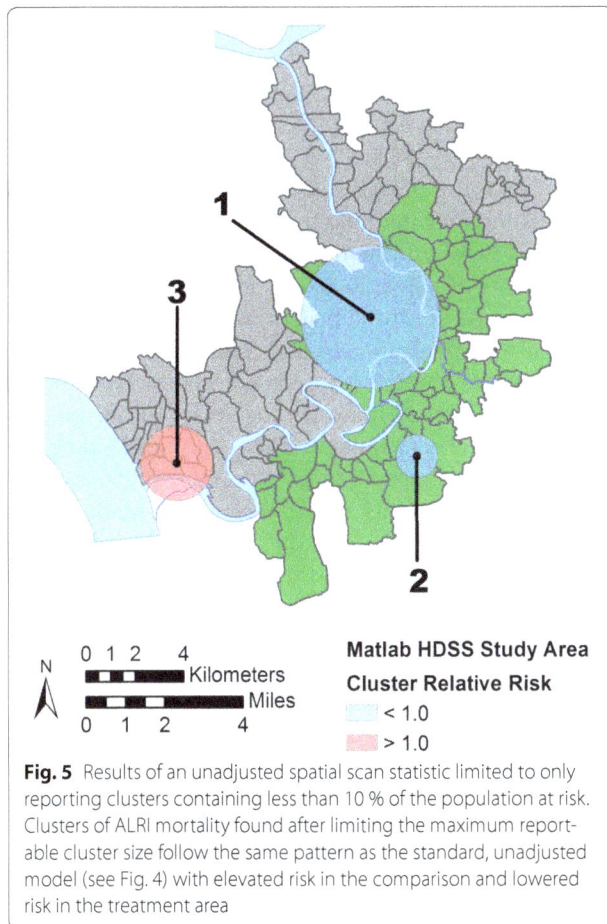

Fig. 5 Results of an unadjusted spatial scan statistic limited to only reporting clusters containing less than 10 % of the population at risk. Clusters of ALRI mortality found after limiting the maximum report-able cluster size follow the same pattern as the standard, unadjusted model (see Fig. 4) with elevated risk in the comparison and lowered risk in the treatment area

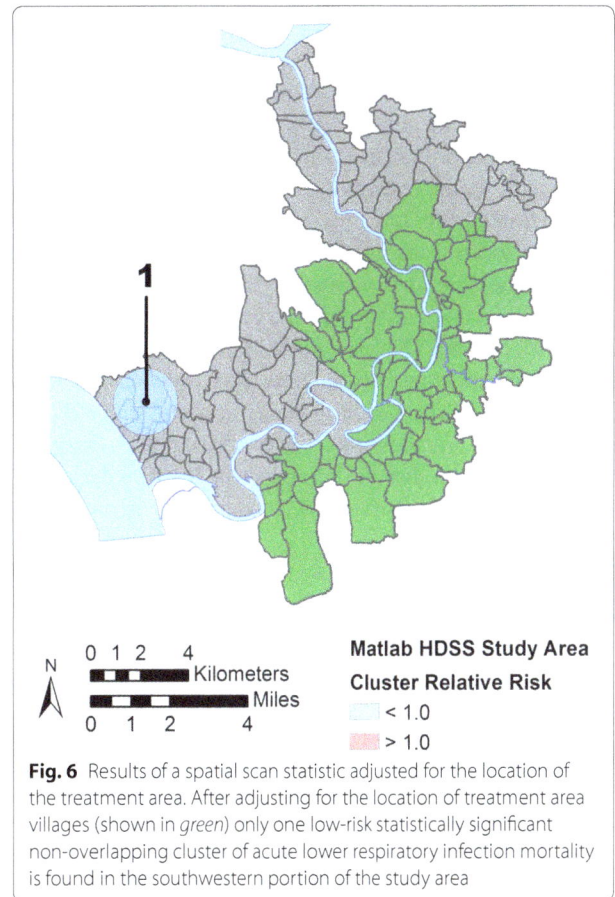

Fig. 6 Results of a spatial scan statistic adjusted for the location of the treatment area. After adjusting for the location of treatment area villages (shown in *green*) only one low-risk statistically significant non-overlapping cluster of acute lower respiratory infection mortality is found in the southwestern portion of the study area

significant but that controlling for the treatment area and population distribution explains much of this local-scale variation.

In the present study, we also hypothesized that exposure to arsenic could be associated with increased ALRI mortality. Recent studies in Matlab and elsewhere have found that arsenic exposure is associated with increases in adverse pregnancy outcomes and infant mortality [65], as well as with harm to the lungs including coughs, cancer, and infections [29, 32–34]. Adding to the biological plausibility for the potential association with ALRI mortality are studies which have shown that arsenic's toxic effects suppress the immune system, particularly in children [20], and damages cellular DNA and chemical receptors in lung tissue providing the opportunity for infections [21, 22]. However, in a zero-inflated negative binomial analysis at the *bari*-level used in this study, increased arsenic levels were not associated ($p = 0.644$) with ALRI mortality in children <2 years.

This study has extended the previous evaluation of the Matlab ALRI control program by Ali et al. [7] by including three additional years of mortality records as well as by incorporating measures of socioeconomic status and arsenic exposure that have not been previously used. *Baris* with higher SES were associated with lower rates of child mortality from ALRI in this study even after controlling for the treatment area effect. A case–control study on child ALRI mortality in Gambia did not find a significant association with SES [9], and, similarly, a prospective cohort study of children under 5 years in Matlab did not find an association with incidence of respiratory infections and various sociodemographic measures [6]. However, other studies have found various measures of social status including income, home ownership, and education to be predictive of respiratory infections in various age groups and country settings [53, 54, 66]. SES may affect respiratory infections by increasing exposure to pathogens in crowded living quarters or by decreasing an individual's immune status due to stress or poor nutrition [58]. The conflicting findings in the literature may be due to differences in the specific measure of SES used in each study. Further work is needed to explore the role of SES in ALRI.

The cost distance to the nearest treatment center was also found to be associated with lower rates of ALRI death, though this finding was only statistically significant in the comparison area. Ali et al. [7] found that decreased access to care as measured by cost distance was associated with reduced mortality rates. While we expected that limiting access to care would increase mortality, this opposite finding is possible evidence of a reporting bias with more distant *baris* less likely to accurately report cases. Studies of diarrheal diseases in Matlab have found a similar pattern of decreased case numbers of diarrheal diseases with increasing distance from the hospital [50, 67].

Previous studies of mortality in Matlab using the spatial scan statistic have found visually similar patterns and areas of locally-clustered mortality related to the placement of the treatment area. In a village-level analysis of all-cause mortality in children under 5 years old between 1998 and 2002, Alam et al. [15] found significant clusters of elevated mortality centered on the northern and southern areas of Matlab as well as a secondary cluster of high risk along the eastern edge of the study area, after adjusting a space–time scan statistic for education and economic status. Using a spatial scan statistic on fetal and infant deaths between 1991 and 2000 and adjusting for age, parity, education, and SES, Sohel et al. [68] found a large cluster of significantly lower rates in central Matlab (coincident with the treatment area), and a smaller, but also significant cluster of elevated rates, in the southwestern portion of the comparison area. Visually these results are remarkably similar to those found in the unadjusted analysis of the present study. Sohel and colleagues [68] suggested that the clustering in fetal and infant mortality could be due to differences in arsenic exposure as they found significantly higher levels of arsenic in the wells used within the higher risk cluster. However, they did not adjust their scan statistic for arsenic level and test whether they could explain their observed spatial variation. Arsenic concentration was found to vary significantly between *baris* in the treatment and comparison areas ($\mu_{treatment} = 186.9$, SD = 183.0 vs. $\mu_{comparison} = 253.1$, SD = 225.3, $p < 0.001$), and a measure of arsenic exposure was incorporated into the final model-adjusted scan statistic; however, as the results of the ZINB model show, our estimate of potential arsenic exposure was not associated with ALRI mortality after adjusting for the differences in the population at risk, treatment area, SES, and cost distance. Therefore, we do not expect that arsenic alone would explain the clustering observed in the present study. The geographic pattern of the ALRI program implementation appears to be crucial for understanding the geographic patterns of child mortality in Matlab.

After adjusting for only the treatment area, which explained the two initial clusters, a new cluster of lower ALRI mortality emerged in the southwestern edge of the study area. This cluster of lower risk was unexpected, and it indicates an area of unexplained variation. The cluster could be the result of underreporting of ALRI deaths due to its location on the far edge of the study area, as discussed above. Another possibility is that these *baris* are receiving care elsewhere (e.g. outside of the Matlab study area) and so are not affected in the same way by the Matlab program placement. Ali et al. [7]. found that reduced ALRI mortality was associated with greater access to local allopathic doctors. Data on the locations of allopathic doctors and care-seeking behaviors were not available for this study. In the final spatial scan test, using the ZINB model to adjust the model, this cluster is no longer significant, indicating that the variation in expected counts has been explained by the addition of the other covariates and model form.

Strengths of this study include the detailed records collected in the demographic surveillance system in Matlab which enables accurate reporting of ALRI deaths and estimates of the population at risk. That these records can be linked in a geographic information system to spatial data on housing locations and tubewells with measured arsenic concentrations further enhances this study and allows for additional environmental and contextual variables to be considered. A limitation of this study is the arsenic exposure measure. The arsenic data come from 2002 to 2003 and are applied to the earlier study period of 1989–1996, which may bias the exposure estimate if arsenic varies over time. Evidence from several studies in Bangladesh, though limited, suggests that arsenic levels in wells are generally consistent over time [42, 51, 52]; however, it is not known which specific wells existed and were used by households during the study period. As arsenic contamination became more well-known in the 1990s, wells installed between 1996 and the arsenic survey in 2002 were likely deeper to access clean water while older wells which may have been broken or removed by 2002 (but were in use during the ALRI program) were typically shallower and, thus, more likely to be contaminated. These potential changes in wells over the years between our study period and arsenic survey would likely bias the arsenic exposure downward and averaging all tubewells belonging to a *bari* also potentially reduces the estimated exposure measure. These steps likely produce a conservative estimate of a *bari's* true arsenic exposure and may explain the lack of a significant association between arsenic exposure and ALRI mortality in this study. Other environmental variables could be important to consider. For example we do not have a measure of indoor air pollution, yet this measure may be contributing to the observed SES association. Solid fuel use, which contributes to indoor air pollution and negative health effects, is more likely among poorer households in Matlab [69].

Conclusion

This work provides one of the few examples of using regression models to adjust the spatial scan statistic and thereby incorporate continuous covariates and more complex models forms. Our initial results of adjusting the scan statistic for only treatment area, while explaining some of the larger clusters, produced an unexpected cluster of lower mortality risk. The model-adjusted scan statistic was able to explain this area of variation. Substantively, as acute lower respiratory infections continue to be a major cause of illness and death for children in Bangladesh and around the world, it is important to evaluate the effectiveness of community-based intervention strategies on population health. The results of this study indicate that child mortality form ALRI does cluster spatially in Matlab. However these patterns are largely explained by the placement of the treatment program. These results confirm the findings from previous non-spatial studies that the ALRI control program is effective at reducing mortality, though even in the presence of such an effective control program, household socio-economic status may continue to influence the mortality patterns and this finding requires further study. More broadly, this study demonstrates the importance of geographic studies to highlight areas of significantly elevated or reduced mortality in order to evaluate and improve public health intervention programs.

Abbreviations

AIC: Akaike Information Criterion; ALRI: acute lower respiratory infection; CHW: community health worker; HDSS: health and demographic surveillance system; HG-AAS: hydride generation atomic absorption spectrometry; icddr,b: formerly the International Centre for Diarrhoeal Disease Research, Bangladesh; MCH/FP: maternal and child health, and family planning program; MGIS: Matlab Geographic Information System; PCA: principal component analysis; RR: relative risk; SES: socioeconomic status; ZINB: zero-inflated negative binomial.

Authors' contributions

WJ and ER designed the study. WJ analyzed the data and drafted the manuscript. AR oversaw data design and collection and helped revise the manuscript. All authors read and approved the final manuscript.

Author details

[1] Department of Geography and Environment, University of Southampton, University Road, Southampton SO17 1BJ, UK. [2] Health Systems and Population Studies Division, icddr,b, 68, Shaheed Tajuddin Ahmed Sarani, Mohakhali, Dhaka 1212, Bangladesh. [3] Department of Geography, Division of Epidemiology, The Ohio State University, 1036 Derby Hall, 154 North Oval Mall, Columbus, OH 43212, USA.

Acknowledgements

WJ was supported by the National Science Foundation (Grant No. DGE 1144083). The authors acknowledge the helpful comments of four anonymous reviewers.

Competing interests

The authors declare that they have no competing interests.

Funding

This research was conducted with the support of icddr,b, which is funded by the John D. and Catherine T. MacArthur Foundation (Grant Number-09-93088-000-GSS). icddr,b acknowledges with gratitude the commitment of current donors providing unrestricted support; these include the Australian Agency for International Development (AusAID), the Government of the People's Republic of Bangladesh; the Canadian International Development Agency (CIDA), the Swedish International Development Cooperation Agency (Sida), and the Department for International Development, UK (DFID). This material is also supported by the National Science Foundation Graduate Research Fellowship under Grant No. DGE 1144083. The funders had no role in the design of the study and collection, analysis, and interpretation of data or in writing the manuscript. Any opinion, findings, and conclusions or recommendations expressed in this material are those of the authors(s) and do not necessarily reflect the views of the National Science Foundation or other funders.

References

1. Black RE, Cousens S, Johnson HL, Lawn JE, Rudan I, Bassani DG, et al. Global, regional, and national causes of child mortality in 2008: a systematic analysis. Lancet. 2010;375:1969–87.

2. Lanata CF, Black RE. Acute lower respiratory infections. In: Semba RD, Bloem MW, Piot P, editors. Nutrition and health in developing countries. Totowa: Humana Press; 2008. p. 179–214.

3. Rudan I, Boschi-Pinto C, Biloglav Z, Mulholland K, Campbell H. Epidemiology and etiology of childhood pneumonia. Bull World Health Organ. 2008;86:408–16.

4. Spika JS, Munshi MH, Wojtyniak B, Sack DA, Hossain A, Rahman M, et al. Acute lower respiratory infections: a major cause of death in children in Bangladesh. Ann Trop Paediatr. 1989;9:33–9.

5. Arifeen SE, Saha SK, Rahman S, Rahman KM, Rahman SM, Bari S, et al. Invasive pneumococcal disease among children in rural Bangladesh: results from a population-based surveillance. Clin Infect Dis. 2009;48:S103–13.

6. Zaman K, Baqui AH, Yunus M, Sack RB, Bateman OM, Chowdhury HR, et al. Acute respiratory infections in children: a community-based longitudinal study in rural Bangladesh. J Trop Pediatr. 1997;43:133–7.

7. Ali M, Emch M, Tofail F, Baqui AH. Implications of health care provision on acute lower respiratory infection mortality in Bangladeshi children. Soc Sci Med. 2001;52:267–77.

8. ICDDR,B. Health and demographic surveillance system—Matlab, vol. 42. Dhaka, Bangladesh: International Centre for Diarrhoeal Diseases Research, Bangladesh; 2010.

9. De Francisco A, Morris J, Hall AJ, Schellenberg JRMA, Greenwood BM. Risk factors for mortality from acute lower respiratory tract infections in young Gambian children. Int J Epidemiol. 1993;22:1174–82.

10. Mizgerd JP. Lung infection-a public health priority. PLoS Med. 2006;3:0155–8.

11. Girard MP, Cherian T, Pervikov Y, Kieny MP. A review of vaccine research and development: human acute respiratory infections. Vaccine. 2005;23:5708–24.

12. Sazawal S, Black RE. Effect of pneumonia case management on mortality in neonates, infants, and preschool children: a meta-analysis of community-based trials. Lancet Infect Dis. 2003;3:547–56.

13. Fauveau V, Stewart MK, Chakraborty J, Khan SA. Impact on mortality of a community-based programme to control acute lower respiratory tract infections. Bull World Health Organ. 1992;70:109–16.

14. Nasreen S, Luby SP, Brooks WA, Homaira N, Mamun AA, Bhuiyan MU, et al. Population-based incidence of severe acute respiratory virus infections among children aged <5 years in rural Bangladesh, June–October 2010. PLoS ONE. 2014;9:e89978.

15. Alam N, Zahirul Haq M, Streatfield PK. Spatio-temporal patterns of under-five mortality in Matlab HDSS in rural Bangladesh. Global Health Action. 2010;3:64–9.

16. Smith AH, Lingas EO, Rahman M. Contamination of drinking-water by arsenic in Bangladesh: a public health emergency. Bull World Health Organ. 2000;78:1093–103.

17. Black M. From handpumps to health: the evolution of water and sanitation programmes in Bangladesh, India and Nigeria. New York: United Nations Children's Fund; 1990.

18. Smith AH, Lingas EO, Rahman M. Contamination of drinking-water by arsenic in Bangladesh: a public health emergency. Bull World Health Organ. 2000;78:1093–103.

19. Selgrade MK. Immunotoxicity: the risk is real. Toxicol Sci. 2007;100:328–32.

20. Soto-Peña GA, Luna AL, Acosta-Saavedra L, Conde P, López-Carrillo L, Cebrián ME, et al. Assessment of lymphocyte subpopulations and cytokine secretion in children exposed to arsenic. FASEB. 2006;20:779–81.

21. Kozul CD, Ely KH, Enelow RI, Hamilton JW. Low-dose arsenic compromises the immune response to influenza A infection *in vivo*. Environ Health Perspect. 2009;117:1441–7.

22. Kozul CD, Hampton TH, Davey JC, Gosse JA, Nomikos AP, Eisenhauer PL, et al. Chronic exposure to arsenic in the drinking water alters the expression of immune response genes in mouse lung. Environ Health Perspect. 2009;117:1108–15.

23. Dauphiné DC, Ferreccio C, Guntur S, Yuan Y, Hammond SK, Balmes J, et al. Lung function in adults following in utero and childhood exposure to arsenic in drinking water: preliminary findings. Int Arch Occup Environ Health. 2010;84:591–600.

24. Von Ehrenstein OS, Mazumder DNG, Yuan Y, Samanta S, Balmes J, Sil A, et al. Decrements in lung function related to arsenic in drinking water in West Bengal, India. Am J Epidemiol. 2005;162:533–41.

25. Smith AH, Yunus M, Khan AF, Ercumen A, Yuan Y, Smith MH, et al. Chronic respiratory symptoms in children following in utero and early life exposure to arsenic in drinking water in Bangladesh. Int J Epidemiol. 2013;42:1077–86.

26. Parvez F, Chen Y, Brandt-Rauf PW, Bernard A, Dumont X, Slavkovich V, et al. Non-malignant respiratory effects of chronic arsenic exposure from drinking water among never smokers in Bangladesh. Environ Health Perspect. 2008;116:190–5.

27. Parvez F, Chen Y, Yunus M, Olopade C, Segers S, Slavkovich V, et al. Arsenic exposure and impaired lung function: findings from a large population-based prospective cohort study. Am J Respir Crit Care Med. 2013;188:813–9.

28. Parvez F, Chen Y, Brandt-Rauf PW, Slavkovich V, Islam T, Ahmed A, et al. A prospective study of respiratory symptoms associated with chronic arsenic exposure in Bangladesh: findings from the Health Effects of Arsenic Longitudinal Study (HEALS). Thorax. 2010;65:528–33.

29. Smith AH, Goycolea M, Haque R, Biggs ML. Marked increase in bladder and lunger cancer mortality in a region of Northern Chile due to arsenic in drinking water. Am J Epidemiol. 1998;147:660–9.

30. Smith AH, Marshall G, Yuan Y, Ferreccio C, Liaw J, von Ehrenstein O, et al. Increased mortality from lung cancer and bronchiectasis in young adults after exposure to arsenic in utero and in early childhood. Environ Health Perspect. 2006;114:1293–6.

31. Smith AH, Marshall G, Yuan Y, Liaw J, Ferreccio C, Steinmaus C. Evidence from Chile that arsenic in drinking water may increase mortality from pulmonary tuberculosis. Am J Epidemiol. 2011;173:414–20.

32. Guha Mazumder DN. Arsenic and non-malignant lung disease. J Environ Sci Health A. 2007;42:1859–67.

33. Raqib R, Ahmed S, Sultana R, Wagatsuma Y, Mondal D, Hoque AMW, et al. Effects of in utero arsenic exposure on child immunity and morbidity in rural Bangladesh. Toxicol Lett. 2009;185:197–202.

34. George CM, Brooks WA, Graziano JH, Nonyane BAS, Hossain L, Goswami D, et al. Arsenic exposure is associated with pediatric pneumonia in rural Bangladesh: a case control study. Environ Health. 2015;14:83.

35. Cameron AC, Trivedi PK. Regression analysis of count data. Cambridge: Cambridge University Press; 1998.

36. Kulldorff M. A spatial scan statistic. Commun Stat Theory Methods. 1997;26:1481–96.

37. Fauveau V, Wojtyniak B, Chakraborty J. Sarder a M, Briend A. The effect of maternal and child health and family planning services on mortality: is prevention enough? BMJ. 1990;301:103–7.

38. Koenig MA, Rob U, Khan MA, Chakraborty J, Fauveau V. Contraceptive use in Matlab, Bangladesh in 1990: levels, trends, and explanations. Stud Fam Plann. 1992;23:352–64.

39. Koenig MA, Bishai D, Khan MA. Health interventions and health equity: the example of measles vaccination in Bangladesh. Popul Dev Rev. 2001;27:283–302.

40. Stewart MK, Fauveau V, Parker B, Chakraborty J, Kham SA. Acute respiratory infections in Matlab: epidemiology, community perceptions and control strategies. In: Fauveau V, editor. Matlab: women, children and health. Dhaka, Bangladesh: The International Centre for Diarrhoeal Disease Research, Bangladesh; 1994. p. 187–204.

41. WHO. Technical basis for the WHO recommendations on the management of pneumonia in children at first-level health facilities. Geneva, Switzerland; 1991. Report No.: WHO/ARI/91.20.

42. BGS, DPHE. Arsenic contamination of groundwater in Bangladesh. 2nd ed. In: Kinniburgh DG, Smedley PL, editors. Geological survey (BGS) technical report WC/00/19. Keyworth: British Geological Survey; 2001.

43. ICDDR,B. Arsenic contamination in Matlab, Bangladesh. Health Sci Bull. 2004;2:11–4.

44. Yunus M, Sohel N, Hore SK, Rahman M. Arsenic exposure and adverse health effects: a review of recent findings from arsenic and health studies in Matlab, Bangladesh. Kaohsiung J Med Sci. 2011;27:371–6.

45. Von Brömssen M, Häller Larsson S, Bhattacharya P, Hasan MA, Ahmed KM, Jakariya M, et al. Geochemical characterisation of shallow aquifer sediments of Matlab Upazila, Southeastern Bangladesh—implications for targeting low-as aquifers. J Contam Hydrol. 2008;99:137–49.

46. Paul BK. Arsenic contamination awareness among the rural residents in Bangladesh. Soc Sci Med. 2004;59:1741–55.

47. Paul BK, De S. Arsenic poisoning in Bangladesh: a geographic analysis. J Am Water Resour Assoc. 2000;36:799–809.

48. Emch M. Diarrheal disease risk in Matlab, Bangladesh. Soc Sci Med. 1999;49:519–30.

49. Rahman M, Vahter M, Wahed MA, Sohel N, Yunus M, Streatfield PK, et al. Prevalence of arsenic exposure and skin lesions. A population based survey in Matlab, Bangladesh. J Epidemiol Commun Health. 2006;60:242–8.

50. Carrel M, Escamilla V, Messina J, Giebultowicz S, Winston J, Yunus M, et al. Diarrheal disease risk in rural Bangladesh decreases as tubewell density increases: a zero-inflated and geographically weighted analysis. Int J Health Geogr. 2011;10:41.

51. Cheng Z, van Geen A, Seddique AA, Ahmed KM. Response to comments on "Limited Temporal Variability of Arsenic Concentration in 20 Wells Monitored for 3 Years in Araihazar, Bangladesh". Environ Sci Technol. 2006;40:1718–20.

52. Cheng Z, van Geen A, Seddique AA, Ahmed KM. Limited temporal variability of arsenic concentrations in 20 wells monitored for 3 years in Araihazar, Bangladesh. Environ Sci Technol. 2005;39:4759–66.

53. Crighton EJ, Elliott SJ, Moineddin R, Kanaroglou P, Upshur R. A spatial analysis of the determinants of pneumonia and influenza hospitalizations in Ontario (1992–2001). Soc Sci Med. 2007;64:1636–50.

54. Cohen S, Doyle WJ, Turner RB, Alper CM, Skoner DP. Childhood socioeconomic status and host resistance to infectious illness in adulthood. Psychosom Med. 2004;66:553–8.

55. Emch M, Yunus M, Escamilla V, Feldacker C, Ali M. Local population and regional environmental drivers of cholera in Bangladesh. Environ Health. 2010;9:1–8.

56. Kolenikov S, Angeles G. Socioeconomic status measurement with discrete proxy variables: is principal component analysis a reliable answer? Rev Income Wealth. 2009;55:128–65.

57. Filmer D, Pritchett LH. Estimating wealth effects without expenditure data—or tears: an application to educational enrollments in states of India. Demography. 2001;38:115–32.

58. Cohen S. Social status and susceptibility to respiratory infections. Ann New York Acad Sci. 1999;896:246–53.

59. Loeys T, Moerkerke B, De Smet O, Buysse A. The analysis of zero-inflated count data: beyond zero-inflated Poisson regression. Br J Math Stat Psychol. 2012;65:163–80.

60. R Core Development Team. R: a language and environment for statistical computing. Vienna, Austria: R Foundation for Statistical Computing; 2010.

61. Zeileis A, Kleiber C, Jackman S. Regression models for count data in R. J Stat Softw. 2008;27:1–25.

62. Jackman S. pscl: Classes and methods for R developed in the Political Science Computational Laboratory, Stanford University. Stanford, CA; 2011.

63. Kulldorff M, Information Management Services Inc. SaTScan v8.0: software for the spatial and space-time scan statistics; 2009.

64. Klassen AC, Kulldorff M, Curriero F. Geographical clustering of prostate cancer grade and stage at diagnosis, before and after adjustment for risk factors. Int J Health Geogr. 2005;4:1.

65. Vahter M. Effects of arsenic on maternal and fetal health. Ann Rev Nutr. 2009;29:381–99.

66. Margolis PA, Greenberg RA, Keyes LL, LaVange LM, Chapman RS, Denny FW, et al. Lower respiratory illness in infants and low socioeconomic status. Am J Public Health. 1992;82:1119–26.

67. Carrel M, Voss P, Streatfield PK, Yunus M. Protection from annual flooding is correlated with increased cholera prevalence in Bangladesh: a zero-inflated regression analysis. Environ Health. 2010;9:1–9.

68. Sohel N, Vahter M, Ali M, Rahman M, Rahman A, Streatfield PK, et al. Spatial patterns of fetal loss and infant death in an arsenic-affected area in Bangladesh. Int J Health Geogr. 2010;9:53.

69. Alam DS, Chowdhury MAH, Siddiquee AT, Ahmed S, Hossain MD, Pervin S, et al. Adult cardiopulmonary mortality and indoor air pollution. Global Heart. 2012;7:215–21.

2

Capturing exposure in environmental health research: challenges and opportunities of different activity space models

Tiina E. Laatikainen[*], Kamyar Hasanzadeh and Marketta Kyttä

Abstract

Background: The built environment health promotion has attracted notable attention across a wide spectrum of health-related research over the past decade. However, the results about the contextual effects on health and PA are highly heterogeneous. The discrepancies between the results can potentially be partly explained by the diverse use of different spatial units of analysis in assessing individuals' exposure to various environment characteristics. This study investigated whether different residential and activity space units of analysis yield distinct results regarding the association between the built environment and health. In addition, this study examines the challenges and opportunities of the different spatial units of analysis for environmental health-related research.

Methods: Two common residential units of analysis and two novel activity space models were used to examine older adults' wellbeing in relation to the built environment features in the Helsinki Metropolitan Area, Finland. An administrative unit, 500 m residential buffer, home range model and individualized residential exposure model were used to assess the associations between the built environment and wellbeing of respondent's (n = 844).

Results: All four different spatial units of analysis yield distinct results regarding the associations between the built environment characteristics and wellbeing. A positive association between green space and health was found only when exposure was assessed with individualized residential exposure model. Walkability index and the length of pedestrian and bicycle roads were found to positively correlate with perceived wellbeing measures only with a home range model. Additionally, all units of analysis differed from each other in terms of size, shape, and how they capture different contextual measures.

Conclusions: The results show that different spatial units of analysis result in considerably different measurements of built environment. In turn, the differences derived from the use of different spatial units seem to considerably affect the associations between environment characteristics and wellbeing measures. Although it is not easy to argue about the correctness of these measurements, what is evident is that they can reveal different wellbeing outcomes. While some methods are especially usable to determine the availability of environmental opportunities that promote active travel and the related health outcomes, others can provide us with insight into the mechanisms how the actual exposure to green structure can enhance wellbeing.

Keywords: Activity space, Exposure, Built environment, Wellbeing, Neighborhood, PPGIS

*Correspondence: tiina.laatikainen@aalto.fi
Department of Built Environment, Aalto University, PO Box 14100, 00076 Aalto, Finland

Background

Built environment health promotion has attracted notable attention across a wide spectrum of health-related research over the past decade [1–4]. Several built environment features, such as connectivity, density, walkability, and mixed land use, have been found to be positively associated with both perceived and objectively measured health, physical activity (PA), and active mobility [5–9]. Furthermore, research has shown that green areas have positive wellbeing effects and exposure to natural settings decreases stress and increases positive affect [10–12]. Studies have also found links between walkable neighborhoods and decreases in prevalence of overweight, obesity, and incidence of diabetes [13, 14]. In addition, neighborhood walkability has been linked to increases in cardiorespiratory fitness [15].

However, the results of the prior research about the contextual effects on health and PA are highly heterogeneous [16–18]. The discrepancies between the results can potentially be explained by the diverse use of different spatial units of analysis in assessing individuals' exposure to various environment characteristics [19–23]. The vast majority of previous studies has concentrated on analyzing the built environment features around individuals' residences or "neighborhoods" that have been delineated through administrative units (e.g., census tract, postal code areas) or residential or workplace buffers with varying radii and buffering methods [22, 24]. These units have been a popular way of defining the spatial extent of individuals' exposure to different environmental features, mostly due to their availability and ease of use.

Network and "sausage" buffers that create polygons around individuals' residences based on the street network have become commonly applied spatial units of analysis to define individuals' neighborhoods in public health research [19]. While it is evident that various network buffers are superior to simple administrative units or circular buffers, these units are also still unable to characterize the space within which people actually move around [25]. Despite the advances in the buffer-based units of analysis, these approaches account only for the built environment characteristics around individuals' residences and neglect the spatial realities of where, as well as the temporal aspect of when and how long, individuals are moving around [20, 26]. Due to the static nature of these units of analysis, it is assumed that individuals are exposed solely to the environment around their residency and, thus, manage to capture only a hypothetical individual exposure. According to Kwan [18], this "uncertain geographic context problem (UGCoP)" is one of the reasons why research findings concerning the effects of the built environment on health have been found to be inconsistent.

In their literature review, Leal and Chaix [25] found that 90% of the studies examining the associations between built environment and cardiometabolic risk factors focused their analysis solely on residential environments [25]. The problematic nature of most of these kinds of studies, where the research is limited to static neighborhoods, has also been highlighted within the new mobilities paradigm [27, 28]. The "mobility turn" in social sciences underlines the essential role of person-based and dynamic analysis and stresses a move forward from static spatial approaches [29]. Similarly, studies examining the associations between built environment and health have noted the complexity of defining individuals' spatial exposure and "local" neighborhoods [30].

Recent research has been taking steps toward more dynamic and person-based units of analysis to define the spatiotemporal extents of individuals' neighborhoods and spatial exposure by capturing the notions of activity space [21, 26, 31–33]. These studies account for individuals' actions and mobility behaviors within and exterior to their residences and local neighborhoods to overcome the uncertainty of the geographic context [18, 32]. The studies have used GPS tracking devices as well as online participatory mapping methods to collect data about the spatial extent of individual behavior [20, 26, 32, 33].

Hasanzadeh et al. [33] have developed a versatile model of activity spaces using an individual-based delineation of places of everyday activities. In their study, Hasanzadeh et al. [33] created an individual-based definition of activity spaces that are dynamic in their boundaries. Later Hasanzadeh and colleagues [26] introduced a more spatially sensitive model of individual activity spaces using a notion of place exposure. This individualized residential exposure model (IREM) is based on the understanding that the influencing context is more than a delineated area around an individual's place of residence and everyday activity places. According to Hasanzadeh et al. [26], a more refined picture of activity spaces can be achieved through an estimation of place exposure and its variation throughout an individual's activity space. In their study, Kestens et al. [32] compared activity spaces delineated from GPS tracking with activity spaces delineated from an online participatory mapping questionnaire on regular destinations and concluded that self-reported destinations provided a representative picture of study participants' spatial realities of where they move around.

Despite the notions that the research on the built environment impacts on health and PA yields varying results, only a few studies have compared whether the association between built environment characteristics and health outcomes differs when using various spatial units of analysis in capturing the context. Zenk et al. [22] found evidence that environmental features were related to participants' weight-related behaviors when using modeled activity spaces as units of analysis, but the environmental features of mere residential neighborhoods were not. In their study, Howell et al. [20] assessed how PA and walkability associations vary when different spatial measures were used and reported stronger associations between PA and walkability with activity spaces rather than with the simple home neighborhood unit of analysis. In their international study, Frank et al. [19] compared different buffering methods and concluded that the values of built environment measures differed significantly between detailed, detailed-trimmed, and sausage buffers. Holliday et al. [31] reported that simple residential buffers are an ill-fitting unit of analysis solution without assessing prior to each study if the simple residential neighborhood is an appropriate exposure area to study the health behavior in consideration. In a recent study, Zhao et al. [23] found that activity space measured with either standard deviational ellipse, minimum convex polygon or road network buffer influenced if and how an environmental variable affected obesity. According to Kestens et al. [34], activity spaces created both using GPS and map-based questionnaires can provide a way to overcome the contextual problems and improve our understanding about the mechanisms that connect place to health.

In this study, we seek to build on the previous, yet rather limited, research that have compared whether the associations between the built environment measures and health differ when individual exposure is assessed with various spatial units of analysis including the latest person-based models [19, 31, 32]. The goal of this study is to investigate whether different spatial units of analysis yield distinct results regarding the association between the built environment and health. This study also examines the challenges and opportunities of the different spatial units of analysis for environmental health-related research.

We applied two common residential units of analysis and two novel activity space models to examine older adults' perceived wellbeing in relation to the built environment features in the Helsinki Metropolitan Area (HMA), Finland. In detail, we investigated whether the associations between commonly used built environment measures and perceived wellbeing outcomes differ when using an administrative unit, residential buffer, home range model [33], or IREM [26] for assessing the individual environmental exposure. We also compared how the four different models match with activity spaces delineated from GPS activity spaces collected from a subsample of the study participants. The GPS tracking offers data about human mobility behavior free of self-report bias [34] and, thus, offers a possibility to study the challenges

and opportunities of the different spatial units of analysis based on participatory mapping in comparison to GPS activity spaces.

Methods
Study area and participants
A random sample of 5000 residents of HMA aged between 55 and 75 years received an invitation letter by mail in September 2015 asking them to participate in an online survey. A total of 1139 full or partial responses were received, and after removing incomplete responses, 844 were taken for further analysis. Participants consisted of 447 women and 331 men with a mean age of 64.3 (SD 5.52). The data showed general consistency on most sociodemographic variables within the study region (Table 1). A raffle for five hundred euro gift cards was arranged between all participants. Aalto University's Research Ethics Board approved the study.

The data were collected using a place-based mapping method, public participation GIS (PPGIS), which combines internet maps with traditional questionnaires [35]. PPGIS has offered convenient tools for previous studies investigating human behavior in a context-sensitive way [36–39]. Localization of human experiences and behavioral patterns by participatory mapping tools attaches them to specific physical environmental context [40]. Thus, human behavior and experiences receive geographic coordinates, which allows simultaneous GIS-based analysis of human behavior in relation to the physical environment [35]. In the survey, the respondents used an online interface to mark their everyday errand points (EEPs) on a map. In addition, the respondents indicated which transport mode they used and how frequently they accessed the places. The survey was created with Maptionnaire® tool. With the place-based mapping method, we were able to study older adults' spatial

Table 1 Explanations of the abbreviations for the variables in the equation

Abbreviations	Variables
WB	Wellbeing measure
Gr	Greenness
LUM	Land use mix
W	Walkability
PC	Pedestrian/cycling routes
S	Size[a]
I	Income
AG	Age
G	Gender
EDU	Education
RT	Retirement status

[a] Not included for buffer and administrative unit models

Capturing exposure in environmental health research: challenges and opportunities of different activity...

17

behavior context-sensitively by asking respondents to think about their typical week and mark on the map all sorts of everyday places they visit during the week. Simultaneously, the respondents' personal background characteristics were studied by asking them to answer several questions related to their sociodemographic background.

Additional GPS data were collected to compare and validate how the different models of activity spaces match with the GPS tracks collected from a subsample of participants. A subsample of 100 participants of the PPGIS survey were selected, and an invitation to participate in additional GPS data collection was sent to participants' home addresses in September 2016. The participants were offered a 50 euro gift card for their participation. Twenty-nine participants used GPS devices with built-in accelerometers (Sensedoc ™ 2.0; MAX-M8 Global Navigation Satellite System receiver from u-blox, 2 s epoch, Tri-axial accelerometer, 50 Hz) for eight consecutive days. The participants also kept travel diaries during the same eight-day period. Those participants with valid data for GPS were included in the analysis, thus leaving

a final sample size of 18 individuals. Excluded users were people who reported having an unusual week, traveled extensively outside home surroundings during the study, or had problems using the device. The excluded users did not show any significant differences to the rest of users in terms of socio-demographics.

Activity space models

We implemented and subsequently compared four different spatial units of analysis. While all four units of analysis are individual-based, they differ significantly in terms of their complexity (Fig. 1). All four units of analysis will be referred to here as models of activity spaces, regardless of the complexity and the way they have been delineated. The first models are technically simple while the other two are more individual-specific and therefore come with higher technical complexities.

The first model, administrative boundary, is based on the postal areas and is determined for each individual based on their place of domicile. The second model is a circular buffer around each individual's home. This buffer was implemented using a static radius of 500 m,

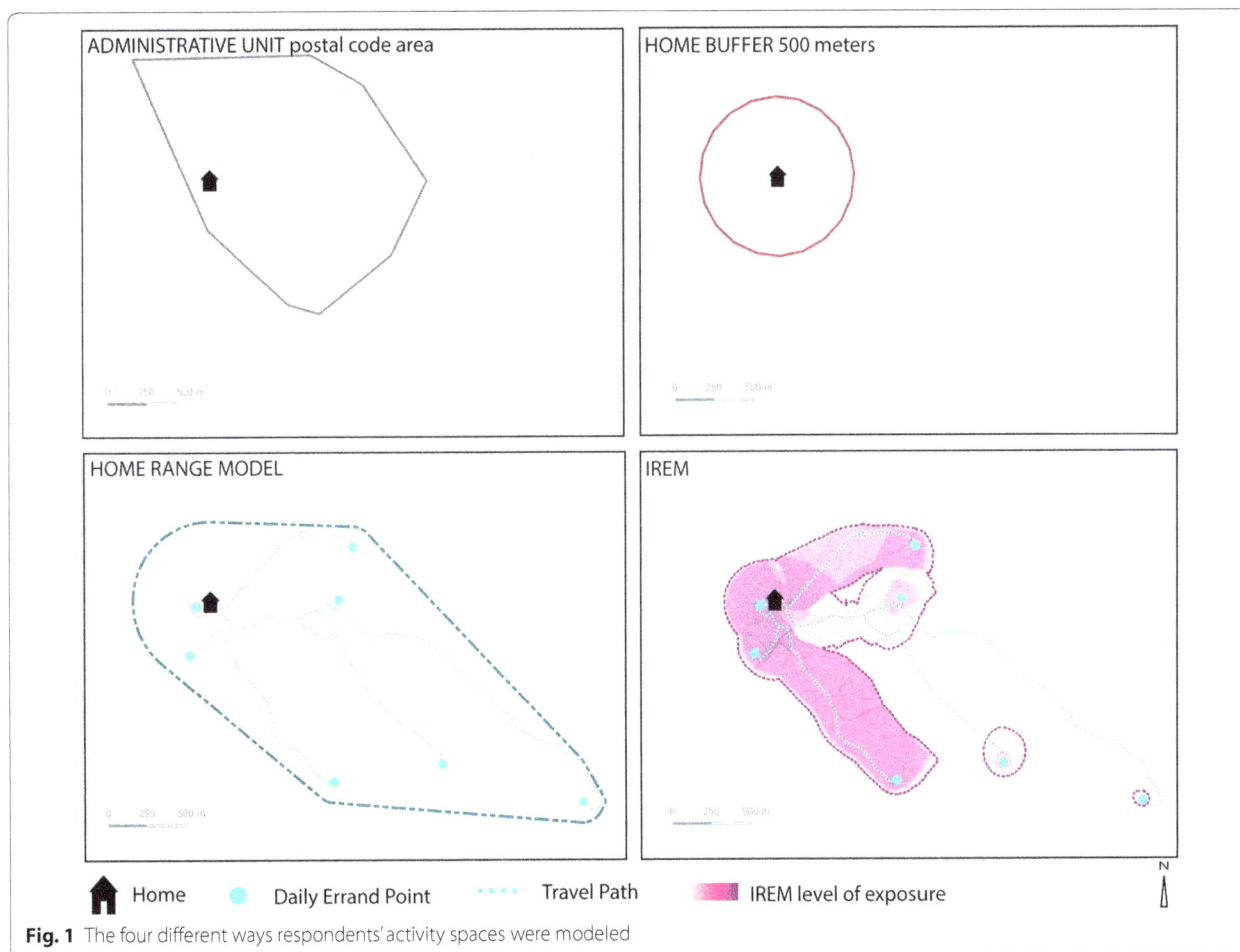

Fig. 1 The four different ways respondents' activity spaces were modeled

which is adopted as a commonly used distance in the literature [33]. The third model used, home range, is an individual-specific boundary method, which was first introduced by Hasanzadeh et al. [33]. Following the criteria suggested in the study, we listed all EEPs based on their distance from the participant's home location. The Jenk's optimization method revealed 4 km as the suitable home range distance for the data set [33, 41, 42]. This distance is based on the first natural break value including at least 80% of EEPs marked by the participants. It should be noted that the optimum number of classes for the Jenk's algorithm was determined using Goodness of Variance Fit (GVF) [42]. In the next step, a convex hull was applied to enclose all EEPs as well as the home point. However, prior to the implementation of convex hulls, buffers were applied to each point marked by the participants. Accordingly, buffers with distances 500 and 140 m were applied to the home locations and EEPs, respectively. According to Hasanzadeh et al. [33], 500 m is the most frequently used distance for defining immediate neighborhoods in literature, and 140 m is identified as a suitable estimation of activity cluster sizes in a data set collected from the same area as the current study. The later distance was calculated in the study as the average diameter of the spatial clusters formed by the aggregate of EEP markings [33].

The fourth model, IREM, is an exposure-based model of activity spaces [26]. Following the IREM criteria, we estimated the level of place exposure for each respondent throughout individual activity spaces using information on home location, visited places, frequency of visits, travel paths, and use of travel modes. In the IREM approach, exposure is expressed by assigning weights for places visited in terms of reported visit times per month with highest frequency of visits assigned to the home location. In addition, IREM estimates the level of exposure by taking into account the travel behavior of each individual. In IREM, the weight assigned to each travel path consists of the geometric average of weights at the origin and destination points and the average speed of the reported travel mode [26]. As an example, an individual who reported a higher frequency of use for a certain path with a non-motorized transportation mode is assumed to have higher exposure to his or her surroundings along their trip route compared to a less-frequently traveling individual who uses motorized transportation modes.

In the last step of creating IREM, an inverse distance function was applied to produce a raster representing the activity space of each individual [26]. The raster is made of square pixels with dimensions 25 m $\times$ 25 m, each containing a value as the estimation of exposure magnitude in its corresponding location. The exposure values are normalized using a sigmoid function with 0 as the minimum exposure and no upper limit defined for highest exposures [26]. The boundary of IREM was defined by the polygon encapsulating the high exposure areas. In this study, high exposure areas were identified as places with exposure values of more than 50% of the individual maximum.

Figure 1 shows an example of all four activity spaces modeled. It should be noted that we did not have any information about the actual travel path in the data set for the home range and IREM modeling. Therefore, the shortest path between each participant's home location and their EEPs was found using the Network Analyst toolbox of ArcGIS 10.5. The transportation mode indicated by the participant for visiting each specific EEP was taken into consideration while choosing the shortest path.

Dependent variables

Four different perceived wellbeing measures were used to test the associations between health and built environment measures. In the survey, the respondents were asked, how would they describe their (1) overall health situation, (2) ability to function, (3) quality of life, and (4) state of happiness at the moment. Respondents were asked to evaluate these four perceived wellbeing measures using a five-point Likert scale that ranged from very bad to very good. According to an extensive review by Kerr and colleagues [3] the evidence is building to suggest that older adults' physical health and functioning is connected to built environment factors. There is also evidence that perceived as well as objectively measured human health is in link with the physical environment characteristics, such as green spaces [10, 12, 43]. The overall health situation and quality of life as well as the happiness measure have been used in previous studies about the contextual effects on perceived health and on gross national happiness [9, 44]. The functional ability was included as an additional measure targeting the specific older age group of the study [3].

Independent variables

The built environment features have been found to be positively associated with health in many studies across the globe [5–9]. Thus, we used five different built environment measures to test their possible associations with perceived health of individuals. We measured amount of green spaces [7, 10, 11], the size of the modeled activity space [22, 26], land-use mix (LUM) [8] and walkability [2, 7] as walkability index and the length of pedestrian and cycling routes. The five measures were derived in GIS for administrative unit, 500 m residential buffer, home range model and IREM.

Greenness

This is a measure showing the amount of green areas within each individual activity space. For the three boundary approaches, namely administrative boundary, buffer, and home range, this was simply calculated as the percentage of land covered by green areas. For IREM, this was defined as the percentage of green exposure, and it was operationalized as the ratio of exposure to green areas to the total exposure within the activity space. Green exposures were determined as the value of exposure to the pixel identified as green, as estimated by IREM.

Size of activity space

This is a geometric measure capturing the total surface of the activity space areas. For IREM, the high-exposure polygon was used to measure the surface.

Land-use mix

Higher mix of land use has been shown to enhance PA because it provides versatility to the built environment and provides a variety of destinations closer to each other [7]. The LUM measure considered four land-use types: residential, commercial, traffic, and green space. Previous studies have also considered entertainment, office, and institutional land uses for the mix measure [45, 46]. We adopted these particular land-use categories for the LUM measure for two reasons: available data sets and they provide the best possible correspondence to the actual built environment in the study area. The formula used to calculate the LUM was modified from the formula used by Frank et al. [46]:

$$H = -1 \left(\sum_{i=1}^{n} pi * \ln(pi) \right) \bigg/ \ln(n)$$

where H is the LUM score, pi is the proportion of land use i among all land-use classes, and n is the number of land-use types. The information concerning land use, including green areas, was calculated from the CORINE dataset which is a raster dataset that provides information on Finnish land cover and land use on 2012. The data of CORINE has been produced as a part of the European Gioland 2012 project by Finnish Environment Institute (SYKE).

Walkability

Walkability was assessed according to the walkability index [45]. Walkability index was calculated as the sum of the z-scores of the four urban form measures [(2 × z-intersection density) + (z-net residential density) + (z-commercial floor area ratio) + (z-land-use mix)]. The measures were drawn from CORINE as well as from Digiroad that is an open road and traffic dataset provided by the Finnish Transport Agency.

Length of pedestrian/cycling routes

This measure was calculated as the total length of pedestrian and cycling routes in meters per square meter of the area of the spatial unit of analysis. For IREM, the high exposure polygon was used for the measurement. The pedestrian and bicycle roads were drawn from Open Street Map which is open geospatial data produced by a community of mappers. The data of OSM is fully open and licensed under the Open Data Commons Open Database License (ODbL) by the OpenStreetMap Foundation (OSMF).

Statistical analyses

The statistical analysis of the different activity space models had three main objectives. The first was to compare the contextual variables obtained with different activity space models in order to examine whether they are significantly different. Paired sample t tests were utilized to examine whether significant differences exist between contextual variables calculated using different activity space models. The significance of comparison results is adjusted for type I error using Bonferroni correction.

Second, we compared how the four activity space models match with the GPS tracks collected from a subsample of participants. To do so, we overlaid the GPS tracks with each model and calculated the percentage of overlap before applying the 4-km locality threshold and then after it.

Third, we conducted four independent regression analyses using multivariate linear regression. Each analysis took all the five activity space-based built environment measures as the independent variables and one of the four wellbeing measures as the dependent variable. All regression models were controlled for gender, age, education level, income, and retirement state. The purpose was to analyze the effect of activity space-based built environment measures on participants' perceived wellbeing and see how the choice of activity space model can affect the significance of observed associations. The model is as follows:

$$\text{WB} = \beta_0 + \beta_1 \text{Gr} + \beta_2 \text{LUM} + \beta_3 \text{W} + \beta_4 \text{PC} + (\beta_5 \text{S})$$
$$+ \beta_6 \text{I} + \beta_7 \text{AG} + \beta_8 \text{G} + \beta_9 \text{EDU} + \beta_{10} \text{RT} + \varepsilon$$

The independent variables of the model are explained in Table 1.

Results
Comparative analysis of activity space extents and measures

As expected, the four models vary significantly in size and shape (Table 2). The results show that the home range model has the most overall overlap with other methods, whereas the buffer approach shares the least overlaps

Table 2 The percentage overlap of the four activity space models (n = 844)

	Administrative unit	Home buffer 500 m	Individual home range	IREM
Administrative unit	–	66.6	46.5	44.4
Home buffer 500 m	26.5	–	22.4	37.3
Individual home range	78.7	100	–	100
IREM	48.2	67.3	40.4	–

among the methods (Fig. 2). Similarly, as Table 3 shows, the home range model has the highest level of consistency with GPS activity space. The home range model covered over half of the total GPS activity space, and the spatial overlap was 40% for IREM. Administrative unit and buffer covered a little less, with mean overlap of 38% for the former and 35% for the latter of the whole GPS activity space. When a 4-km cutoff distance to the GPS activity space was considered, the home range model covered nearly 80% and IREM two-thirds of the GPS activity space. The buffer approach shows the lowest match rate with GPS activity space with an average overlap of around 55% within the 4-km locality threshold (Table 3).

Next, we performed paired sample t tests to examine whether significant differences are evident in the activity-space-based contextual measures obtained from different models. Table 4 summarizes the significance of paired sample t tests for the contextual variables between the activity space models for the 844 participants. As shown, significant differences exist for most of the pairs of the activity space measures. However, there are also pairs of activity space models that do not yield statistically

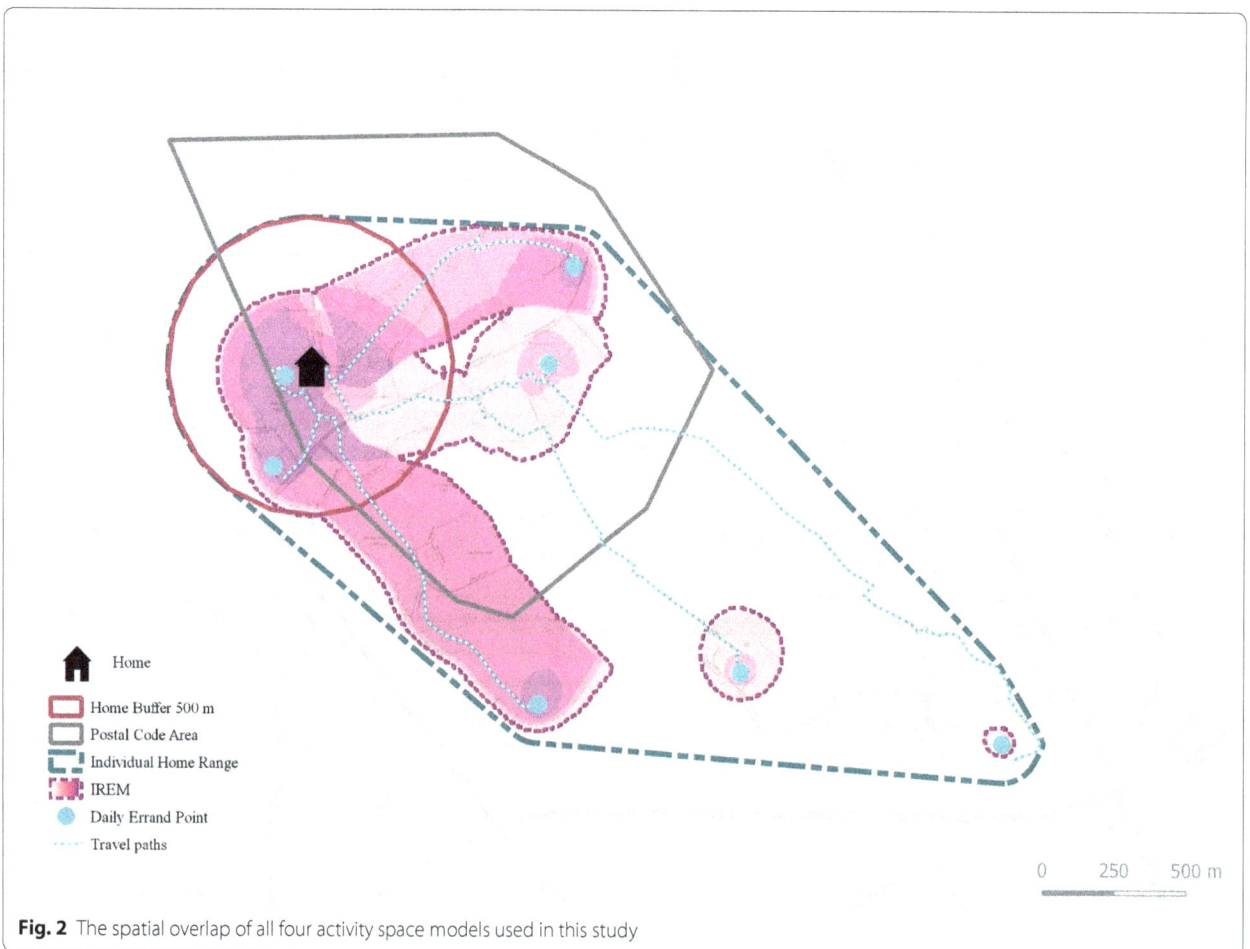

Home
Home Buffer 500 m
Postal Code Area
Individual Home Range
IREM
Daily Errand Point
Travel paths

0   250   500 m

Fig. 2 The spatial overlap of all four activity space models used in this study

Table 3 The spatial overlap of the four activity space models with GPS activity spaces collected from a subsample of the study participants

Method	Mean overlap % (overall)	Mean overlap % within locality threshold (4 km)
Administrative unit	38	59
Home buffer (500 m)	35	55
Individual home range	56	79
IREM	40	65

Table 4 The significance of paired sample *t* tests for the contextual variables between the four activity space models

	Admin. unit	Buffer	Home range	IREM
Greenness				
Admin		< 0.001	< 0.001	< 0.001
Buffer	< 0.001		< 0.001	< 0.001
HR	< 0.001	< 0.001		< 0.001
IREM	< 0.001	< 0.001	< 0.001	
Size of activity space				
Admin		< 0.001	< 0.001	< 0.001
Buffer	< 0.001		< 0.001	< 0.001
HR	< 0.001	< 0.001		< 0.001
IREM	< 0.001	< 0.001	< 0.001	
Land use mix				
Admin		0.797	0.801	0.803
Buffer	0.797		1.000	1.000
HR	0.801	1.000		1.000
IREM	0.803	1.000	1.000	
Walkability index				
Admin		< 0.001	< 0.001	0.803
Buffer	< 0.001		1.000	1.000
HR	< 0.001	1.000		< 0.001
IREM	0.803	1.000	< 0.001	
Pedestrian roads				
Admin		< 0.001	< 0.001	< 0.001
Buffer	< 0.001		< 0.001	0.002
HR	< 0.001	< 0.001		< 0.001
IREM	< 0.001	0.002	< 0.001	

A significance level of 0.05 (with adjustment for multiple comparison *p* < 0.008) is used to judge whether two measures are significantly different. The italicized values are statistically significant

significantly different measurement outcomes. Measurement of LUM does not significantly vary between any pairs of activity space models. Further, the value for walkability index does not significantly vary between some pairs of activity space models. The walkability index calculated using IREM appears to be significantly different from the one obtained using the home range model. Nevertheless, it does not seem to be significantly different from values obtained from the buffer and administrative boundary activity space model.

Regression analysis of health measures

In this section, we report the results of the regression analysis that explored how the contextual variables derived with different activity space models are associated with different aspects of health. To demonstrate whether the choice of activity space model influences the results, we compare the regression analysis results based on the significant associations found using the four activity space models.

Table 5 summarizes the results of the regression analysis based on different activity space models. The coefficients found to be statistically significant (Table 5) vary greatly between different activity space models. Some of the associations found via different activity space models contradict with each other. Greenness was found to be positively associated with several domains of health when using IREM as the activity space model; however, an opposite trend (significant negative associations) was found when home buffer and, in one case, when administrative boundary were used as activity space models.

The size of activity space appears to be positively associated with several aspects of health when measured via IREM. It is noteworthy that the size of postal areas is based on administrative preferences, and circular buffers have arbitrary and static areas. Accordingly, the notion of size when using these two approaches was deemed irrelevant and, therefore, left out of the regression analysis.

Positive associations were found between the length of pedestrian and cycling routes within an activity space and walkability index of an activity space with different aspects of wellbeing. These associations were best found using the home range model. LUM was not found to be statistically significantly associated with wellbeing measures in most cases.

Discussion

The aim of this study was to examine whether the associations between the built environment measures and health differ when individual exposure is assessed with several different spatial units of analysis. Earlier studies have concluded that the mixed results of the impact of the built environment on health can be at least partly due to the diverse use of different spatial units of analysis aiming to capture the individual spatial exposure [18–20, 23, 31]. There are only a few studies that have truly intended to study and overcome the contextual problems related to place exposure [23, 32].

Table 5 The association of contextual variables derived from different activity space models with different aspects of health

| | Greenness | | | | Land use mix | | | | Walkability | | | | P/C routes | | | | Size | | | |
	Administrative unit	Buffer	Home range	IREM	Administrative unit	Buffer	Home range	IREM	Administrative unit	Buffer	Home range	IREM	Administrative unit	Buffer	Home range	IREM	Administrative unit	Buffer	Home range	IREM
Health	_−0.25_	–	–	0.01	–	–	–	–	–	–	0.10	–	_0.11_	–	_0.13_	–	NA	NA	–	_0.10_
Func	_−0.03_	–	–	0.09	_0.15_	–	–	0.10	–	–	–	–	0.08	–	0.09	–	NA	NA	–	–
QOL	_−0.17_	0.08	–	0.09	–	–	–	–	–	–	0.12	–	–	–	_0.19_	–	NA	NA	–	_0.14_
Happiness	−0.1	–	–	–	–	–	–	–	_0.18_	0.09	0.10	–	–	–	_0.19_	–	NA	NA	–	_0.14_

AU administrative unit, *BF* buffer, *HR* home range, *IR* IREM

Only the coefficients significant at level *p* < 0.05 are shown in the table and those that are significant at level *p* < 0.01 are underlined

We compared two common residential and two novel activity space models as units of analysis to investigate whether differences exist in the associations between built environment features and perceived individual wellbeing outcomes. According to the results, all units of analysis differed from each other in terms of size, shape, and how they capture different contextual measures. These findings support the existence of the uncertain geographic context problem when examining the association between the built environment and human health [18]. In addition, we found that the associations between commonly used built environment measures and perceived wellbeing outcomes differed when using an administrative unit, residential buffer, home range model, and IREM for assessing the individual environmental exposure.

The four studied units of analysis—administrative unit, 500-m residential buffer, home range model [33], and IREM [26]—varied significantly in their size and shape. Thus, all four models are very distinct from each other. In general, administrative units and residential buffers manage to capture only a hypothetical individual exposure as these methods presume that individuals are exposed solely to the environment around their residency or within administrative boundaries. Both are static models and do not capture the dynamic nature of everyday human behavior [23, 26]. The administrative unit covered less than half and buffer only around one-third of the area that the home range model and IREM captured, which was shown when the different models were overlapped with each other. The uncertain geographic context problem is evident for these kinds of static spatial units of analysis that cannot capture individuals' true daily activities [23]. In contrast, the dynamic and people-based spatial models that use place-based data collected with online participatory mapping methods manage to capture the notions of activity spaces in a more individualized way [21, 26, 32, 33]. The home range model had the most overall overlap with other models. The home range model is an individual-specific boundary method created to capture individual activity spaces. Thus, the home range model captures the complete geographic area where individuals report themselves moving around. However, the individual home range model fails to capture varying levels of place exposure as it does not account for any temporal aspects. In contrast, IREM captures the areas where an individual is exposed to the physical environment according to the reported activities, frequency of visitations, and modes of transport used. Thus, the areal coverage of IREM is smaller than in home range models, but its capability to capture precise individual exposure is superior to any other models studied here.

Comparison of the four different spatial units of analysis with activity spaces delineated from GPS tracking demonstrated parallel results. The overall mean spatial overlap between the four studied models and a GPS activity space was highest for the novel people-based models. The home range model covered nearly 80% of the GPS activity space when a 4-km cutoff distance was applied to the GPS activity space. In comparison, the buffer covered only half of the same space. These results are in line with a study by Kestens et al. [32] where they found that both GPS and map-based questionnaires provide novel and suitable ways to collect daily mobility data and improve the exposure assessment of context-specific health research. Yet, it is noteworthy that GPS data collections are highly costly and time consuming. Thus, online map-based questionnaires can provide cost-efficient solutions for health research to delineate individual activity spaces in studies where context plays a significant role.

The differences of the contextual measures obtained from different models reassert the results of previous studies [20, 23]. We found significant differences in most built environment measures calculated using different activity space models. The amount of green space, the size of the activity space, and the length of pedestrian and bicycle roads differed significantly between all the activity space models. In their study, Zhao et al. [23] also found evidence that built environment measures differed between several activity space models. Nevertheless, there were a few exceptions in our results. LUM did not significantly vary between any pairs of activity space models. This might be because of the land use characteristics of the study area, which were rather mixed within the whole HMA in general. The conventional single-use zoning does not exist similarly in the study area when compared to North America where LUM has been commonly used as a well-fitting measure in environmental health studies. Additionally, a recent large international comparison found LUM not being related to PA [7]. Further, walkability index did not significantly differ between the static models and the activity space models. This might be related to the residential self-selection bias [47], where people who prefer walking may seek out to both live in and move around in walkable areas. In this case, respondents who prefer walking and active lifestyles seek to live in areas that are highly walkable (captured by administrative unit and home buffer) and move around in highly walkable areas (captured by individual home range model and IREM).

The associations between commonly used built environment measures and perceived wellbeing outcomes differed when using an administrative unit, residential buffer, home range model, and IREM for assessing the individual environmental exposure. The association between green space, LUM, walkability index, length of pedestrian and cycling routes, and wellbeing was assessed with all four different models. Additionally, the association between the size of the exposure model and health was assessed.

Only two very distinct models showed any results between the green space and health. When the individual exposure was assessed with IREM, a positive association between green space and health was found. For the administrative unit, a negative association was found. Thus, the amount of green space was found positively associated with respondents' perceived overall health, functional capability, and quality of life when the exposure was assessed with a unit of analysis that accounts for the true individual exposure and activities undertaken in a certain place. On the other hand, the amount of green space was found negatively associated with respondents' perceived wellbeing measures when administrative unit was used as a spatial unit of analysis. Thus, higher green area proportions around the residency decreased the perceived wellbeing. This is a rather contradictory result compared to previous studies on nature, green space and health [48, 49]. These results suggest that the true exposure to green instead of availability of green spaces are important to wellbeing. Thus, the accessibility, quality, and desirability instead of quantity of green spaces could be the focal aspects in planning healthy cities [50]. Additionally, these results can be explained by the fact that residential areas with vast green land uses in HMA are mostly fringe suburban areas surrounded by large forests and are highly car-oriented and less connected than the core urban areas. Thus, it might be that the quality of certain green areas instead of quantity of green space around one's home matters to the wellbeing of the people living in HMA [9].

LUM was positively associated with perceived functional capability when measured with administrative unit but not with any other unit of analysis or any other perceived health measure. LUM alone is perhaps not an applicable measure because its association with health, PA, and neighborhood satisfaction has shown no significant associations [7, 51]. Once LUM is combined with other urban structural measures, such as building and residential density, it forms a more applicable measure to capture the true mixed character of the urban areas, which is not limited only to the horizontal mix of land uses but extends also to the mix of vertical urban space [52].

Walkability index and the length of pedestrian and bicycle roads were found to have a positive correlation with most of the perceived wellbeing measures when studied with the home range model as a unit of analysis.

Thus, the more walkable the complete geographical area of the activity space is, the healthier, functionally more capable, and happy the respondents perceive themselves. Interestingly, no association was found between walkability index and perceived health when IREM was used as a unit of analysis. This discrepancy between the two activity space measures warrants further investigation because the results suggest that true exposure to walkable environments does not associate with health but that it is the availability and supply of highly walkable environments that associates with perceived health. Future studies investigating how walkability potential of activity spaces affect PA behavior of individuals compared to the exposure to walkable physical environments would continue to advance the understanding of the built environment relationship with health behavior.

By using the novel activity space models, future research could capture the various health promotive aspects of (urban) environments. The health impacts of the environment are complex, as the environment can affect all the physical, mental, and social health and wellbeing of individuals as well as the whole society [2, 6, 53, 54]. However, different characteristics of the environment can support mental health [10] compared to those that support physical health [7]. Exposure to green areas have been shown to reduce stress levels, and at the same time, well-connected, walkable, and dense urban environments support PA. These characteristics of the physical environment and their association to individuals' wellbeing can be captured with the different spatial modelling techniques.

In line with previous research, the size of activity space was found to be positively associated with different aspects of wellbeing. This is related to the actual exposure measurement because the size shows statistically significant associations with wellbeing only when it is measured with IREM. Given the more concentrated characteristic of IREM, and the fact that the use of active travel modes contribute positively to the exposure to the surrounding areas, this association could be attributed to the greater extent of active travel. Active mobility is an important source of daily PA for many people and, thus, may improve general health [55–59]. A similar conclusion cannot be drawn from less concentrated activity space models, such as home range, because a bigger size of activity space in these models is more likely to be associated with car use, which is found to impede PA [60].

This study aimed at investigating the challenges and opportunities of different spatial units of analysis—not determining which one should be used. Our results show that different models of activity spaces result in considerably different measurements of built environment. In turn, the differences derived from the use of different spatial units seem to considerably affect the associations between environment characteristics and wellbeing measures. Although it is not easy to argue about the correctness of these measurements, what is evident is that they can tell us different things. While some methods can be used to determine the availability of certain environmental opportunities, others can provide us with insight into their relevance based on the actual exposure. Therefore, one might argue that the choice of spatial unit should be made based on the context and the contents of a study. Nevertheless, our findings suggest that over-simplistic and static residential units of analysis, such as administrative unit and home buffer, may not be suitable approaches for measuring the activities of individuals and, thus, capturing individual environmental exposure [23].

Furthermore, a growing body of research has used GPS data to capture the notions of activity spaces and the true environmental exposure of human behavior [22, 61, 62]. However, the resources, costs, and time that GPS data collection and acquisition demands often make it impractical for studies requiring large data sets. The activity spaces generated from a participatory mapping survey showed general consistency with the GPS activity spaces in this study and a study by Kestens et al. [32]. Thus, studying environmental exposure through participatory mapping seems accurate and precise compared to GPS but is less demanding, costly, and time consuming.

Some limitations of this research need to be acknowledged. This study examined only the association between the physical environment and perceived wellbeing, but other various background factors, such as jobs, family situations, and socioeconomic status, also play a role in individuals' health. Previous studies have shown that demographic variables can mediate the relationships between health behavior and environmental variables [9]. Future research is warranted to investigate the multi-level influences of sociodemographic, built environment, and individual exposure variables on health. This study analyzed only a limited number of simple built environment variables in relation to perceived wellbeing. Using more complete and complex built environment variables may reveal more in-depth associations between the environment and health. Moreover, the comparisons made with GPS tracks are only based on a few participants. Future studies could benefit from a broader comparison based on a larger subsample of participants. In addition, the data used for this study were collected only from older adults aged 55–75. It would be interesting to see future studies exploring the presence of similar patterns in other age groups.

Conclusions

The notion of the uncertain geographic context problem has been linked to the conventional spatial units of analysis used in multidisciplinary research fields studying the questions of health geographics. In this study, we applied two common residential and two novel activity space models as units of analysis to investigate whether there exist differences in the associations between built environment features and perceived individual health outcomes. According to the results of this study, different spatial units of analysis yield distinct results regarding the association between the built environment and health. Walkability index and the length of pedestrian and bicycle roads were found to positively correlate with perceived wellbeing measures only when the spatial context was captured with a home range model [33]. In contrast, a positive association between green spaces and perceived wellbeing was found when the individual exposure was assessed with IREM, which is a novel dynamic and people-based spatial model using data collected through online participatory mapping method to capture the notions of activity spaces [25].

This study investigated the challenges and opportunities of different spatial units of analysis and concludes that there are several suitable units of analysis that can be used to capture the human exposure. While one cannot simply argue about the correctness of a certain unit of analysis, what is evident is that they can tell us different things. The essential challenge that the broad field of health geographics needs to overcome is the comparability of different studies and results; using diverse, not standardized spatial units of analysis and measures makes comparisons hard if not impossible. However, as the results of this and previous studies show, researchers should not rely only on the easy and over-simplistic spatial units of analysis [18, 20, 22, 23, 32]. For a better assessment of contextual effects, researchers should more carefully consider different spatial units and evaluate their implications for the research outcomes.

Authors' contributions
TL collected the original dataset, prepared the data for the analysis, contributed in the interpretation of the results, and was a major contributor in writing the manuscript. KH analyzed and interpreted the spatial and statistical data regarding different activity space models and contributed in writing the manuscript. MK contributed in writing the manuscript. All authors read and approved the final manuscript.

Acknowledgements

The authors would like to thank Finnish academy for funding the PLANhealth Project (13297753) which is has been the primary source of funding for this research. This research is also partially funded by Finnish Ministry of education and culture and Aalto University. The authors would like to thank the anonymous reviewer's for their comments, as well as Mary Lukkonen for the valuable language editing. The authors are also thankful to the OpenStreet-Map© contributors.

Competing interests

The authors declare that they have no competing interests.

Funding

Finnish academy PLANhealth Project (13297753). Finnish ministry of education and culture ActivAGE project funding.

References

1. Ding D, Gebel K. Built environment, physical activity, and obesity: what have we learned from reviewing the literature? Health Place. 2012;18:100–5.
2. Giles-Corti B, Vernez-Moudon A, Reis R, Turrell G, Dannenberg AL, Badland H, et al. City planning and population health: a global challenge. Lancet. 2016. https://doi.org/10.1016/S0140-6736(16)30066-6.
3. Kerr J, Rosenberg D, Frank L. The role of the built environment in healthy aging: community design, physical activity, and health among older adults. J Plan Lit. 2012;27:43–60.
4. Wang Y, Chau CK, Ng WY, Leung TM. A review on the effects of physical built environment attributes on enhancing walking and cycling activity levels within residential neighborhoods. Cities. 2016;50:1–15.
5. Adams MA, Ding D, Sallis JF, Bowles HR, Ainsworth BE, Bergman P, et al. Patterns of neighborhood environment attributes related to physical activity across 11 countries: a latent class analysis. Int J Behav Nutr Phys Act. 2013;10:34.
6. Frank L, Giles-Corti B, Ewing R. The influence of the built environment on transport and health. J Transp Health. 2016;3:423–5. https://doi.org/10.1016/j.jth.2016.11.004.
7. Sallis JF, Cerin E, Conway TL, Adams MA, Frank LD, Pratt M, et al. Physical activity in relation to urban environments in 14 cities worldwide: a cross-sectional study. Lancet. 2016;387:2207–17.
8. Saelens BE, Handy SL. Built environment correlates of walking: a review. Med Sci Sports Exerc. 2008;40(7 Suppl):S550–66. https://doi.org/10.1249/MSS.0b013e31817c67a4.
9. Kyttä M, Broberg A, Haybatollahi M, Schmidt-Thomé K. Urban happiness: context-sensitive study of the social sustainability of urban settings. Environ Plan B: Plan Des. 2016;43(1):34–57.
10. Tyrväinen L, Ojala A, Korpela K, Lanki T, Tsunetsugu Y, Kagawa T. The influence of urban green environments on stress relief measures: a field experiment. J Environ Psychol. 2014;38:1–9.
11. Thompson CW, Roe J, Aspinall P, Mitchell R, Clow A, Miller D. More green space is linked to less stress in deprived communities: evidence from salivary cortisol patterns. Landsc Urban Plan. 2012;105:221–9. https://doi.org/10.1016/j.landurbplan.2011.12.015.
12. Bratman GN, Daily GC, Levy BJ, Gross JJ. The benefits of nature experience: improved affect and cognition. Landsc Urban Plan. 2015;138:41–50.
13. Glazier RH, Creatore MI, Weyman JT, Fazli G, Matheson FI, Gozdyra P, et al. Density, destinations or both? A comparison of measures of walkability in relation to transportation behaviors, obesity and diabetes in Toronto, Canada. PLoS ONE. 2014;9:e85295. https://doi.org/10.1371/journal.pone.0085295.
14. Creatore M, Glazier R, Moineddin R, AI E. Association of neighborhood walkability with change in overweight, obesity, and diabetes. JAMA. 2016;315:2211–20. https://doi.org/10.1001/jama.2016.5898.
15. Hoehner CM, Handy SL, Yan Y, Blair SN, Berrigan D. Association between neighborhood walkability, cardiorespiratory fitness and body-mass index. Soc Sci Med. 2011;73:1707–16. https://doi.org/10.1016/j.socscimed.2011.09.032.
   James P, Berrigan D, Hart JE, Hipp JA, Hoehner CM, Kerr J, et al. Effects of buffer size and shape on associations between the built environ-
16. ment and energy balance. Health Place. 2014;27:162–70. https://doi.org/10.1016/j.healthplace.2014.02.003.
17. Wilks D, Besson H, Lindroos K, Ekelund U. Objectively measured physical activity and obesity prevention in children, adolescents and adults: a systematic review of prospective studies. Obes Rev. 2011;12:e119–29. https://doi.org/10.1111/j.1467-789X.2010.00775.x.
18. Kwan M-P. The uncertain geographic context problem. Ann Assoc Am Geogr. 2012;102:958–68.
19. Frank L, Fox EH, Ulmer JM, Chapman JE, Kershaw SE, Sallis JF, et al. International comparison of observation-specific spatial buffers: maximizing the ability to estimate physical activity. Int J Health Geogr. 2017;16:4.
20. Howell NA, Farber S, Widener MJ, Booth GL. Residential or activity space walkability: What drives transportation physical activity? J Transp Health. 2017;7:160–71.
21. Perchoux C, Chaix B, Brondeel R, Kestens Y. Residential buffer, perceived neighborhood, and individual activity space: New refinements in the definition of exposure areas—the RECORD cohort study. Health Place. 2016;40:116–22.
22. Zenk SN, Schulz AJ, Matthews SA, Odoms-Young A, Wilbur J, Wegrzyn L, et al. Activity space environment and dietary and physical activity behaviors: a pilot study. Health Place. 2011;17:1150–61. https://doi.org/10.1016/J.HEALTHPLACE.2011.05.001.
23. Zhao P, Kwan M-P, Zhou S. The uncertain geographic context problem in the analysis of the relationships between obesity and the built environment in Guangzhou. Int J Environ Res Public Health. 2018;15:308.
24. Feng J, Glass TA, Curriero FC, Stewart WF, Schwartz BS. The built environment and obesity: a systematic review of the epidemiologic evidence. Health Place. 2010;16:175–90.
25. Leal C, Chaix B. The influence of geographic life environments on cardiometabolic risk factors: a systematic review, a methodological assessment and a research agenda. Obes Rev. 2011;12(3):217–30.
26. Hasanzadeh K, Laatikainen T, Kyttä M. A place-based model of local activity spaces: individual place exposure and characteristics. J Geogr Syst. 2018.
27. Hannam K, Sheller M, Urry J. Mobilities, immobilities and moorings. Mobilities. 2006;1(1):1–22.
28. Faist T. The mobility turn: a new paradigm for the social sciences? Ethn Racial Stud. 2013;36:1637–46. https://doi.org/10.1080/01419870.2013.812229.
29. Sheller M, Urry J. The new mobilities paradigm. Environ Plan A Econ Space. 2006;38:207–26.
30. Chaix B. Geographic life environments and coronary heart disease: a literature review, theoretical contributions, methodological updates, and a research agenda. Annu Rev Public Health. 2009;30:81–105.
31. Holliday KM, Howard AG, Emch M, Rodriguez DA, Evenson KR. Are buffers around home representative of physical activity spaces among adults? Health Place. 2017;45:181–8.
32. Kestens Y, Thierry B, Shareck M, Steinmetz-Wood M, Chaix B. Integrating activity spaces in health research: comparing the VERITAS activity space questionnaire with 7-day GPS tracking and prompted recall. Spat Spatiotemporal Epidemiol. 2018;25:1–9.
33. Hasanzadeh K, Broberg A, Kyttä M. Where is my neighborhood? A dynamic individual-based definition of home ranges and implementation of multiple evaluation criteria. Appl Geogr. 2017;84:1–10.
34. Sallis JF, Saelens BE. Assessment of physical activity by self-report: status, limitations, and future directions. Res Q Exerc Sport. 2000;71:1–14.
35. Brown G, Kyttä M. Key issues and research priorities for public participation GIS (PPGIS): a synthesis based on empirical research. Appl Geogr. 2014;46:122–36. https://doi.org/10.1016/j.apgeog.2013.11.004.
36. Brown G, Raymond CM. Methods for identifying land use conflict potential using participatory mapping. Landsc Urban Plan.

2014;122:196–208.

37. Brown G, Schebella MF, Weber D. Using participatory GIS to measure physical activity and urban park benefits. Landsc Urban Plan. 2014;121:34–44.

38. Kytta AM, Broberg AK, Kahila MH. Urban environment and children's active lifestyle: SoftGIS revealing children's behavioral patterns and meaningful places. Am J Health Promot. 2012;26:e137–48.

39. Schmidt-Thome K, Wallin S, Laatikainen T, Kangasoja J. Kyttä M. J Community Inform: Exploring the use of PPGIS in self-organizing urban development: case softGIS in Pacific Beach; 2014. p. 10.

40. Kyttä M, Broberg A, Tzoulas T, Snabb K. Towards contextually sensitive urban densification: location-based softGIS knowledge revealing perceived residential environmental quality. Landsc Urban Plan. 2013;113:30–46.

41. Jenks GF. The data model concept in statistical mapping. Int Yearb Cartogr. 1967;7:186–90.

42. Hasanzadeh KIASM. Individualized activity space modeler. SoftwareX. 2018;7:138–42.

43. Cummins S, Stafford M, Macintyre S, Marmot M, Ellaway A. Neighbourhood environment and its association with self rated health: evidence from Scotland and England. J Epidemiol Community Health. 2005;59(3):207–13.

44. Pennock M, Ura K. Gross national happiness as a framework for health impact assessment. Environ Impact Assess Rev. 2011;31:61–5.

45. Frank LD, Sallis JF, Saelens BE, Leary L, Cain L, Conway TL, et al. The development of a walkability index: application to the neighborhood quality of life study. Br J Sports Med. 2010;44:924–33.

46. Frank LD, Schmid TL, Sallis JF, Chapman J, Saelens BE. Linking objectively measured physical activity with objectively measured urban form: findings from SMARTRAQ. Am J Prev Med. 2005;28(2):117–25. https://doi.org/10.1016/j.amepre.2004.11.001.

47. Cao X, Mokhtarian PL, Handy SL. Examining the impacts of residential self-selection on travel behaviour: a focus on empirical findings. Transp Rev. 2009;29:359–95. https://doi.org/10.1080/01441640802539195.

48. Korpela K, Nummi T, Lipiäinen L, De Bloom J, Sianoja M, Pasanen T, Kinnunen U. Nature exposure predicts well-being trajectory groups among employees across two years. J Environ Psychol. 2017;1(52):81–91.

49. Sugiyama T, Carver A, Koohsari MJ, Veitch J. Advantages of public green spaces in enhancing population health. Landsc Urban Plan. 2018;31(178):12–7.

50. Corburn J. City planning as preventive medicine. Prev Med. 2015;77:48–51. https://doi.org/10.1016/j.ypmed.2015.04.022.

51. Van Dyck D, Cardon G, Deforche B, De Bourdeaudhuij I. Do adults like living in high-walkable neighborhoods? Associations of walkability parameters with neighborhood satisfaction and possible mediators. Health Place. 2011;17:971–7. https://doi.org/10.1016/j.healthplace.2011.04.001.

52. Laatikainen TE, Broberg A, Kyttä M. The physical environment of positive places: exploring differences between age groups. Prev Med (Baltim). 2017;95:S85–91.

53. Ward Thompson C, Aspinall PA. Natural environments and their impact on activity, health, and quality of life. Appl Psychol Health Well-Being. 2011;3:230–60.

54. Goenka S, Andersen LB. Urban design and transport to promote healthy lives. Lancet. 2016;388.

55. Perchoux C, Chaix B, Cummins S, Kestens Y. Conceptualization and measurement of environmental exposure in epidemiology: accounting for activity space related to daily mobility. Health Place. 2013;21:86–93. https://doi.org/10.1016/j.healthplace.2013.01.005.

56. Pucher J, Buehler R, Bassett DR, Dannenberg AL. Walking and cycling to health: a comparative analysis of city, state, and international data. Am J Public Health. 2010;100:1986–92.

57. Shephard RJ. Is active commuting the answer to population health? Sports Med. 2008;38:751–8.

58. de Hartog JJ, Boogaard H, Nijland H, Hoek G. Do the health benefits of cycling outweigh the risks? Environ Health Perspect. 2010;118:1109–16.

59. Milton S, Pliakas T, Hawkesworth S, Nanchahal K, Grundy C, Amuzu A, et al. A qualitative geographical information systems approach to explore how older people over 70 years interact with and define their neighbourhood environment. Health Place. 2015;36:127–33.

60. Saunders LE, Green JM, Petticrew MP, Steinbach R, Roberts H. What are the health benefits of active travel? A systematic review of trials and cohort studies. PLoS ONE. 2013;8:e69912.

61. Hirsch JA, Winters M, Ashe MC, Clarke P, McKay H. Destinations that older adults experience within their GPS activity spaces relation to objectively measured physical activity. Environ Behav. 2016;48:55–77. https://doi.org/10.1177/0013916515607312.

62. Chaix B, Meline J, Duncan S, Merrien C, Karusisi N, Perchoux C, et al. GPS tracking in neighborhood and health studies: a step forward for environmental exposure assessment, a step backward for causal inference? Health Place. 2013;21:46–51.

3

Development of a spatial sampling protocol using GIS to measure health disparities in Bobo-Dioulasso, Burkina Faso, a medium-sized African city

Daouda Kassié[1,2], Anna Roudot[1], Nadine Dessay[3], Jean-Luc Piermay[4], Gérard Salem[1,5] and Florence Fournet[6,7*] ⓘ

Abstract

Background: Many cities in developing countries experience an unplanned and rapid growth. Several studies have shown that the irregular urbanization and equipment of cities produce different health risks and uneven exposure to specific diseases. Consequently, health surveys within cities should be carried out at the micro-local scale and sampling methods should try to capture this urban diversity.

Methods: This article describes the methodology used to develop a multi-stage sampling protocol to select a population for a demographic survey that investigates health disparities in the medium-sized city of Bobo-Dioulasso, Burkina Faso. It is based on the characterization of Bobo-Dioulasso city typology by taking into account the city heterogeneity, as determined by analysis of the built environment and of the distribution of urban infrastructures, such as healthcare structures or even water fountains, by photo-interpretation of aerial photographs and satellite images. Principal component analysis and hierarchical ascendant classification were then used to generate the city typology.

Results: Five groups of spaces with specific profiles were identified according to a set of variables which could be considered as proxy indicators of health status. Within these five groups, four sub-spaces were randomly selected for the study. We were then able to survey 1045 households in all the selected sub-spaces. The pertinence of this approach is discussed regarding to classical sampling as random walk method for example.

Conclusion: This urban space typology allowed to select a population living in areas representative of the uneven urbanization process, and to characterize its health status in regards to several indicators (nutritional status, communicable and non-communicable diseases, and anaemia). Although this method should be validated and compared with more established methods, it appears as an alternative in developing countries where geographic and population data are scarce.

Keywords: Health disparities, Spatial sampling, Typology, Medium-sized city, Bobo-Dioulasso

Background

Urbanization is a phenomenon that modifies the environment and living conditions on all continents. Since 2007, more than half of the world population live in cities and this percentage is expected to increase to almost 70% in 2050 [1], and to 50% for West Africa from now to 2030. Many cities in developing countries experience an unplanned growth that, as a result, exposes the populations to numerous environmental risks with complex and still poorly known health consequences.

Cities are dense (concentration of populations), open (high mobility due to, for instance, migrations from and

*Correspondence: florence.fournet@ird.fr
[6] MIVEGEC, Institut de Recherche pour le Développement, 911, Avenue Agropolis, BP 64501, 34394 Montpellier Cedex 5, France
Full list of author information is available at the end of the article

to rural environments) and heterogeneous environments. This heterogeneity is not linked only to the uneven distribution of infrastructures [2, 3]. It is also caused by the urbanization process on its own. Indeed, a city is not built in the same way if it develops in a plain or in the middle of mountains, or if it is traversed by low-lying grounds or close to the seaside, or if its growth is controlled or not. Several studies have shown that the irregular urbanization and patchy infrastructure of cities have many consequences on health [3–5], by producing different health risks and uneven risk of exposure to specific diseases [6]. Many of these studies were conducted in big cities, although urbanization occurs more and more in medium-sized cities [7]. These places have the disadvantages of cities (unplanned growth, pollution) and also of rural areas (under-equipment) and their consequences on health have been not fully investigated [8].

The study of urban health disparities is complex for different reasons. First of all, the health status of a population is influenced not only by individual factors, but also by a multitude of genetic, social, demographic, cultural, physical, economic and also political determinants that interact with each other [9]. Therefore, due to the urban heterogeneity, it is clear that a prevalence given for the whole city will mask intra-urban differences that are not without consequences on the population quality of life [2, 4]. For instance, infant deaths are less frequent in Nairobi than in rural areas of Kenya; however, this urban mean value hides substantial variations within the city. Indeed, the mortality rate of deprived areas is much higher than that of the whole city [1].

Consequently, the need of working at the micro-local scale becomes obvious [10]. However, a major issue is to know how to capture this urban diversity and how to analyse health in the light of such diversity. The quantitative and qualitative characterization of urbanization remains a black box, particularly in low-income countries. Although in many cities, the centre is distinguished from the peripheries, this dichotomy is not always present. Moreover, it cannot be reduced to a gradient that translates a progressively stronger urbanization from the periphery towards the centre, for example. In the cities of developing countries, often a high-quality house stands alongside a very precarious house. According to Grafmeyer [11], a city is at the same time a territory and also a population, a framework collective life, a collection of physical objects and a cluster of relationships. Indeed, although a city is the results of a long-term construction, it cannot be dissociated from those that are building it. Therefore, the urban space should be considered as the support, product and subject of social relationships [4].

In developing country settings, old censuses as well as lack of health surveillance and geographic data limit

survey design options. In these situations, approaches require to propose new sampling frames. Expanded programme on immunization (EPI) method may be a solution but is often difficult to apply in urban settings [12]. Alternatives based on adaptation of EPI method [13], or on purposeful selection of clusters guided by knowledge of the spatial arrangement of key population characteristics [14] could be proposed. But the challenge remains to develop a method allowing sampling of specific subspaces which illustrate the urban diversity, and of populations who participate to this diversity while providing approaches applicable to other contexts.

To determine the effect of the production of an urban space on the health in a medium-sized city, we developed a multi-stage sampling method adapted to our objective. Our aim was to investigate the health status of Bobo-Dioulasso (Burkina Faso) populations at the intra-city scale, in view of presenting concrete proposals to the municipal authorities, healthcare and urban planning policy-makers. The chosen methodological approach combined the use of different tools with qualitative approaches that allowed the fine characterization of the urban space of Bobo-Dioulasso relative to health questions. The obtained city typology was used to select study areas that are representative of different urbanization modes, assuming that population health status would be different. The health status was described based on different indicators of communicable (malaria and dengue) and non-communicable diseases (blood hypertension and diabetes), nutritional status and anaemia. This choice was justified by the growing evidence of a double burden of diseases in cities of developing countries [15].

The different steps of this approach are presented as well as the results in terms of choice of sub-spaces and surveyed populations.

Methods
Study site
The city of Bobo-Dioulasso is in the West of Burkina Faso, in the middle of Houet province of which it is the main city (Fig. 1).

Bobo-Dioulasso has been showing relatively important and constant growth rates (4.7% per year, on average) since its discovery by colonialists, with the exception of some key periods, particularly 1985–1996. During this period, all the efforts were focused on Ouagadougou, which was the showcase of the Sankarist urban policy, and Bobo-Dioulasso was left outside the fast evolutionary dynamics [16, 17]. This expansion was not without consequences on the urban planning. An irregular distribution of healthcare services in space and time in Bobo-Dioulasso was observed. The installation of healthcare structures did not always follow the major phases of

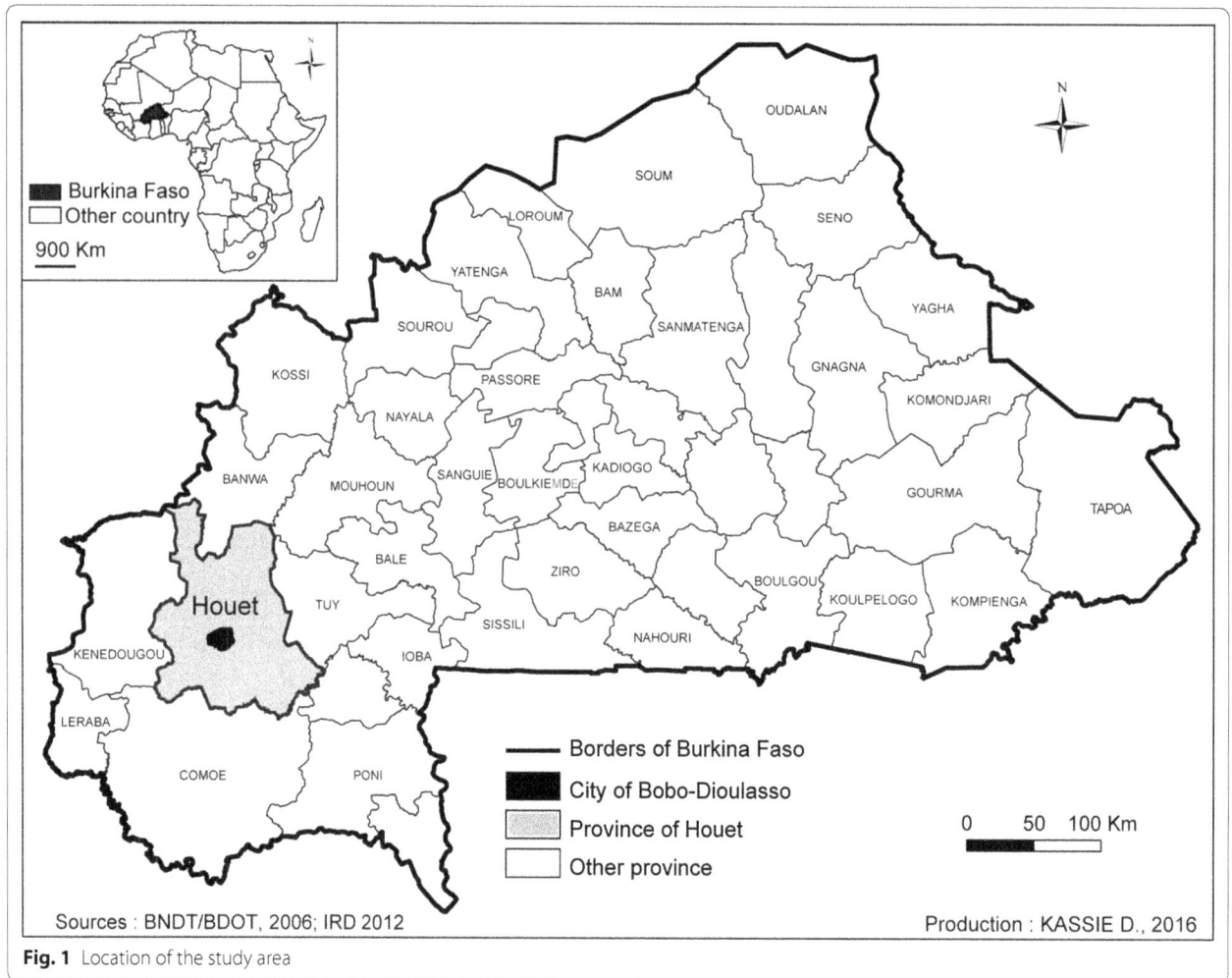

Fig. 1 Location of the study area

urban growth due to the different policies started by the State and international institutions. Thus, the number of healthcare structures rose from four before 1960 to 52 in 2012, without an even coverage of the entire urban space [18] (Fig. 2). Similarly, differences concerning the access to drinking water were observed, with inexistent rates of connection in non-regularized settlements and variable rates in regularized areas (Fig. 3).

Data sources

The literature on the history, social organization and urbanization of Bobo-Dioulasso was reviewed. Aerial photographs from 1952 to 1987 (Institut Géographique National, in English French National Geographic Institute), and aerial photographs of 1994 (Institut Géographique du Burkina, in English: Burkina Faso Geographical Institute) were used to retrace the city growth in time and space. These photographs were georeferenced and then mosaics were generated for each year.

The satellite images used for this study corresponded to: (1) two SPOT 5 images of 2004 and 2007 at high definition acquired in multi-spectral (M) at 10 m and panchromatic (P) mode from the ISIS programme of CNES (the French space agency). For 2004, the spatial resolution for the P mode image was 5 m and for 2007 it was 2.5 m (generated from two images at 5 m acquired simultaneously); (2) one Pléiades satellite image at very high resolution of 2012 also from CNES. Its resolution was 2.8 m for the M mode and 0.7 m re-sampled to 0.5 m for the P mode. The images obtained with the optic system SPOT 5 present the advantage of covering a large geographical area (60 km). The Pléiades images cover a reduced area (20 km), but allow the detection of objects smaller than 1 m.

The 2012 cadastral map of Bobo-Dioulasso was obtained from the National Water and Sanitation Office (Office National de l'Eau et de l'Assainissement, ONEA) of the city.

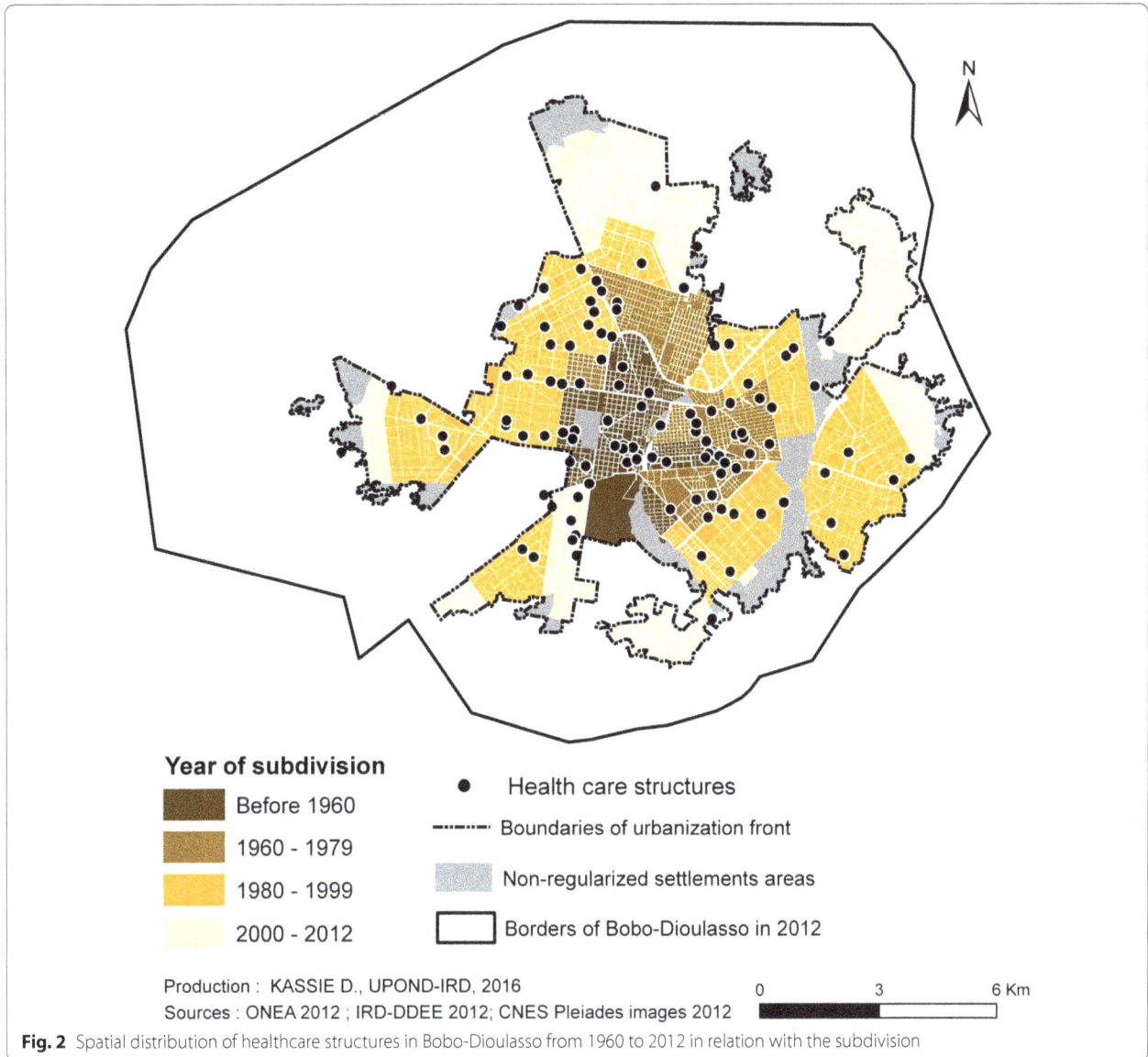

Fig. 2 Spatial distribution of healthcare structures in Bobo-Dioulasso from 1960 to 2012 in relation with the subdivision

Methodological approach

The methodological approach was developed to meet different objectives: (a) to establish the urban growth and the displacement of the urbanization front by visual interpretation of photographs for the following years: 1952, 1958, 1964, 1980, 1987, 1994 and of scenes for the following years: 2004, 2007 and 2012; (b) to divide the city in homogeneous spatial units based on the size and the organization of the built environment, the configuration of the road network, and the presence of vegetation by visual interpretation of the scene of 2012; (c) to extract the city's fabric, the vegetation and the road network from the satellite image of 2012 to produce a spatial database that should facilitate the analysis of health

disparities (Table 1); (d) to produce a typology of the city based on spatial analysis (principal component analysis and hierarchical ascendant classification).

The definition of spatial units inside which health status was surveyed allowed to throw of classical administrative division like districts or census blocks, which did not necessary ensure to evaluate how neighbourhoods may affect individual or population health [19, 20].

Urban growth and identification of AHU by visual photo-interpretation

From 1952 to 2012, the mosaics of aerial photographs and remote sensing images were visually interpreted to delimit the urbanization front and to determine the

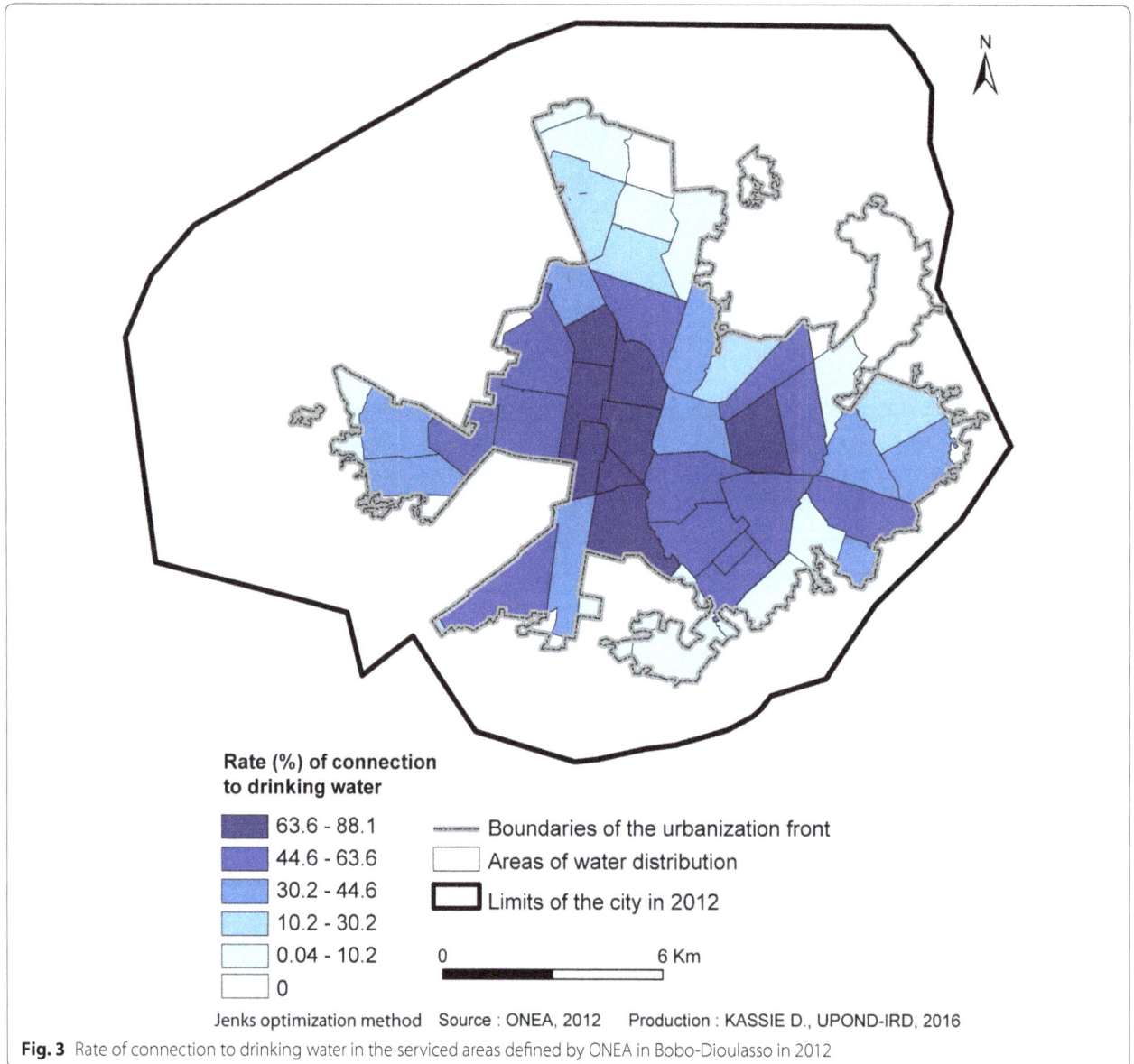

Rate (%) of connection to drinking water

- 63.6 - 88.1
- 44.6 - 63.6
- 30.2 - 44.6
- 10.2 - 30.2
- 0.04 - 10.2
- 0

— — Boundaries of the urbanization front
☐ Areas of water distribution
☐ Limits of the city in 2012

0   6 Km

Jenks optimization method   Source : ONEA, 2012   Production : KASSIE D., UPOND-IRD, 2016

Fig. 3 Rate of connection to drinking water in the serviced areas defined by ONEA in Bobo-Dioulasso in 2012

growth of the urban space. The urban fabric morphology was then analysed to obtain fine and precise information on the shapes of subsets within the city. This analysis took into account simultaneously the built space, the space covered by vegetation and the road network [21–24]. Hence, the space will appear in the shape of urban subsets that are characterized by their coherence and unity. This was realized with the Pléiades images of 2012 by visual interpretation and led to delineate morphologically similar spaces called areas of homogeneous units (AHU). These spatial units were delimitated around urban blocks comprising a variable number of plots.

This approach gave a structured and synthetic vision of the urban fabric by putting it in the global context. It allowed the categorization of a city in different urban fabrics that could be charted, thus producing a good image of what could be observed in the field. Therefore, this segmentation allowed studying the space continuity and the areas where it breaks up.

Supervised classification of the urban morphology at very high spatial resolution

The aims of this classification were: (a) to move from the photo-interpretation towards a generic method, (b) to put in place a stratified sampling method in order to optimize the use of classes that have a direct or potential link with health as sampling criteria for the areas to be surveyed.

Table 1 Overview of aerial photographs and remote sensing datasets

Providers	Datasets	Date	Spatial resolution	Type of analysis
IGN France	5 Aerial photographs	1952	1/15,000	Analysis of the urban growth (photo-interpretation)
	9 Aerial photographs	1958	1/15,000	
	6 Aerial photographs	1964	1/26,000	
	5 Aerial photographs	1980	1/20,000	
	9 Aerial photographs	1987	1/20,000	
IGB	11 Aerial photographs	1994	1/20,000	
CNES	1 SPOT panchromatic image	2004	5 m	
	1 Multispectral Image	2004	10 m	
	1 SPOT panchromatic image	2007	2.5 m	
	1 Multispectral image	2007	10 m	
CNES	2 Pléiades high resolution panchromatic images	2012	0.5 m	Analysis of the urban growth and identification of the AHU (photo-interpretation, supervised classification of the urban morphology)
	2 Pléiades high resolution Multispectral images	2012	2 m	

The supervised classification by maximum similarity was performed starting from the Pléiades image of 2012. Two classes were added to the already identified thematic classes: water collections (water puddles, river, ponds) and bare soil (sand, laterite). Asphalted roads were differentiated within the road network class.

Different indexes were calculated: Normalized Vegetation Index, Humidity Index and Brightness Index. The confusions identified based on the confusion matrix were corrected after integration of the results in a geographic information system (GIS). This is the class "clouds" when confused with the class "urban" and the class "building" when attached to the wrong urban component. These corrections were implemented manually.

The results of these post-treatments allowed calculating the density of vegetation and of built surfaces in each AHU and then using these density values for spatial analyses, specifically the principal component analyses (PCA) and hierarchical ascendant classification (HAC).

Field surveys were also carried out to localize the urban infrastructures (healthcare structures, schools, water fountains, traffic lights, markets, coach stations) and to validate the satellite image-based analyses. They were completed with surveys in the healthcare structures to collect additional information on the structure type and opening year.

Finally, these data were completed by surveys based on the statements of responsible people at the town hall, ONEA, waste management service, associations, media and traditional and religious rulers.

Generation of a town typology

Its objective was to select in a robust manner the urban sub-spaces in which the population will be surveyed. A sampling method that combined PCA and HAC was applied on the AHU identified at the precedent stage to generate the city typology. This allows improving the sampling quality compared with the simple random sampling technique[1] by taking into account simple, objective and measurable criteria [23], such as the built surfaces or those covered by vegetation. A similar method was used in Dakar to analyse socio-economic disparities [25].

PCA generates new artificial variables and graphic representations that allow visualizing the relationships between variables or between individuals (spatial units), as well as the possible existence of relationships between groups of individuals or between groups of variables. It detects and reduces the number of correlated variables to be used for HAC. HAC objective is to find, in several steps, the closest classes and then to merge them till only one class remains [26]. Several variables that discriminate the urban space were retained to identify via PCA and HAC the sub-spaces that represent diversified urbanization processes where the health status may vary. The chosen variables measured health vulnerability (building density, level of infrastructures, risk of flooding, age of the district) or the access to urbanization (access to healthcare structures and to drinking water). They could be expressed by a mean (e.g., mean building density within the AHU), by a percentage (e.g., portion of the AHU at risk of flooding) or even by a standard deviation (e.g., standard deviation of the rate of connection to the drinking water network within the AHU).

These analyses generated a typology of Bobo-Dioulasso that could be used to select urban sub-spaces for health

---

[1] Simple random sampling is a type of probability sampling in which observations are selected randomly within a population with a known sampling probability or fraction. (http://documentation.statsoft.com/STATISTICA-Help.aspx?path=Glossary/GlossaryTwo/S/SimpleRandomSamplingSRS).

surveys. Within each class identified by the HAC, a sub-space was randomly selected. Only one sub-space was selected in each class as the objective was to compare the health disparities between the different classes, and not between different AHU belonging to a same class.

Spatial and demographic sampling for the health survey
After the identification of the four AHU to be surveyed, several spatial random sampling without replacement allowed selecting plots within each AHU using the cadastral map of 2012. This method ensures the comparability of the data collected in the different AHU. The Pléiades image and the cadastral map of 2012 were used to identify and eliminate from the sampling, uninhabited plots dedicated to administrative or commercial usage. In regular areas, plots were randomly selected using the 'Sampling Design Tool' of ArcGIS 10. For non-regular areas, without delimited plots, houses were digitalized by referring to the roof and their geographical coordinates were integrated in the GIS for the sampling.

Ripley's K-function which is typically used to compare a given point distribution with a random distribution, was used to test the spatial distribution of the selected households in each AHU [18]. The point distribution is tested against the null hypothesis that the points are distributed randomly and independently. We used a common transformation of the K-Function, often referred to as L(d) which is implemented in ArcGIS. When the observed K value is larger than the expected K value for a particular distance, the distribution is more clustered than a random distribution at that distance (scale of analysis). When the observed K value is smaller than the expected K, the distribution is more dispersed than a random distribution at that distance.

The geographical coordinates of the randomly selected plots or digitalized houses were integrated in Garmin eTrex 10 handheld GPS units. Surveyors had to find these concessions by using the procedure 'Go to' of the GPS unit and with the help of maps on which these plots were shown. Each survey sub-space was subdivided in three parts and each part was attributed to a surveyor who had to cover it completely. This technique avoided having all the selected households in a single part of the study area.

To be easily identified by the populations, each surveyor had a badge and a work kit (GPS unit, map with the randomly selected points, forms for data collection, etc.). As one or more households may live inside a same plot or a same house in non-regularized areas, the surveyor counted the number of households and identified those eligible for the survey before selecting one by random sampling. A household was eligible if it included at least one eligible child (6–59 months of age) and one eligible adult (35–59 years of age) (Fig. 4).

First, the surveyor needed to collect the household head's authorization for the household participation in the survey after eligibility verification. In the case of absence or doubts on the age of the people to be surveyed, the surveyor took an appointment. After three unsuccessful appointments, the household was abandoned and replaced by another household in the random sampling list for that sub-space.

All collected and analysed geographical data[2] (aerial photographs, satellite images, geographical coordinates of urban infrastructures) were integrated in a geodatabase with a map projection WGS84 UTM 30 N (Fig. 5).

In order to observe significant differences between AHU at the 5% threshold with a precision of 2.6% based on a prevalence of 5% (which was the smallest expected prevalence for diabetes in adults), a sample size of 250 adults and 250 children (and then 250 households) was calculated. The same number of adults and children were chosen in each AHU to allow the comparability between AHU by multivariate analysis. This method permitted to determine if the same risk factors were associated to the same health indicator in each AHU.

Results
Between the beginning of its colonization and the independence, the population of the second city of Burkina Faso, which is presented as the economic capital, increased from 3000 to 50,000 inhabitants, to reach 230,000 inhabitants in 1975, 310,000 in 1996 and 490,000 in 2006 [27]. This growth led to a radial extension of the city without specific building densification due to the absence of physical constraints. According to the urban growth analysis based on aerial photographs and satellite images, the city surface increased from 10.7 km^2 in 1952 to 95.7 km^2 in 2012 (Fig. 6). Analysis of the urban morphology showed that Bobo-Dioulasso could be divided in 125 AHU that were well differentiated and that could be easily distinguished on the basis of the density of buildings, vegetation and roads (Fig. 7).

The spatial analyses based on AHU allowed dividing the city in five classes that explained almost 50% of the total variance (Fig. 8). Class 1 (C01; in dark blue) corresponded to peripheral areas under development, but with few infrastructures (both regularized and non-regularized settlements). Class 2 (C02; in light blue) included areas of different age, sometimes distant from the city centre, but globally well-equipped in infrastructures. Class 3 (C03; in green) grouped together central areas that were urbanized long ago, densely built and well

---

[2] Data were analysed with the Envi (image analysis), ArcGIS (database and mapping) and Philcarto (statistical cartography) software programmes.

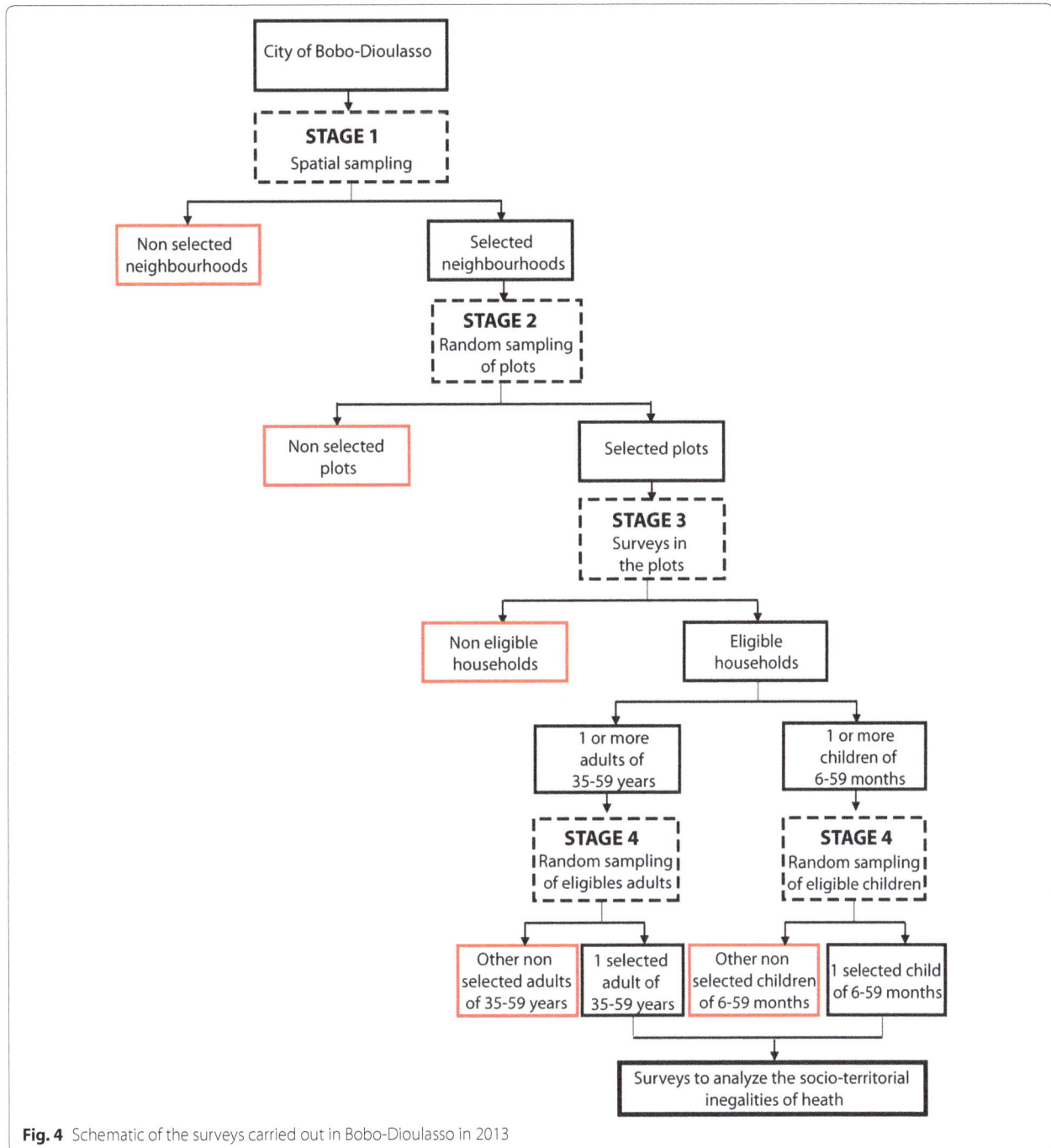

Fig. 4 Schematic of the surveys carried out in Bobo-Dioulasso in 2013

equipped. Class 4 (C04; in pink) corresponded to peripheral AHU under development and with low population density. Class 5 (C05; in olive green) included the recent peripheral areas under development and well equipped.

As there was not enough population to be included in the Class 4, it was not considered for the population survey. Finally, four AHU were randomly selected for the population survey to describe the health disparities:

Yéguéré (CO1), Dogona (CO2), Tounouma (CO3) and Secteur 25 (CO5). They were characterized by very different conditions of urbanization, position within the city, time of creation and access to healthcare structures (Fig. 8 and Table 2).

Finally, 3400 eligible plots were selected by several spatial random sampling without replacement, among the 8812 plots identified from the Pléiades mosaic image

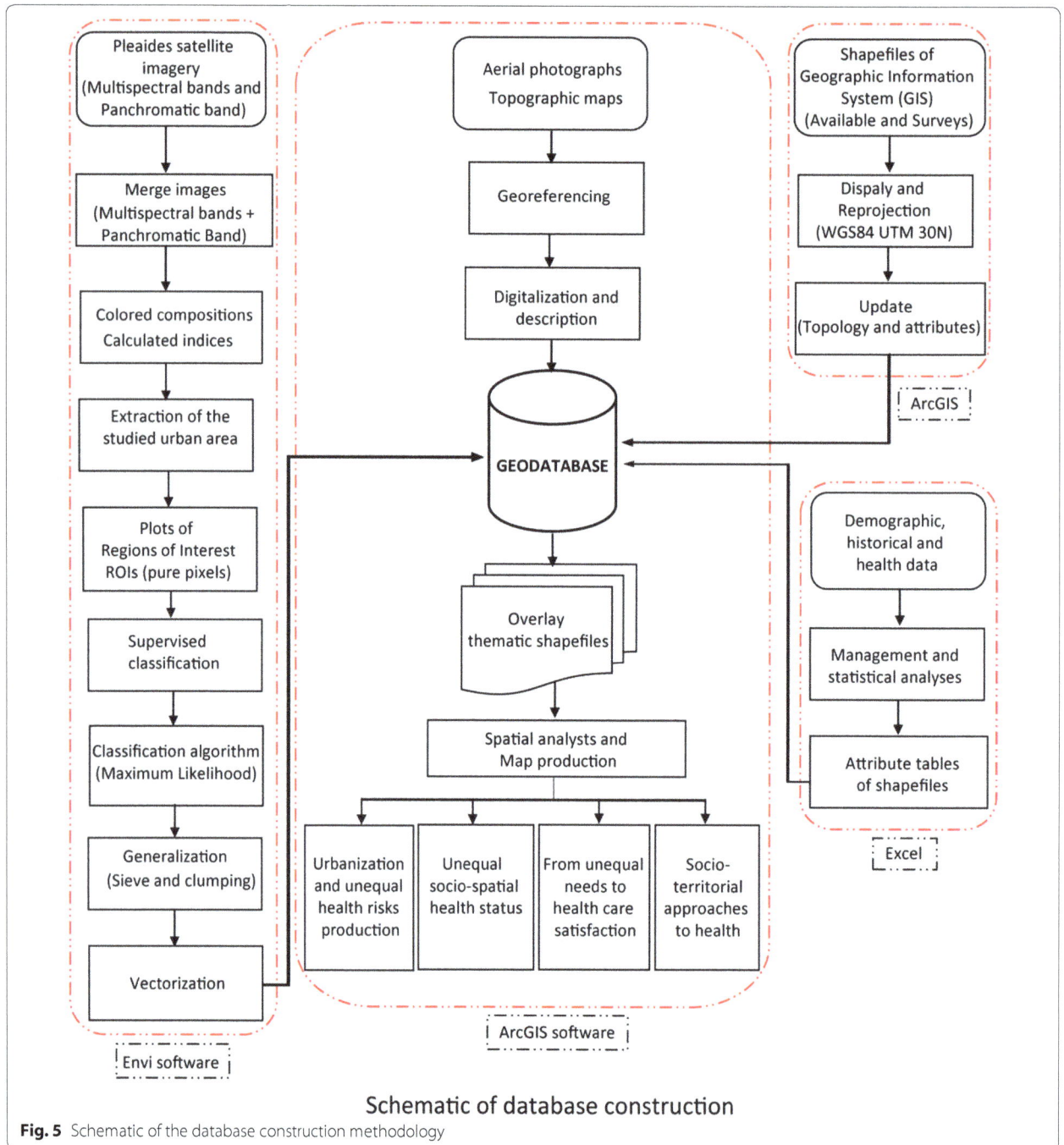

Fig. 5 Schematic of the database construction methodology

(Table 3). A first random selection of 350 plots for each sub-space was carried out to offset the problems of uninhabited plots, wrong plot identification in the satellite images, absence of people, possible refusal and non-eligibility of households (single-member, non eligible children or adults). Additional random samplings were carried out after the removal of already visited plots to achieve the aim of 250 households by AHU.

In the eligible plots (1084), 1320 households (1320/2192; 60.2%) were included in the survey. Finally, 1045 households were surveyed (Table 4 and Fig. 9).

The analysis of the spatial distribution of the surveyed households by Ripley's K function showed that in Dogona, households were not randomly distributed. Within 300 m radius, the households appeared concentrated. The spatial structuring of the area which is

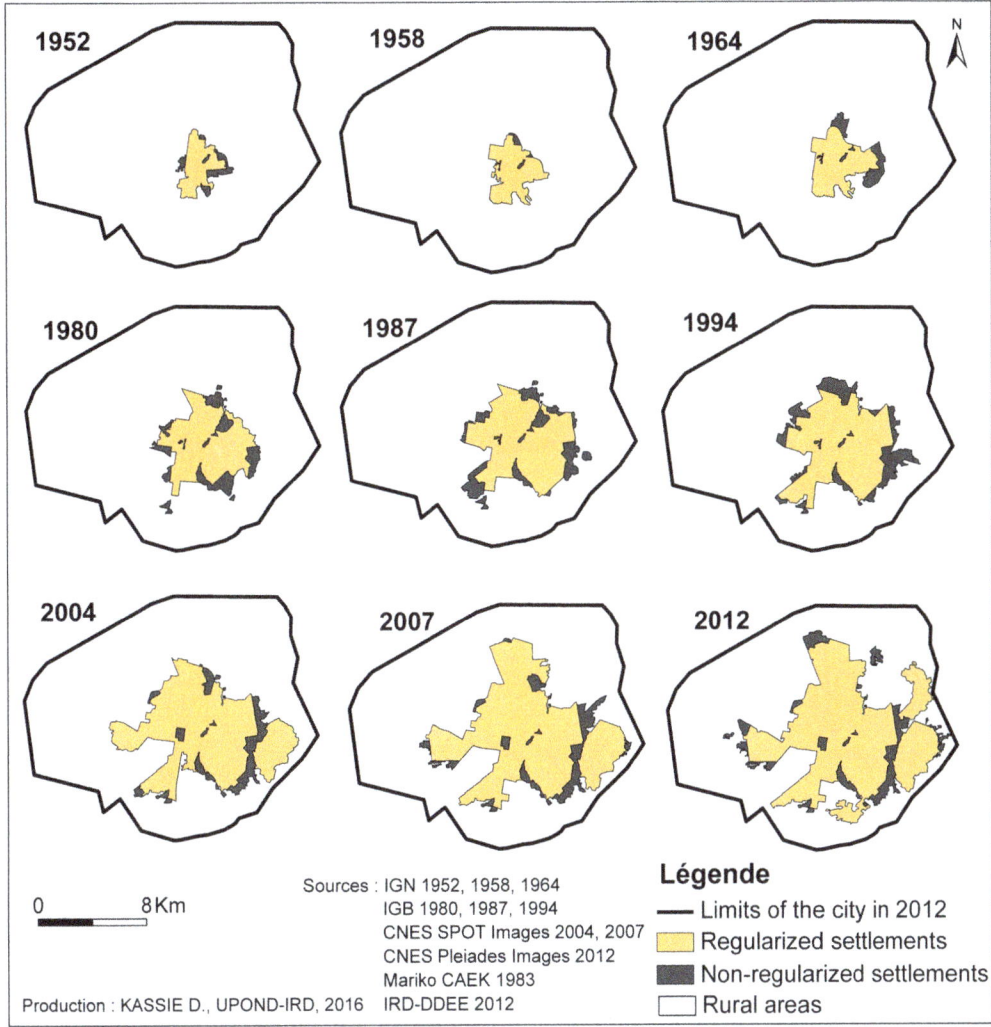

Sources : IGN 1952, 1958, 1964
IGB 1980, 1987, 1994
CNES SPOT Images 2004, 2007
CNES Pleiades Images 2012
Mariko CAEK 1983
Production : KASSIE D., UPOND-IRD, 2016   IRD-DDEE 2012

Légende
— Limits of the city in 2012
▢ Regularized settlements
▇ Non-regularized settlements
▢ Rural areas

0   8 Km

Year	1952	1958	1964	1980	1987	1994	2004	2007	2012
RSA (Km2)	8.3	12.2	14.7	27.7	36.3	41.7	61.0	74.2	83.2
NRSA (Km2)	2.4	0.6	4.0	8.5	10.5	13.0	9.2	10.5	12.5
Combined area (Km2)	10.7	12.9	18.7	36.1	46.8	54.8	70.2	84.7	95.7

RSA = Regularized Settlements Areas
NRSA = Non-regularized Settlements Areas

Fig. 6 Expansion of Bobo-Dioulasso from 1952 to 2012

divided by two rivers might explain this situation. In the other districts, the households could be considered as dispersed. In Dogona, analysis of the morbidity should take into account the spatial aggregation of households, while in the other districts a concentration of cases could not be related to the sampling (Fig. 10).

Finally, 860 adults (35–59 years of age) and 883 children (6–59 months of age) were surveyed (Table 5).

The number of surveyed men was lower than that of women, but the difference was not significant with respect to the data registered during the demographic and health survey carried out in Burkina Faso in 2010 ($p = 0.25$) [28].

Discussion

The objective of the study carried out in Bobo-Dioulasso was to highlight health disparities linked to differential urbanization due to non-homogeneous urbanization processes. Therefore, this sampling method was developed with the aim of identifying sub-spaces as different

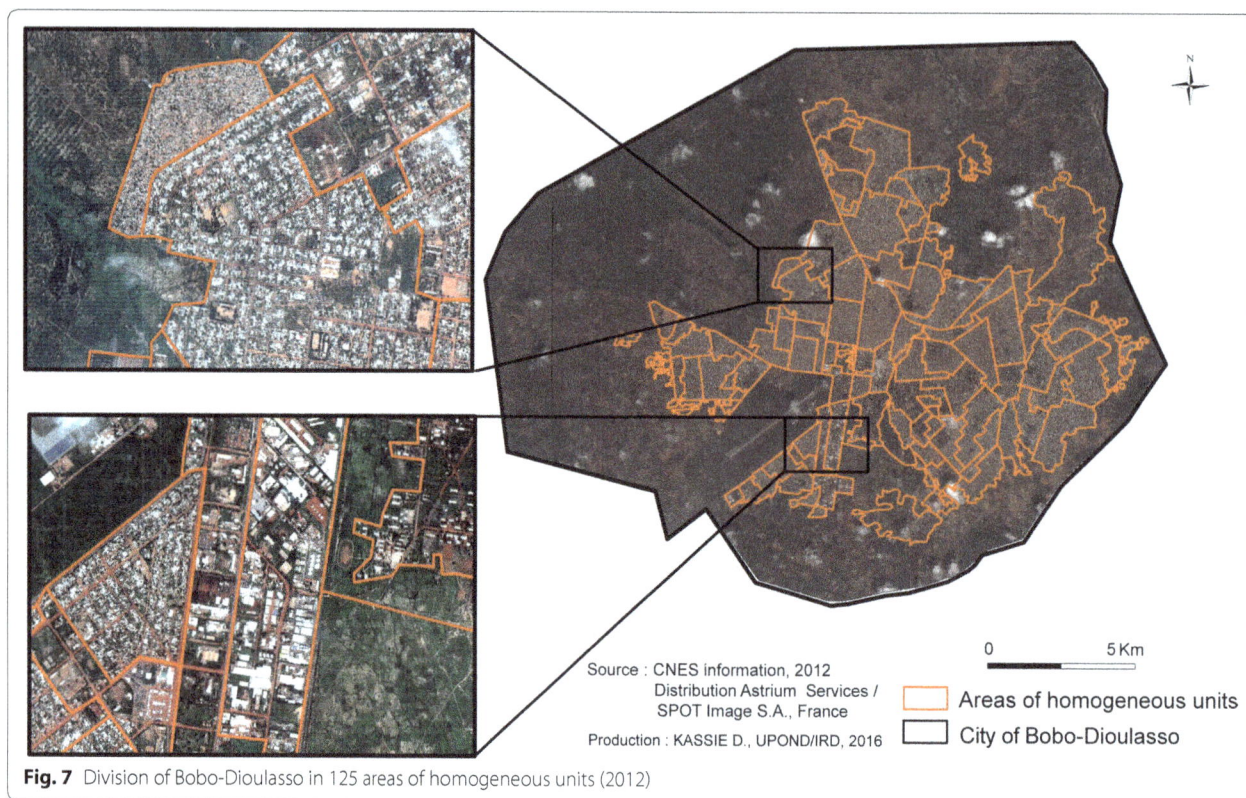

Fig. 7 Division of Bobo-Dioulasso in 125 areas of homogeneous units (2012)

Source : CNES information, 2012
Distribution Astrium Services /
SPOT Image S.A., France

Production : KASSIE D., UPOND/IRD, 2016

0   5 Km

☐ Areas of homogeneous units
☐ City of Bobo-Dioulasso

as possible, starting from the hypothesis that the health status of populations living in different environments is different. Thus, five different types of urbanization could be characterized. They were then used to guide the approach for the analysis of the health status within Bobo-Dioulasso through the selection of four sub-spaces that are representative of the urban diversity. The results show that a multifactorial approach, which includes the use of spatial information on the urbanization process, the urban morphology and the access to infrastructures, allows meeting this objective [29].

Several studies have demonstrated the value of the spatial sampling methods for population health surveys in developing countries where little information is available [30–33].

In such approaches, surveyors must follow a standardized procedure to find the randomly generated points in the field and select the nearest household or group of households for surveying [13, 34]. In Bobo-Dioulasso, the households could be located at their exact geographic position and the surveyor had to move to another random point integrated in his GPS unit in case of ineligibility or refusal. The randomly points to survey may be generated within different methods. Escamilla et al. [33] used Google Earth imagery to digitalize household structures in a rural area and then to produce a random

sample from the list of generated households. In our study, we rather used the plot centres (regular areas) or the house coordinates (irregular areas). Lowther et al. [30] applied a similar method for a health survey in an urban area in Zambia. They showed that this method offered an alternative sampling technique which allowed besides the reduction of the selection bias of the households. All these studies highlighted the accuracy of such approaches as well as their time and cost efficiency.

Our method showed its feasibility in regularized areas, such as the district of Tounouma, but also in non-regularized areas, such as the district of Yéguéré. It could be applied also in other cities. Moreover, the typology of Bobo-Dioulasso could be used in other studies, or even for the development of a system for demographic monitoring.

Although the techniques of multifactorial analysis and classification allow a good synthesis of the information and the distribution of the whole space in different classes, the question of the choice of the spatial unit to privilege within the identified classes remains essential. In Bobo-Dioulasso, the good knowledge of the area and the qualitative surveys carried out before these analyses could guide our choice. It should be also noted that the digitalization of all the houses of the non-regular subspace is time consuming. In addition, this sampling frame

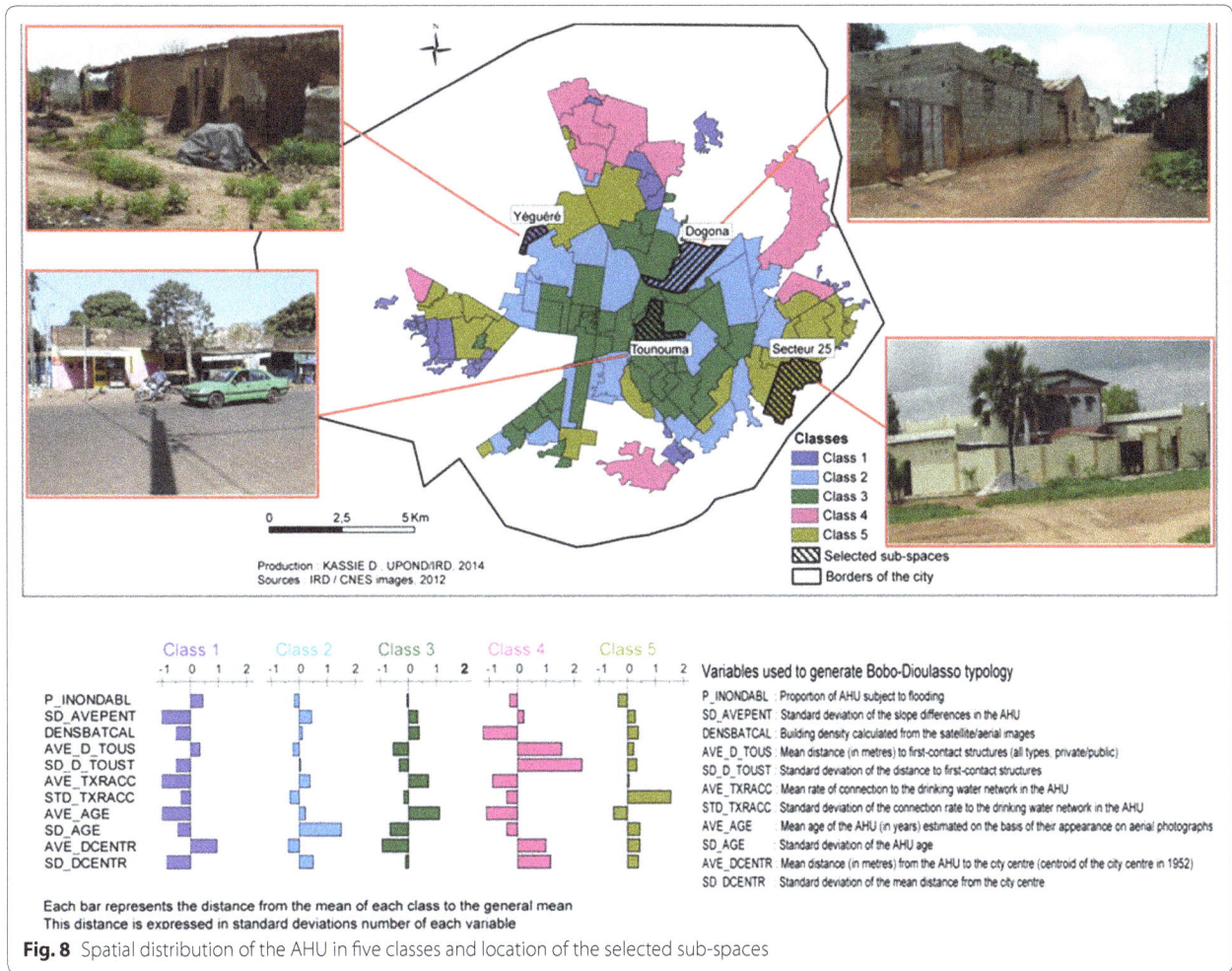

Each bar represents the distance from the mean of each class to the general mean
This distance is expressed in standard deviations number of each variable

Fig. 8 Spatial distribution of the AHU in five classes and location of the selected sub-spaces

Table 2　Features of the chosen sub-spaces

Sub-space	Age of the neighbour-hood (years)	Parcel-ling by-law	Proximity to centre[a] (m)	Proximity to health infra-structures (m)
Tounouma	>55	Yes	1000	750
Dogona	51	Yes	300	900
Secteur 25	17	Yes	600	900
Yéguéré	26	No	500	1000

[a] Barycentre of the town in 1952

Table 3　Distribution of plots in the sub-spaces under study

Sub-space	Plots on the Pléiades mosaic image	Inhabited plots	Randomly selected plots	Eligible plots
Dogona	2310	2124	700	262
Secteur 25	3281	2852	1400	290
Tounouma	600	600	600	298
Yéguéré	2621	2621	700	234
Total	8812	8197	3400	1084

Table 4　Distribution of the surveyed households in the different sub-spaces

Sub-space	Number of visited households	Number of eligible households	Number of surveyed households
Dogona	500	279	235
Secteur 25	490	329	290
Tounouma	964	479	286
Yéguéré	238	234	234
Total	2192	1320	1045

may require a training for the use of GPS units and the reading of maps. In terms of tools and material, we must stress that the development of this sampling method required the acquisition of relatively expensive data (aerial photographs and especially satellite images), the use of expensive software programmes, such as ArcGis, and specific skills for the analyses. Some of these costs could be reduced by using open-source software, such as QGis, and data provided by the OpenStreetMap community

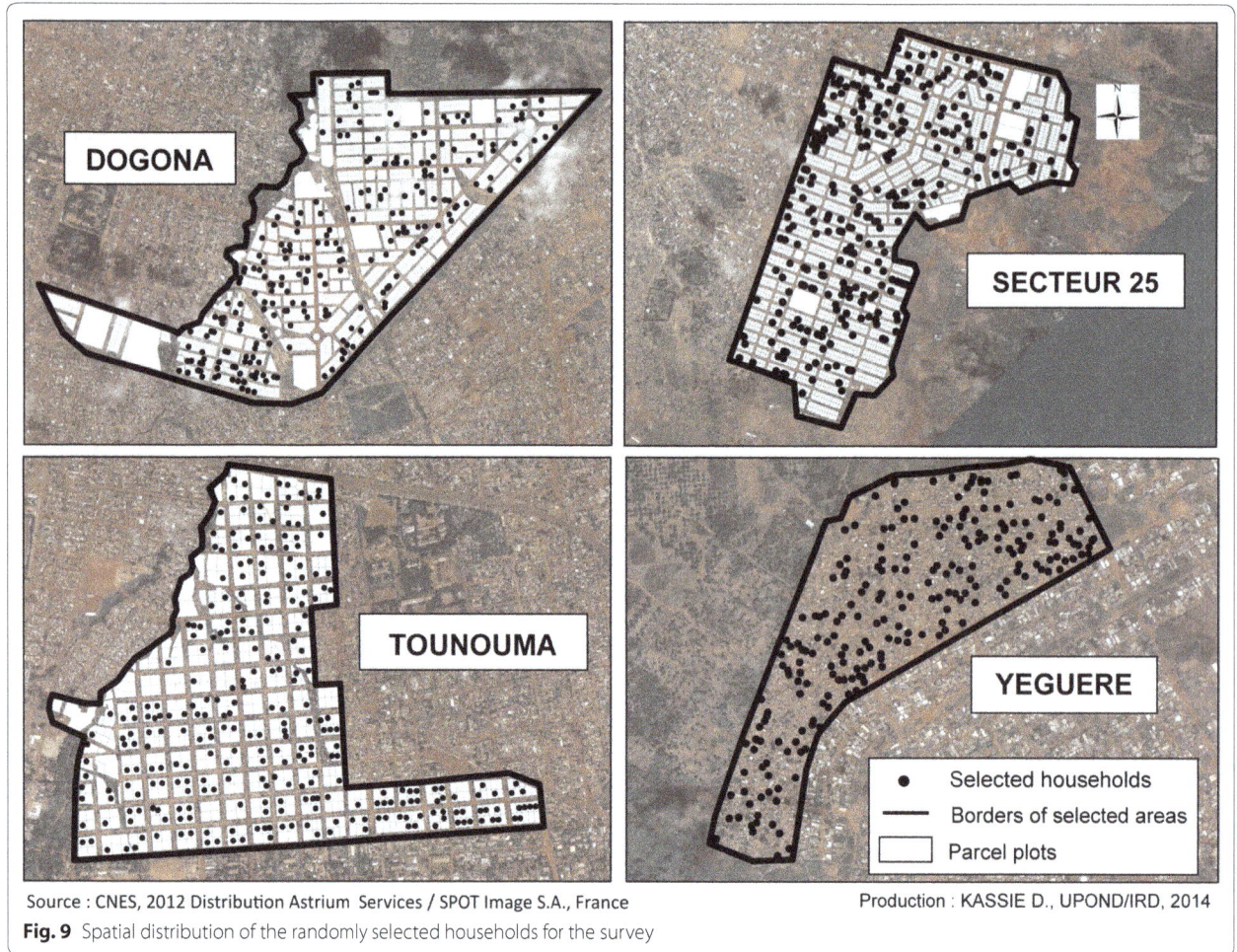

Source : CNES, 2012 Distribution Astrium Services / SPOT Image S.A., France   Production : KASSIE D., UPOND/IRD, 2014

Fig. 9 Spatial distribution of the randomly selected households for the survey

and by using free-of-charge satellite images, for instance Sentinel-2 imagery.

Conclusion

Different sampling methods can be used to carry out cross-sectional population surveys (i.e., stratified and non-stratified random, by purposeful sampling, cluster sampling). Overall, the aim of such methods is to obtain a good representativeness of the space or of the population that seems impossible to reach in the context of a city due to its complexity. Moreover, these methods cannot be always implemented without multiplying the bias, particularly in low-income countries, due to the lack of data availability and quality. More often they were aggregated at the scale of the whole city or of specific administrative zones (urban sectors, areas serviced by drinking water or waste collection) that were not always overlapping and that were not necessarily appropriate for studying health questions.

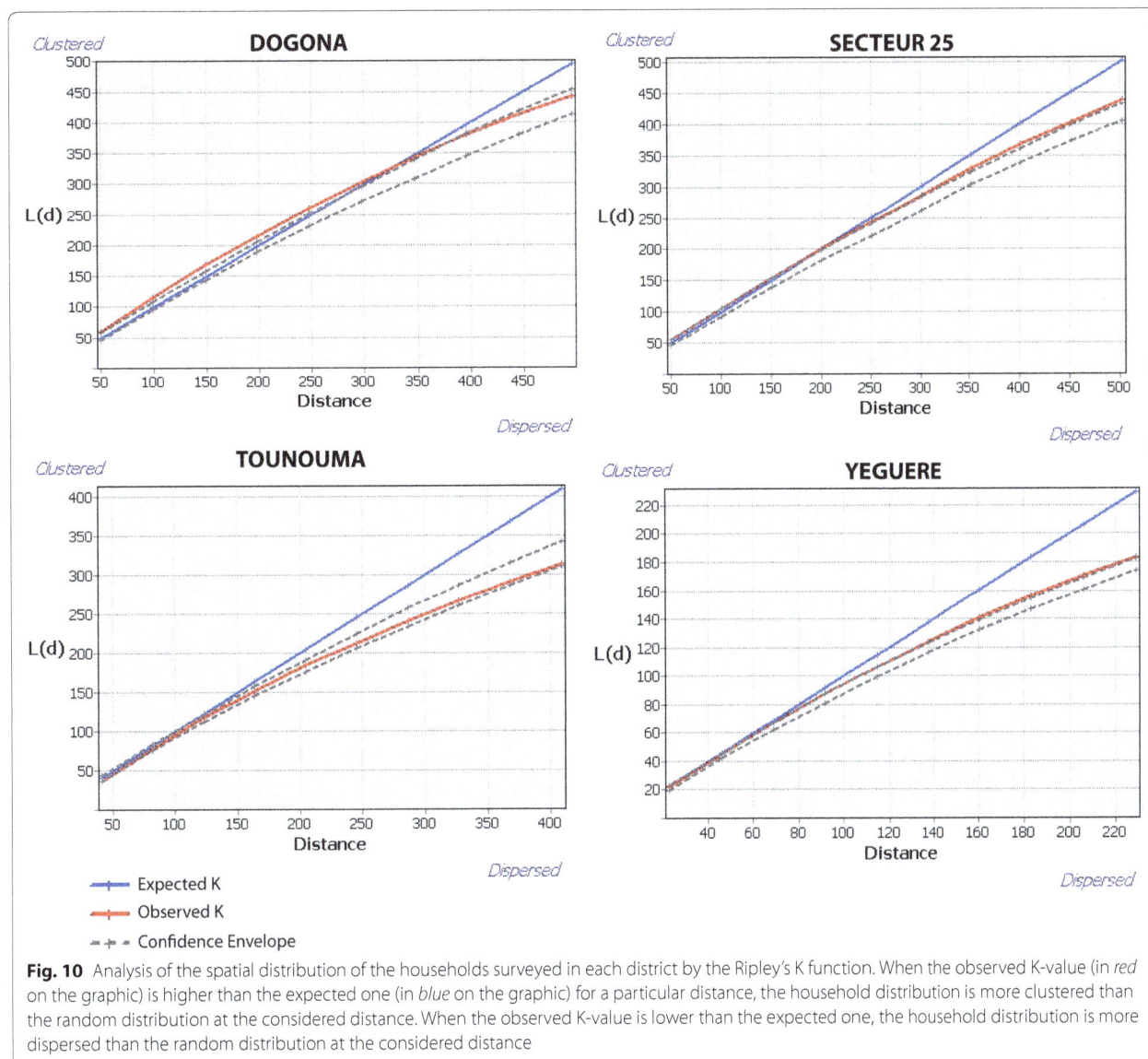

Fig. 10 Analysis of the spatial distribution of the households surveyed in each district by the Ripley's K function. When the observed K-value (in *red* on the graphic) is higher than the expected one (in *blue* on the graphic) for a particular distance, the household distribution is more clustered than the random distribution at the considered distance. When the observed K-value is lower than the expected one, the household distribution is more dispersed than the random distribution at the considered distance

Table 5 Distribution of surveyed adults and children in the different sub-spaces

Sub-space	Men	Women	Total	Boys	Girls	Total
Dogona	84	109	193	103	99	202
Secteur 25	79	136	215	119	105	224
Tounouma	111	142	253	119	129	248
Yéguéré	104	95	199	113	96	209
Total	378	482	860	454	429	883

However, our approach shows that alternatives to sample an urban population in a low-income country exist. It was applied in Saint-Louis of Senegal as part of the SANTINELLES project in which this study fitted [35].

Abbreviations
HAC: hierarchical ascending classification; AHU: area of homogeneous units; GIS: geographic information system; CNES: Centre National d'Etudes Spatiales; GPS: global positioning system; IGB: Institut Géographique du Burkina; IGN: Institut Géographique National; ONEA: Office National de l'Eau et de l'Assainissement; PCA: principal component analyses; SANTINELLES: SANTé, INégalités villES; UPOND: Université Paris Ouest Nanterre la Défense.

Authors' contributions

GS and FF developed the design of the study. KD conceived the sampling approach. KD and AR realized the spatial analysis, and KD interpreted the results. ND oversaw the remote sensing analysis and JLP supervised the qualitative analysis. KD and FF drafted the manuscript. GS, JLP and ND assisted with the manuscript preparation. All authors read and approved the final manuscript.

Author details

[1] Université Paris Ouest Nanterre La Défense, 200 Avenue de la République, 92000 Nanterre, France. [2] CIRAD, ASTRE, CIRAD TA C-22/E, Campus International de Baillarguet, 34398 Montpellier Cedex 5, France. [3] ESPACE DEV, Institut de Recherche pour le Développement, Maison de la Télédetection, 500 rue Jean-François Breton, 34093 Montpellier Cedex 5, France. [4] Université De Strasbourg, 4 Rue Blaise Pascal, 67081 Strasbourg, France. [5] CEPED, Institut de Recherche pour le Développement, 19 Rue Jacob, 75006 Paris, France. [6] MIVEGEC, Institut de Recherche pour le Développement, 911, Avenue Agropolis, BP 64501, 34394 Montpellier Cedex 5, France. [7] Institut de Recherche en Sciences de la Santé, 01 BP 545, Bobo-Dioulasso, Burkina Faso.

Acknowledgements

We thank the Maison de la télédétection for its help with the analyses of satellite images. We also thank the population of Bobo-Dioulasso as well as the authorities of the town hall and of the Health Ministry for their support in the survey implementation.

Competing interests

The authors declare that they have no competing interests.

Funding

The Agence Nationale de la Recherche (ANR12-INEG-007) supported data collection analysis, interpretation of the data and the writing of the manuscript. CNRS (PEPS107-IE) funded satellite images which were purchased from the ISIS programme of CNES.

References

1. WHO/UN-Habitat. Hidden cities: unmasking and overcoming health inequities in urban settings. Geneva, Switzerland, 2010.
2. Fournet F, Rican S, Salem G. Environnement urbain et santé. In: Dorier-Apprill E, editor. Ville et environnement. Paris: SEDES; 2006. p. 345–64.
3. Fournet F, Meunier-Nikiema A, Salem G. Ouagadougou (1850–2004): une urbanisation différenciée. Marseille: IRD; 2008.
4. Salem G. La santé dans la ville: géographie d'un petit espace dense: Pikine (Sénégal). Paris: Karthala – ORSTOM; 1998.
5. Vallée J. Urbanisation et santé à Vientiane (Laos). Les disparités spatiales de santé dans la ville. https://tel.archives-ouvertes.fr/tel-00377209/fr/ (2008). Accessed 15 Apr 2010.
6. Vallée J. Les disparités spatiales de santé en ville: l'exemple de Vientiane (Laos). Cybergeo Eur J Geogr [On line], Espace, Société, Territoire, document 477. http://cybergeo.revues.org/22775 (2009). Accessed 12 Feb 2013.
7. Satterthwaite D. Outside the large cities: the demographic importance of small urban centres and large villages in Africa, Asia and Latin America. Human Settlements Working Paper Series Urban Change: 3; 2006.
8. Bertrand M, Dubresson A. Petites et moyennes villes en Afrique noire. Paris: Karthala; 1997.
9. MacIntyre PD, Baker SC, Clément R, Donovan LA. Sex and age effects on willingness to communicate, anxiety, perceived competence, and L2 motivation among junior high school French immersion students. Lang Learn. 2003;53(Suppl 1):137–66.
10. Vlahov D, Galea S. Urbanization urbanicity, and health. J Urban Health. 2002;79(supplement 1):S1–12.
11. Grafmeyer Y. Sociologie urbaine. Paris: Nathan; 1994.
12. Bostoen K, Bilukha OO, Fenn B, Morgan OW, Tam CC, ter Veen A, Checchi F. Methods for health surveys in difficult settings: charting progress, moving forward. Emerg Themes Epidemiol. 2007;4:13.
13. Grais RF, Rose AMC, Guthmann J-P. Don't spin the pen: two alternative methods for second-stage sampling in urban cluster surveys. Emerg Themes Epidemiol. 2007;4:8.
14. Vallée J, Souris M, Fournet F, Bochaton A, Mobillion V, Peyronnie K, Salem G. Sampling in health geography: reconciling geographical objectives and probabilistic methods. An example of a health survey in Vientiane (Lao PDR). Emerg Themes Epidemiol. 2007;4:6.
15. Kuate Defo B. Demographic, epidemiological, and health transitions: are they relevant to population health patterns in Africa? Glob Health Action. 2014;7:22443.
16. Fourchard L. De la ville coloniale à la cour africaine: Espaces, pouvoirs et sociétés à Ouagadougou et à Bobo-Dioulasso (Haute-Volta) fin XIXè siècle-1960. Paris: L'Harmattan; 2002.
17. Le Bris E. Ouagadougou. In: Dureau F, Dupont V, Lelièvre E, Lévy JP, Lulle T, editors. Métropoles en mouvement: une comparaison internationale. Paris: Anthropos - IRD; 2000.
18. Meunier-Nikiema A, Karama BF, Kassié D, Fournet F. Ville et dynamique de l'offre de soins: Bobo-Dioulasso (Burkina Faso). Revue Francophone sur la santé et les territoires. https://rfst.hypotheses.org/meunier-nikiema-aude-karama-fatou-kassie-daouda-fournet-florence (2015).
19. Caughy MO, Leonard T, Beron K, Murdoch J. Defining neighborhood boundaries in studies of spatial dependence in child behavior problems. Int J Health Geogr. 2013;12:24.
20. Amat-Roze JM. La territorialisation de la santé: quand le territoire fait débat. Hérodote. 2011;4(143):13–32.
21. Salem G, Marois C. De l'analyse à la description: morphologie de l'habitat, dynamique spatiales et paysages urbains à Pikine (SENEGAL). Séminfor. 1991.
22. Frankhauser P. La morphologie des tissus urbains et périurbains à travers une lecture fractale. Rev Géogr l'Est. 2005;45(3–4):145–60.
23. Fouad AO. Morphologie urbaine et confort thermique dans les espaces publics: Etude comparative entre trois tissus urbains de la ville de Québec. Maîtrise en science de l'architecture. Faculté des études supérieures de l'Université Laval, Canada. www.grap.arc.ulaval.ca/diffusion/maitrise-memoire.html (2007). Accessed Jan 2014.
24. Pham TS. Morphologie urbaines, dispositifs techniques et pratiques sociales: cas des quartiers de ruelles hanoiens. Thèse de doctorat de Géographie, aménagement, urbanisme. Institut National des Sciences Appliquées de Lyon. https://tel.archives-ouvertes.fr/tel-00797324/ (2010). Accessed Nov 2014.
25. Borderon M, Oliveau S, Machault V, Vignolles C, Lacaux J-P, N'Donky A. Qualifier les espaces urbains à Dakar, Sénégal. Cybergeo Eur J Geogr [Online]. Cartographie, Imagerie, SIG, document 670. http://cybergeo.revues.org/26250 (2014). Accessed 17 Sept 2015.
26. Pumain D, Saint-Julien T. L'analyse spatiale. Localisation dans l'espace. Paris: Armand Colin; 2008.
27. INSD. Recueil des concepts, définitions, indicateurs et méthodologies utilisés dans le Système statistique national. Ouagadougou: Institut National de la Statistique et de la Démographie; 2008.
28. INSD. Enquête Démographique et de Santé et à Indicateurs Multiples du Burkina Faso 2010. Calverton: INSD et ICF International; 2012.
29. Fournet F, Kassié D, Dabiré RK, Salem G. Processus d'urbanisation et inégalités de santé: l'exemple d'une ville moyenne africaine, Bobo-Dioulasso (Burkina Faso). Dynamiques environnementales, Environnement et santé:

où en est la géographie? 2016; 36:128–42.

30. Lowther SA, Curriero FC, Shields T, Ahmed S, Monze M, Moss WJ. Feasibility of satellite image-based sampling for a health survey among urban townships of Lusaka, Zambia. Trop Med Int Health. 2009;14(1):70–8.

31. Kondo MC, Bream KDW, Barg FK, Branas CC. A random spatial sampling method in a rural developing nation. BMC Public Health. 2014;14:338.

32. Siri JG, Lindblade KA, Rosen DH, Onyango B, Vulule JM, Slutsker L, Wilson ML. A census-weighted, spatially-stratified household sampling strategy for urban malaria epidemiology. Malar J. 2008;7:39.

33. Escamilla V, Emch M, Dandalo L, Miller WC, Martinsona F, Hoffman I. Sampling at community level by using satellite imagery and geographical analysis. Bull World Health Organ. 2014;92:690–4.

34. World Health Organization. Training for mid-level managers: the EPI coverage survey. Geneva: WHO Expanded Programme on Immunization; 1991.

35. Vialard L, Squiban C, Fournet F, Salem G, Foley EE. Toward a socio-territorial approach to health: health equity in West Africa. Int J Environ Res Public Health. 2017;14(1):106.

4

Gardening in the desert: a spatial optimization approach to locating gardens in rapidly expanding urban environments

Elizabeth A. Mack[1]*, Daoqin Tong[2] and Kevin Credit[1]

Abstract

Background: Food access is a global issue, and for this reason, a wealth of studies are dedicated to understanding the location of food deserts and the benefits of urban gardens. However, few studies have linked these two strands of research together to analyze whether urban gardening activity may be a step forward in addressing issues of access for food desert residents.

Methods: The Phoenix, Arizona metropolitan area is used as a case to demonstrate the utility of spatial optimization models for siting urban gardens near food deserts and on vacant land. The locations of urban gardens are derived from a list obtained from the Maricopa County Cooperative Extension office at the University of Arizona which were geo located and aggregated to Census tracts. Census tracts were then assigned to one of three categories: tracts that contain a garden, tracts that are immediately adjacent to a tract with a garden, and all other non-garden/non-adjacent census tracts. Analysis of variance is first used to ascertain whether there are statistical differences in the demographic, socio-economic, and land use profiles of these three categories of tracts. A maximal covering spatial optimization model is then used to identify potential locations for future gardening activities. A constraint of these models is that gardens be located on vacant land, which is a growing problem in rapidly urbanizing environments worldwide.

Results: The spatial analysis of garden locations reveals that they are centrally located in tracts with good food access. Thus, the current distribution of gardens does not provide an alternative food source to occupants of food deserts. The maximal covering spatial optimization model reveals that gardens could be sited in alternative locations to better serve food desert residents. In fact, 53 gardens may be located to cover 96.4% of all food deserts. This is an improvement over the current distribution of gardens where 68 active garden sites provide coverage to a scant 8.4% of food desert residents.

Conclusion: People in rapidly urbanizing environments around the globe suffer from poor food access. Rapid rates of urbanization also present an unused vacant land problem in cities around the globe. This paper highlights how spatial optimization models can be used to improve healthy food access for food desert residents, which is a critical first step in ameliorating the health problems associated with lack of healthy food access including heart disease and obesity.

Keywords: Community gardens, Vacant land, Spatial optimization, Food access, Food deserts, Urbanization, Urban agriculture

*Correspondence: emack@msu.edu
[1] Department of Geography, Environment and Spatial Sciences, Michigan State University, Geography Building, 673 Auditorium Rd, Room 202, East Lansing, MI 48824, USA
Full list of author information is available at the end of the article

Introduction

The World Bank notes that developing countries have large amounts of unused land, which run the risk of marginalizing a growing number of urban poor [1]. Cities in countries around the globe including Afghanistan [2], India [3] and Brazil [4] are urbanizing rapidly and experiencing symptoms of rapid growth including lack of food access and unused vacant land. Urban agriculture initiatives are a promising solution to the vacant land and food security problem in global cities, and urban residents around the world are pursuing urban gardening initiatives [5]. These gardening initiatives are not only important for establishing communities that are more connected and have better access to food systems, they also represent an important piece of the puzzle in solving the growing global health issue of obesity given the link between lack of access to quality food and health [6–9].

The United Nations estimates that in 2014, 54% of the world's population lived in urban areas, and this number is projected to increase to 66% by 2050 [10]. Rising rates of urbanization mean diminished connections to food sources as agricultural land disappears [3] and local food sources disappear in favor of superstores that meet consumer demand for standardized, unblemished food products [11–13]. The shift in size, scale, and location of food outlets over the past 60 years—from small, urban neighborhood stores to large suburban superstores—is a global phenomenon that is increasingly prevalent in the food economics of the developed world [12]. Locales where residents do not have access to and/or cannot afford healthy food are commonly referred to as "food deserts".

While there has been a wealth of research dedicated to understanding the location of food deserts [14, 15] and the benefits of urban gardens [16–18] few studies have linked these two strands of research together to analyze whether urban gardening activity may be a step towards addressing issues of food access for residents of food deserts. To better understand the neighborhood context of urban gardening activity and its spatial linkages with food deserts, this study analyzes the locations of food deserts and urban gardening activity. The key contribution of the study is the use of a garden siting technique, the maximal covering location model, to propose alternative urban garden sites and improve food access for area residents. The potential utility of this type of analytical approach is demonstrated for Phoenix, Arizona, which is rapidly urbanizing and has a vacant land problem. This technique can be applied however to any urban environment where the necessary data are available. In this respect, siting gardens on vacant land is a particularly promising tool for improving food access and urban food security in cities around the globe.

Background: food access and food deserts

Food access is a precursor to healthy food consumption and healthy food consumption is associated with better health [19–22]. While the food environment is not the sole driver of food consumption practices, studies do find linkages between healthy food access and the quality of human health [7, 8, 23, 24]. Given the health implications associated with food access, several studies have endeavored to identify neighborhoods, especially low-income neighborhoods, with inadequate access to healthy food [25]. These studies find that changes in food retailing practices, with small independent retailers slowly replaced by large superstores, have changed the landscape of food access [26, 27], leaving urban residents with fewer food choices. This retailing change makes suburban locations more attractive because of the land area required for larger stores and the reduced expense of land in suburban areas [26]. It is important to note that this consolidation of food outlets also impacts rural residents when local neighborhood stores close due to competition from larger retailers [15]. While a majority of the literature on food deserts emphasizes this issue in an urban context [28–30], more recent work has uncovered that the hinterlands of metropolitan areas have residents that suffer from lack of access to healthy food [25], as well as residents in suburban [31] and rural areas [15, 26, 32]). Sharkey et al. [33] note that food access in rural locations is particularly important to analyze given the compounding challenges of distance and transportation access in rural environments. Work also highlights the importance of considering temporal aspect of food access related to changes in public transportation schedules and the operating hours of food stores [34]. Farber, Morang, and Widener [35], note that the operating hours of public transportation can impact travel times, which then impacts peoples' ability to patronize food outlets.

Despite the amount of attention dedicated to food access, there is a lack of consensus on the definition of food deserts [26, 36, 37]. Table 1 provides several examples of food desert definitions, and highlights the sources of variation in how these are defined. Some definitions define a particular distance that constitutes good food access [14, 38, 39]. Some definitions explicitly refer to low-income neighborhoods or groups [15, 30, 40] while others do not [14, 38]. Other sources of variation in food desert definitions include the explicit mention of transit times [41] and/or specific mention of a particular type of food outlet used to determine food access.

In addition to variations in food desert locations and counts stemming from basic definitional issues, Bao and Tong [42] point out inconsistencies in the findings of food desert studies that are related to differences in the spatial scale and level of data aggregation. Studies have

Table 1 Definitions of food deserts used in previous studies

Definition	Geography	Study
Term *first used* in UK to describe "rapidly decreasing number of grocers in urban, low income neighborhoods after World War II"	Urban areas	[40, p. 3]
Spatial disparity in access to retail food stores	Urban areas	[82]
Areas "where cheap and varied food is only accessible to those who have private transport or are able to pay the costs of public transport"	Urban areas	[83, p. 65]
Areas with barriers to food access based on "ability" (physical barriers), "assets" (financial barriers), or "attitudes" (state of mind)	Urban areas	[84, p. 241]
"Economic and physical access constraints perceived and experienced by disadvantaged consumers in an area of compound social exclusion and poor food retail access"	Urban areas	[85, p. 2084]
Empirical definition—minority neighborhoods with lower access to healthy food destinations within 5-min travel times	Urban areas	[41]
"Places where the transportation constraints of carless residents combine with a dearth of supermarkets to force residents to pay inflated prices for inferior and unhealthy foods at small markets and convenience stores"	Urban areas	[44, p. 352]
"Socially-distressed neighbourhoods with relatively low average household incomes and poor access to healthy food"	Urban areas	[30, p. 1]
"Urban areas with 10 or fewer stores and no stores with more than 20 employees"	Urban areas	[29, p. 372]
"Poor urban areas, where residents cannot buy affordable, healthy food"	Urban areas	[76, p. 436]
Locales situated more than 10 miles (16 km) from a supermarket	Rural	[14, 38]
"Socio-economically disadvantaged areas with relatively low household incomes and poor geographical access to nutritious, affordable food sources"	Not specified	[15, p. 2]
"Areas of relative exclusion where people experience physical and economic barriers to accessing health food"	Not specified	[27, p. 138]
A low-income tract where at least 33% of the population is greater than 1 mile (1.61 km) (in an urban area) or greater than 10 miles (16 km) (in a rural area) from the nearest supermarket, supercenter, or large grocery store	Urban and rural areas	[39]
"Low-income, urban neighborhoods, often centrally located, with inadequate physical or economic access to healthy food"	Urban areas	[25, p. 204]

also found that the choice of study area matters, and that not all locations have a food desert problem. For example, Apparicio et al. [43] found no evidence of a food desert problem in Montréal, which suggested the need for other mechanisms beyond improved healthy food access to resolve diet-related health problems for Montréal residents.

Background: urban gardens

Several studies of alternative means of food access have analyzed small food stores as a means of solving the food desert problem [6, 41, 44]. Mobile vans have also been suggested as a means of providing food insecure neighborhoods with fresh fruits and vegetables [45]. Other studies have suggested that building a strong local food economy through farmer's markets and direct sales from farms could be an important strategy in the fight against obesity [46]. This approach includes the use of community gardens as a mechanism for providing access to nutritious foods [47]. Locally grown food has a long history as an alternative means of food access in urban environments, and studies have noted that in the United Kingdom and the United States, gardens are a notable feature of the urban landscape, although the intensity of gardening activities varies over time [48].

Throughout the history of the United Kingdom, allotment gardens served as an important source of employment and food [48]. In the United States, urban gardens were part of the social reform movements in the 1890s, and were also an important source of food during the Great Depression [49, 50]. In both World Wars, urban gardens served as an alternative food source. During World War II in particular, "victory gardens" were an important source of fresh food for U.S. residents so food stuffs could be sent to troops abroad [49]. Post-WWII, urban gardening efforts experienced a comparative lull until the 1970s, when gardens become a component of urban revitalization efforts [49]. Starting in the 1970s, federal programs such as the United States Department of Agriculture's (USDA) Urban Garden Program continued to support gardening activities in urban environments [48]. Today, in cities around the globe—from Puerto Maldonado, Peru to Canberrra, Australia to Mumbai, India—organizations and urban residents are now growing food in urban environments [5].

Because of rising rates of urbanization and growing interest in urban food production globally, studies have begun to incorporate farmer's markets and community gardens into analyses of food deserts. It has been noted that studies that do not consider these sources of fresh foods will overestimate inequities in food access [51]. Studies have also found that community gardens are a viable source of food for low-income people and can provide additional benefits to neighborhoods by improving the attitudes and outlooks of residents [16, 17]. As regards access and consumption of healthy food, Litt et al. [17] found that community gardeners were more likely to consume fruits and vegetables than were home gardeners and non-gardeners.

Given the importance of local, healthy food sources, researchers have also begun to examine the potential for cultivating food within urban environments [52, 53]. These studies use a wide range of tools including geographic information systems (GIS), remote sensing, and site suitability techniques. For example, Kremer and DeLiberty [52] combined GIS and remote sensing techniques to examine the availability of urban land in Philadelphia, Pennsylvania for garden activity. Site suitability analysis was used to propose locations for urban gardens in cities ranging from Hanoi, Vietnam [54] and Chittendon County, Vermont [55]. In Portland, Oregon and Vancouver, Canada, Mendes et al. [56] conducted a visual assessment of parcels, including tree canopy and built environment characteristics, to identify the most suitable government-owned land on which to pursue urban agriculture projects. Finally, participatory mapping has been used to visualize relationships in local food systems [57] and locate healthy food retail outlets [58]. This approach draws upon the knowledge of experts to understand and restructure aspects of local food systems.

While these techniques represent important advancements to understanding and improving urban food systems, they are not without drawbacks. Studies have found that remote sensing techniques do not accurately identify garden locations because of their small size and heterogeneous layouts, which produce non-uniform visual patterns [53]. Site suitability techniques are an improvement over remote sensing techniques because they are capable of incorporating multiple variables above and beyond land use, but are perhaps more accurately viewed as an initial screening process that helps to find suitable areas for gardens. From this perspective, spatial optimization models represent a potential improvement over site suitability analyses. This brand of optimization model can be viewed as a type of site selection analysis with additional considerations, that include: (1) the number of gardens to site due to budget constraints, (2) a more accurate way to account for multiple factors, and (3) the spatial relationship among gardens (and between neighborhoods and gardens). Thus, spatial optimization models not only have the site-identifying capacity of site suitability analyses, but they also have the added capability of providing information about the spatial configuration of sites,

in conjunction with a sense of tradeoffs about the number of gardens to be cited and the population of interest serviced by these gardens. Because of the enhanced analytical capabilities of these models, they can be used to analyze how urban gardens may be distributed better to resolve issues of access for food desert residents.

Methods
Study area
Maricopa County, which contains the majority of the Phoenix metropolitan area, is the study area for this analysis. Figure 1 depicts the distribution of urban, suburban, and rural areas across the metropolitan area. Dark colors represent the most tracts while lighter colors represent comparatively rural tracts. These 2010 Rural–Urban Commuting Area (RUCA) categories of the urban–rural continuum were obtained from the United States Department of Agriculture (USDA) and contain 10 categories of tracts ranging from the most urbanized (code 1) to the most rural tracts (code 10). Based on this classification scheme, the majority of tracts (95%) across Phoenix are classified as part of the metropolitan area core. Only two tracts are classified as rural. Interestingly, tracts that are classified as having high levels of commuting to the urban core are located mostly in the West Valley of Phoenix in communities such as Glendale, El Mirage, and Surprise.

These high commuting tracts highlight the sprawling nature of the metropolitan area [59, 60], which means that residents are more likely to drive to everyday activities than residents in older, more walkable metropolitan areas. In this context, several locations across Maricopa County represent less centrally located communities, where issues of adequate access to healthy foods are perhaps exacerbated [25]. This issue of sprawl is not unique to Phoenix but is characteristic of cities across the globe. Another feature of the metropolitan area that is characteristic of rapidly urbanizing cities is a vacant land problem [61–63] with over 10,000 acres of unused land [63]. While a lot of this land is on the urban fringe, satellite imagery also highlights many examples of vacant lots in built-up portions of the study area. Recently, City of Phoenix officials have attempted to find temporary uses for vacant land and community gardens represent one of these proposed land uses [61]. For example, as part of the Phoenix Renews project, a 15-acre vacant lot at the intersection of Central Avenue and Indian School Road was proposed as the location of an urban community farm. Unfortunately, the owner of the lot defaulted on payments and had to return the land to the U.S. Department of the Interior [64]. This closure means that local gardeners who started growing crops will lose their plots, and must find a location elsewhere. Given the potential for gardens to alleviate poor access to healthy foods, finding

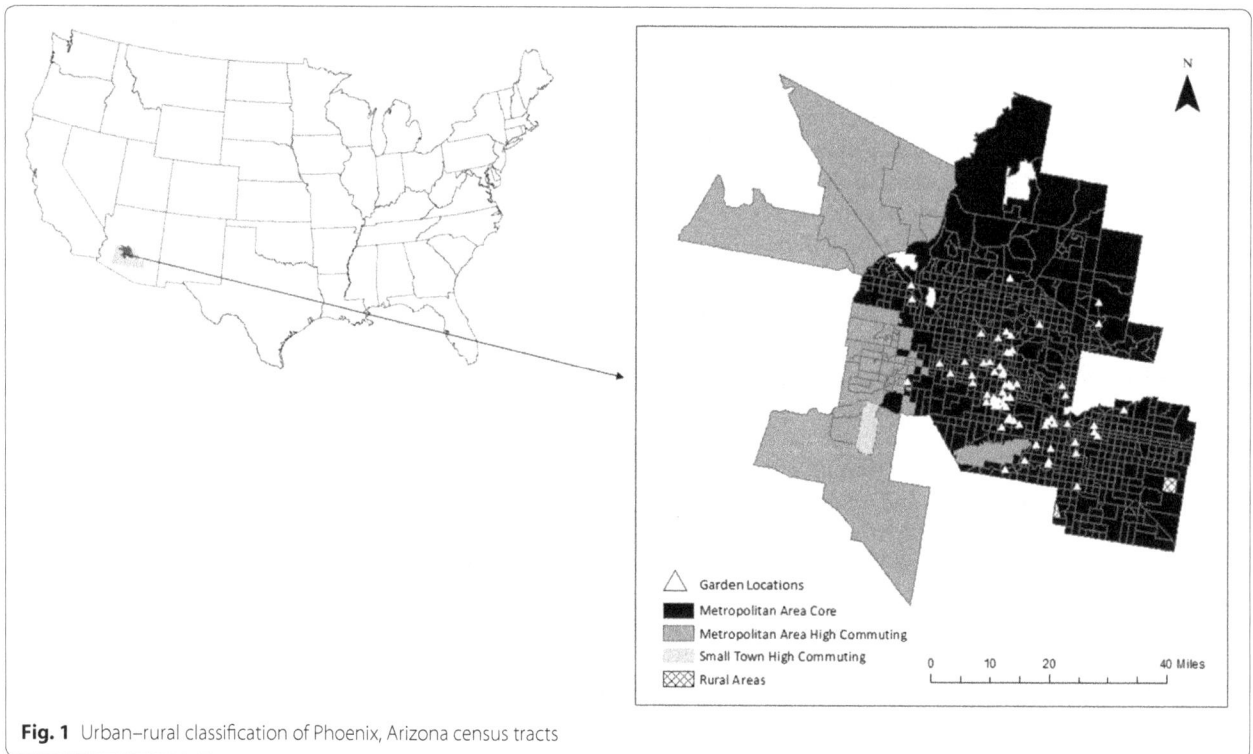

Fig. 1 Urban–rural classification of Phoenix, Arizona census tracts

suitable locations for community gardens is no easy task, but perhaps a necessary step to move towards a more comprehensive resolution to the vacant land problem in Phoenix, and to simultaneously improve food access for residents.

Data

Given the complex swathe of factors to consider in siting gardens, this study will analyze current sites of urban gardening activities with an emphasis on their neighborhood context. It will then propose new locations for urban gardening activity to improve access for food desert residents. To provide a more comprehensive perspective on urban garden locations, several variables are used to characterize the neighborhood environment. To do this, a variety of data including housing, land use, zoning, demographic, and socio-economic characteristics were collected at the census tract level based on the precedent of prior studies [25, 30, 43]. From this perspective, special attention was devoted to collecting information about economic disadvantage given the link between socio-economic status (SES) and access to healthy food [25, 28, 39]. Table 2 contains summary information about these data.

Garden data

Urban garden locations are derived from a list obtained from the Maricopa County Cooperative Extension

(MCCE) office at the University of Arizona which provided the name and address for gardens across the county. Information from this database was verified from aerial imagery on Google Maps, which provided historical images of garden locations in some cases. When necessary, contacts with garden managers were also used to verify the start and end date of the gardens to ascertain whether they were active or inactive. The address of active gardens was also verified because some gardens had moved since their initial start date. When garden managers could not be contacted, in-person visits were made to the address for the garden listed in the database to verify the status of the garden. Above and beyond information in this database, efforts were made to triangulate and supplement data from the MCCE list with information from the American Community Garden Association (ACGA) website and city government websites. Out of the 99 garden locations identified, 77 gardens locations were verified within the boundaries of the Phoenix metropolitan area. Of these 77 gardens, 68 were active at the time the data were collected. However, both active and inactive gardens will be used in the analysis that follows to understand both past and current trends in garden locations given the transient nature of urban gardening activity [49].

Once the addresses of garden locations were verified, they were geocoded and matched to their relevant census tract in order to integrate garden data with data collected

Table 2 Description of data and data sources

Variable	Description	Data source
Land use	Parcel data about land use data for 2014 in 16 categories: i.e., industrial, single family residential, commercial, office	Maricopa Association of Governments (MAG)
Food desert	Tract level data about food access reported in 2013	United States Department of Agriculture (USDA)
Median home value	Median value of owner-occupied housing units (current dollars)	2014 American Community Survey: 5-year estimates (2010–2014)
Percent owner occupied	Percent of housing units that are owner occupied	2014 American Community Survey: 5-year estimates (2010–2014)
Percent vacant housing units	Percent of housing units that are vacant	2014 American Community Survey: 5-year estimates (2010–2014)
Median contract rent	Renter-occupied housing units paying cash rent (current dollars)	2014 American Community Survey: 5-year estimates (2010–2014)
Percent Black	Percent of the population that is Black	2014 American Community Survey: 5-year estimates (2010–2014)
Percent Hispanic	Percent of the population that is Hispanic	2014 American Community Survey: 5-year estimates (2010–2014)
Percent bachelor's	Population aged 25 and older with a bachelor's degree or higher	2014 American Community Survey: 5-year estimates (2010–2014)
Percent food stamps	Percent of households receiving Food Stamps/SNAP in the past 12 months	2014 American Community Survey: 5-year estimates (2010–2014)
Percent no healthcare	Percent of the population with no healthcare	2014 American Community Survey: 5-year estimates (2010–2014)
Percent under 18 with no healthcare	Percent of the population under 18 with no healthcare	2014 American Community Survey: 5-year estimates (2010–2014)
Percent unemployment	Percent of the population 16 years and older that is unemployed	2014 American Community Survey: 5-year estimates (2010–2014)
Food outlets	2010 point level food outlet data aggregated to census-tracts	ESRI Reference USA
Percent of workers who drove alone to work	Percentage of workers 16 and over who drove alone to work in tract	2014 American Community Survey: 5-year estimates (2010–2014)
Percent of workers commuting using non-auto modes	Percentage of workers 16 and over who commuted to work using public transit, bicycle, or walking in tract	2014 American Community Survey: 5-year estimates (2010–2014)
Less than 15 min travel time to work	Percentage of commuters with a commute time of less than 15 min in tract	2014 American Community Survey: 5-year estimates (2010–2014)
30 min or more travel time to work	Percentage of commuters with a commute time of greater than 30 min in tract	2014 American Community Survey: 5-year estimates (2010–2014)

from other sources. Census tracts were then assigned to one of three categories: tracts that contain a garden, tracts that are immediately adjacent to a tract with a garden, and all other non-garden/non-adjacent census tracts. The adjacency category was used to identify tracts that are proximal to a tract with a garden, as opposed to a binary breakdown of tracts into those with and without a garden. This category is important to consider because these tract residents are still nearby a source of fresh fruits and vegetables. In the analysis that follows, 75 of the 77 garden sites were located in Census tracts that fell within the boundaries of Phoenix area neighborhoods. Thus, these 75 gardens will serve as the basis for the ANOVA comparison of garden-oriented neighborhoods

and non-garden oriented neighborhoods. For the spatial optimization analysis, all 77 gardens will be used because the analysis assigns gardens to tracts based on a threshold distance of 1 mile (1.61 km).

Food outlet and food desert information

In addition to information about garden locations, healthy food outlet information from the ESRI Reference USA dataset was compiled using the definition of food outlets from Raja et al. [41]. Based on this study, point-level information about outlets selling healthy food was compiled and aggregated to census tracts. These data include the following types of food outlets: supermarkets, natural food stores, meat and fish stores, specialty food stores, and fruit and vegetable stores.[1] Bakeries and dairy stores were excluded from the analysis because their food offerings could not be classified as healthy: most of the dairy stores in this database were verified as selling frozen yogurt.

Census tract information about food deserts was obtained from the United States Department of Agriculture (USDA). Since the USDA provides several definitions of food deserts, the definition used in this study defines food deserts as Census tracts with low access to supermarkets or larger grocery stores where low access means residents are more than 1 mile (1.61 km) from food outlets in urban areas and more than 10 miles (16.09 km) from food outlets in rural areas [65].

Demographic and socio-economic data

Contextual information about the demographic and socio-economic profile of Phoenix area residents was compiled from the National Historic Geographic Information System (NHGIS) Database, which contains American Community Survey (ACS) estimates for census tracts between 2010 and 2014. Demographic information collected from this database includes information about race/ethnicity, educational attainment, as well as the poverty status and income level of households.

Housing, land use and zoning information

Housing and land use information were also collected to provide a sense of the types of housing and land uses in and around tracts with gardens. Information about home value and occupancy status were obtained from the NHGIS archive of ACS data 2010–2014 5-year estimates. Parcel level information about land use across the metropolitan area was obtained from the Maricopa Association of Governments (MAG) database as of 2014. A critical aspect of this database is the information about vacant developable land, which is important to identify given the vacant land problem discussed above, and because these vacant land parcels represent potential urban garden locations. Parcel data were aggregated to the census tract level to get a sense of the amount of a particular land use (in square miles) within each census tract. To incorporate information about travel time for residents, tract-level data from the ACS 2010–2014 5-year estimates on commuting mode and travel time to work were also gathered.

Analytical approach

Analysis of variance (ANOVA) is used to determine whether there are statistical differences between the three categories of tracts described above (contain a

garden, adjacent to a garden, not adjacent/does not contain a garden) based on the contextual data summarized in Table 2. This portion of the analysis is needed to test the following three hypotheses:

H1 Households in tracts with a garden, or nearby a garden, will have higher socioeconomic status than households in tracts without gardens.

H2 Tracts with gardens, or nearby a garden, will have different land uses than tracts without a garden.

H3 Tracts without gardens will have poor access to other types of food sources than tracts with gardens, or nearby a garden.

These hypotheses are important to test, because they can help characterize important economic, land use and food access differences between the three types of tracts. If for example, there are no differences in food access between the three categories of tracts, a reconfiguration of current garden locations is not necessary to improve access for residents.

After analyzing the neighborhood context of urban gardens, location models are used to identify potential sites for future garden activity. Here, it is important to remember that this analytical approach is different from prior remote sensing and site suitability techniques for identifying garden locations because it not only identifies potential sites for gardens based on particular criteria, but it also provides a sense of the number of gardens needed to cover a given population of interest (in this case, residents of food deserts).

Location analysis and modeling has been used to support locational decisions in a wide range of applications [66], including emergency service planning [67, 68], school district design [69, 70] and wireless device placement [71] to name a few. Building on the fact that food deserts are demarcated based on distance thresholds, and the goal of the analysis is to service the food desert population, two covering models were considered for this particular study: the location set covering problem [67] and the maximal covering location problem [72]. Different from other types of location models, covering models examine service efficiency using a coverage standard that is often based on travel distance or time: demand is considered covered if it is within the coverage standard of a service provider. Recently, Bao et al. [42] developed a variant of the maximal covering location model to strategically site independent food stores for addressing food desert issues.

In our study, coverage provided by a community garden will be assessed based on whether a food desert is located within the 1-mile travel distance as defined by the USDA.

---

[1] Note this definition of healthy food outlets is more comprehensive than that of the USDA, which bases its definition of food deserts on access to supermarkets [39].

The location set covering model can be used to produce output that would specify the minimum number of gardens needed to ensure that no food desert is left uncovered, while the maximal covering location problem can be used to prescribe the spatial configuration of urban gardens that maximizes the coverage of food deserts when the number of gardens to site is fixed due to a budget constraint.

The model selected to implement in this paper is the maximal location covering problem [72], because it is infeasible to cover all food deserts due to the limited vacant land available. The output of the maximal covering location model is the location of and coverage of food desert residents provided by a given number of gardens. The output from this spatial optimization model also provides geographic information about proposed garden sites, and a tradeoff curve which contains the number of gardens to be sited on the x-axis and the population residing in food deserts covered by the specified number of gardens on the y-axis. From this tradeoff curve, it is possible to understand tradeoffs in the number of gardens located and the percentage of food desert residents covered.

Given the potential for urban gardens to serve as an affordable source of fresh fruits and vegetables for residents in food deserts, the goal of the optimization analysis will be to locate gardens based on two criteria: to cover as many residents in food deserts as possible and to locate these gardens on vacant land within the Phoenix metropolitan area. The location model is specified below.

Maximal covering location problem

$$\text{Maximize} \sum_i w_i y_i \tag{1}$$

Subject to

$$\sum_{j \in N_i} x_j \geq y_i \quad \forall i \tag{2}$$

$$\sum_j x_j = p \tag{3}$$

$$x_j \in \{0, 1\} \quad \forall j \tag{4}$$

$$y_i \in \{0, 1\} \quad \forall i \tag{5}$$

where i index of food deserts, j index of vacant land, w_i population in food desert i

$N_i = \{j | d_{ij} \leq D\}$ consists of all the candidate site j that if converted can serve food desert i (i.e., the travel distance from i to j is within D the low-access threshold used for defining food deserts). p: the number of community gardens to site

Objective (1) aims to maximize the food desert population to be covered. Constraint (2) specifies that a food desert is considered covered only when there is at least one urban garden that is located within the coverage threshold D. Given that the food deserts in this study are located in urban areas, we define the coverage threshold D to be 1-mile (1.61 km) travel distance in order to be consistent with the definition of food deserts provided by the USDA. Constraint (3) specifies the number of urban gardens to be sited. Constraints (4) and (5) impose binary integer conditions on decision variables x and y that dictate whether vacant land is selected or not, and whether a food desert is covered or not, respectively.

Results

Before undertaking the spatial optimization analysis to pinpoint proposed garden sites, an analysis of the location of past and present gardens sites is conducted. This portion of the analysis is important because it provides information about the spatial distribution of garden sites, their neighborhood context, and their proximity to food desert locations across the metropolitan area. Figure 2 displays the locations of existing gardens (see Additional file 1 for a shapefile of these gardens). This graphic highlights that the majority of gardens (66%) are located in the city limits of Phoenix in areas that include the historic Encanto district, Maryvale, and South Mountain. Other cities, including Tempe, Mesa, and Chandler, also have garden activity, but the majority is highly centralized in the old urban core. Figure 2 also shows the hotspots of healthy food outlets by census tract, which was produced by aggregating the healthy food outlet point locations from the ESRI Reference USA database to census tracts. The local Moran [73] was used to identify hotspots of healthy food outlets. These are tracts with a high level of healthy food outlet clustering.[2]

While the figure does not present a formal test of spatial dependence between garden locations and healthy food outlet hotspots, it does provide some support for prior work showing that gardens cluster near healthy

$$x_j = \begin{cases} 1 & \text{if vacant land } j \text{ is selected for the conversion to a community garden} \\ 0 & \text{otherwise} \end{cases}$$

$$y_i = \begin{cases} 1 & \text{if food desert } i \text{ is covered} \\ 0 & \text{otherwise} \end{cases}$$

[2] Hotspots are defined as tracts corresponding to the high–high and high–low output of the local Moran. Census tracts are drawn to include roughly 4000 people [81]; thus, mapping a density measure or per capita number of food outlets in Fig. 1 would be redundant.

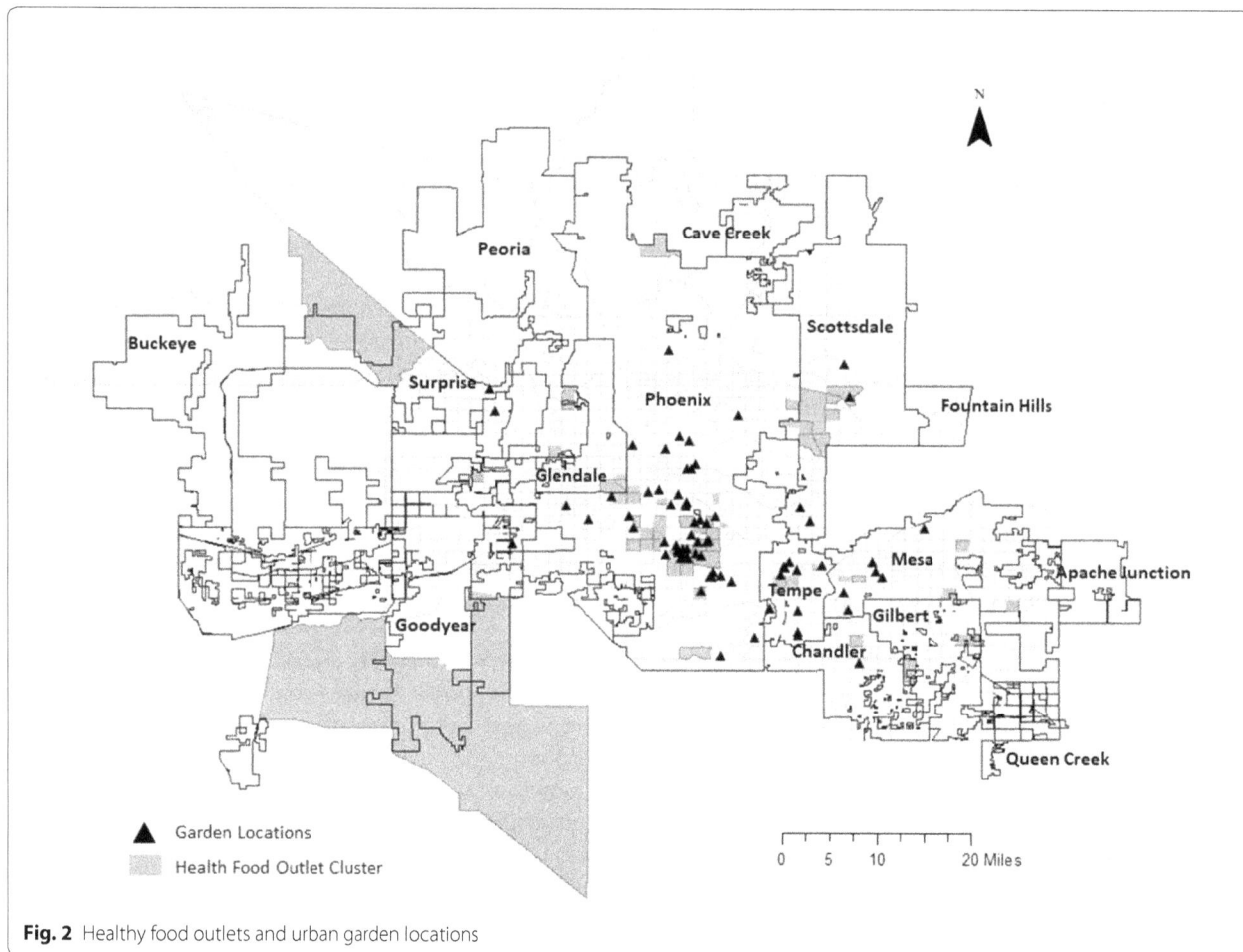

Fig. 2 Healthy food outlets and urban garden locations

food outlets [51]. As the ANOVA results below indicate, these areas are also more likely to be commercial neighborhoods that are zoned to allow retail uses. This means the current locations of gardens do not help residents in food deserts because they are already located in areas with access to healthy food stores. In general, the majority of gardens are located near the central city areas of Phoenix, Tempe, and Mesa. There are also several gardens in the more residential areas of North Phoenix, Scottsdale, and Mesa that are not located near clusters of healthy food outlets, but these are generally the exception.

Neighborhood context of garden locations

These differences in garden locations raise questions about the neighborhood context of garden sites. To provide some resolution on the extent that neighborhoods with gardens are different from those without gardens, analysis of variance (ANOVA) was conducted to statistically test for neighborhood differences based on five sets of characteristics: demographics, socio-economic status, land use characteristics, housing type, food outlet type, and commuting characteristics. Given the relatively low number of garden-containing census tracts (75 out of 880 in the study area, or 8.5% of tracts), garden-adjacent census tracts were also included in the analysis (34.3% of tracts) in order to evaluate the neighborhood context of communities with gardens. Garden-adjacent tracts are also important to identify since they are closer to garden locations—and thus more likely to receive some supplementary benefit—than other tracts in the metropolitan area.

Table 3 presents summary results of this analysis and highlights significant differences between census tracts with gardens, tracts adjacent to those with gardens, and tracts without gardens. Detailed ANOVA results may be found in Additional file 2 included at the end of this paper. In terms of interpreting the information in Table 3, each variable is listed next to the tract type with the *highest value* of that variable; for example, industrial, neighborhood commercial, educational, office, and medical land uses are all statistically different between the tract

Table 3 Highest values of various characteristics for no garden, garden-adjacent, and garden-containing tracts

Tract type	Land use characteristics	Food deserts	Housing	Socio-demographics	Food outlets	Urban design and transportation
Contains garden	Industrial	Low access low income share at 1/2-mile (0.8 km)	% Vacant housing units	% Black	# Supermarkets	
	Neighborhood commercial			% Hispanic	# Convenience outlets	
	Educational			% Food stamps	# Bakeries	
	Office				# Restaurants	
	Medical				# Other grocery outlets	% Drove alone to work
					# Fruit and vegetable outlets	% Non-auto commuters
						% < 15 min commute
						% ≥ 30 min commute
Garden-adjacent	Multi-family residential				# Specialty food outlets	
					# Meat and fish outlets	
No gardens	Single-family residential low density	Low access kids' share at 1/2-mile (0.8 km)	Median home value	% Bachelor's		
	Single-family residential medium density		% Owner occupied			
	Single-family residential high density					
	Developable agriculture					
	Developable land					
	Developing residential					

Table shows only results significant at the 10% level or better

types, *and* have higher percentages in garden-containing tracts. Similarly, garden-adjacent tracts show the highest percentage of multi-family residential land use. In terms of demographics, urban garden tracts and tracts adjacent to gardens are more racially and ethnically diverse; tracts with gardens have a higher percentage of Black and Hispanic residents than do non-garden tracts. They also have lower levels of educational attainment. In terms of other measures of socio-economic status, garden tracts and tracts adjacent to gardens have a higher percentage of persons who are unemployed, on food stamps, and without healthcare.

Aside from demographic and socio-economic differences, there are also interesting differences in land uses amongst the three categories of tracts analyzed, particularly for tracts with gardens and tracts adjacent to garden tracts. These tracts have less land dedicated to residential land, but more land area dedicated to medical, office, and educational uses than tracts without gardens. As for the characteristics of nearby food outlets, gardens and tracts neighboring garden tracts have higher access to a variety of food outlets including restaurants, supermarkets, and convenience stores. Interestingly tracts with gardens also had the lowest share of workers commuting to work by driving alone, the highest share of workers commuting by non-auto modes (transit, walking and cycling), the highest percentage of residents with a commute under 15 min, and the lowest percentage of residents with a commute of 30 min of more.

Figure 3 displays the locations of gardens and food deserts in the metropolitan area. It highlights that many gardens are not located in food deserts; in fact, only 24 out of the 75 gardens (32%) are located in food desert tracts. Also, of the 68 active urban gardens identified at the time of this analysis, only nine cover food deserts with a population of 27,290, corresponding to just 8.4%

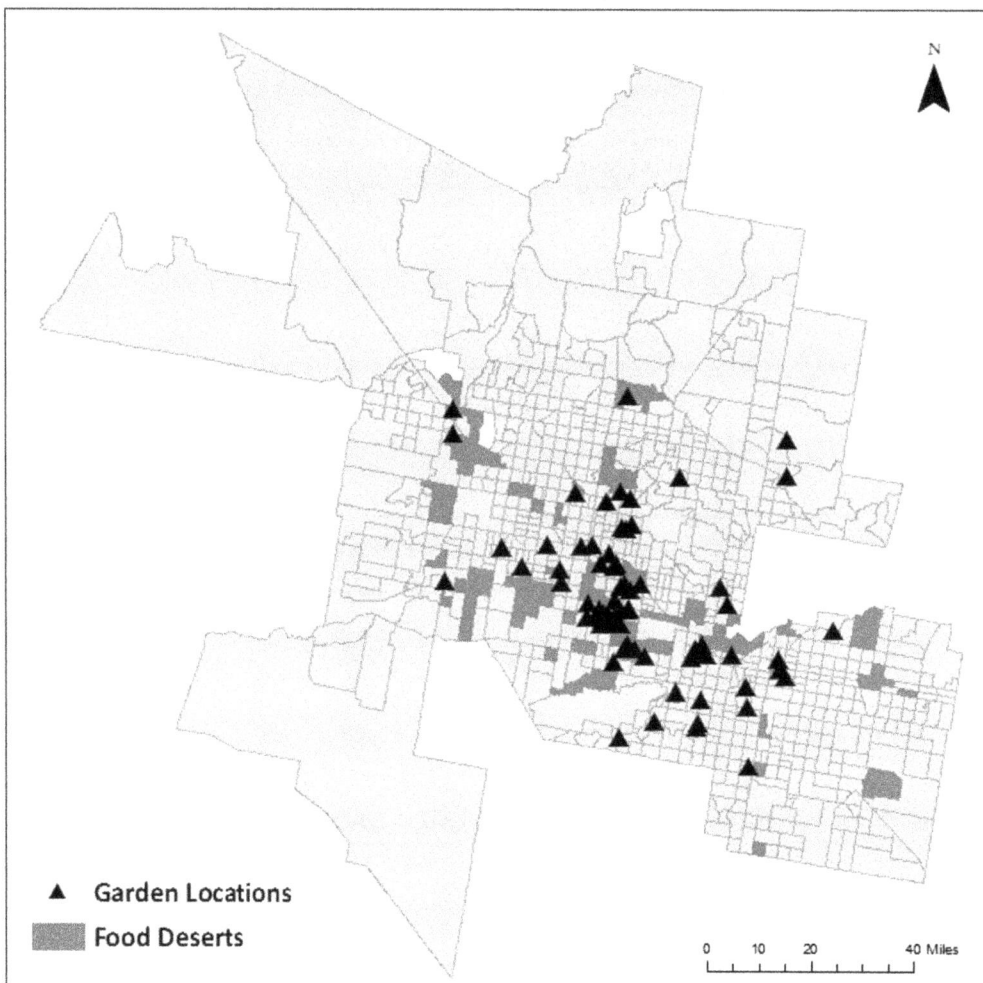

Fig. 3 Urban garden and food desert locations

of all food desert residents. Several of the uncovered food deserts are located in exurban locations to the West of downtown Phoenix in neighborhoods such as El Mirage and Glendale. Uncovered food deserts are also evident in the east of the metropolitan area in Mesa. Based on this distribution of gardens, it appears future garden sites could be located more strategically to cover residents in food desert locations.

Siting urban gardens

To analyze how gardens could be distributed better, a maximal covering spatial optimization model was used to identify gardens sites to provide better coverage for food desert residents. To do this, only vacant land classified as developable was considered; military and native community lands were excluded. Land considered too small for community gardens (< 5000 ft^2) was also excluded. This threshold of 5000 ft^2 is based

on recommendations that to achieve a critical mass of gardeners, the total size of a garden should be a minimum of 3000–3500 ft^2 so that it may contain 10–12 good sized garden plots [74]. A size of 5000 ft^2 would accommodate this number of plots and also provides space for a toolshed and community garden activities.

The analysis resulted in 5947 pieces of vacant land selected to serve as potential urban garden sites. The coverage assessment was performed based on the travel distance from a food desert to a candidate garden site using ESRI's Network Analyst and the region's street network. During the distance calculation, vacant land was represented using the geometric centroids and food deserts were converted to points using their population centers. The maximal covering location problem introduced in the previous section was then solved to identify which vacant land sites can serve the food deserts not served currently by existing gardens.

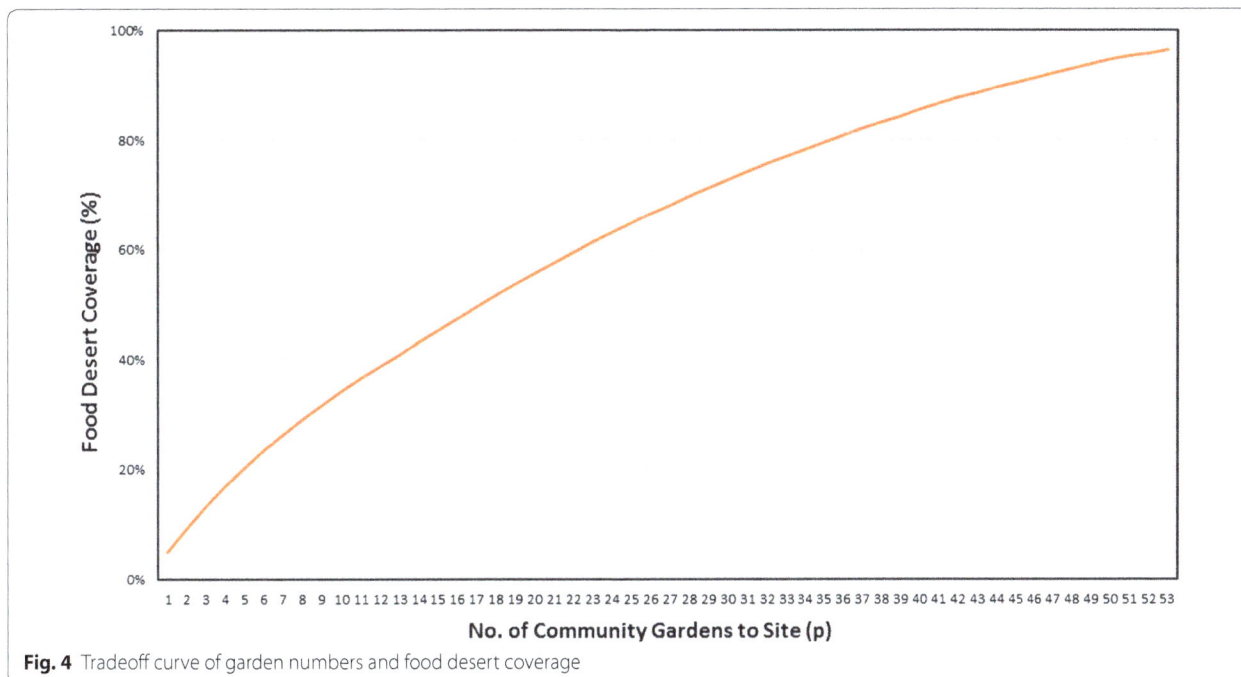

Fig. 4 Tradeoff curve of garden numbers and food desert coverage

Figure 4 presents a tradeoff curve that summarizes the results of this analysis. On the x-axis of this graph is the number of gardens, and the y-axis represents the percentage of food desert residents covered by siting p number of community gardens. The tradeoff curve provides important insights for planners and government agencies to better allocate limited funds for food project planning. Similar to many other maximal coverage location problem applications, marginal coverage achieved decreases with the number of facilities sited. For example, siting 25 urban gardens achieves coverage of about 65% of the food desert population whereas an increase of gardens to twice that number (50 gardens), achieves 30% more coverage. Constrained by the location of the vacant land available, it is infeasible to achieve complete coverage of all 68 food deserts not covered by existing gardens. This is because three food deserts are left uncovered due to the lack of available land closer to food desert sites. The best coverage possible can be obtained by siting 53 urban gardens, providing maximal coverage of 65 food deserts with 96.4% of the food desert population covered (Additional file 3). This is a vast improvement over the current distribution of gardens; the 68 active community garden sites only cover 8.4% of food desert populations. A map of the 53 proposed garden sites along with food desert locations is shown in Fig. 5. Several of the proposed sites (45%) are located in the city limits of Phoenix. Proposed garden sites to the west of Phoenix include the communities of El Mirage, Glendale, Sun City, and Peoria. To the southeast of Phoenix, other proposed garden sites are located in Tempe, Chandler, and Mesa.

Discussion

Across the world, urbanization continues at a rapid pace. As agricultural land is converted to other uses and people become disconnected from traditional food sources, access to healthy food is a growing issue for urban residents worldwide. Given the health implications associated with the lack of access to healthy food [9, 75, 76], this study set out to demonstrate how spatial optimization models may be used to better locate urban gardens to improve access for residents and to resolve the issue of unused vacant land simultaneously. This technique is demonstrated here for the Phoenix Arizona metropolitan area but can also be applied to any city globally where food access and vacant land issues are present. As mentioned previously, several cities in countries around the globe, such as Afghanistan, India, and Brazil, are currently experiencing similar problems associated with rapid rates of urbanization.

Analytical results reveal important demographic, socio-economic, and land use differences between tracts with or near urban gardens and tract without or not near urban gardens. Tracts with or near gardens are more racially and ethnically diverse and also contain characteristics of low socio-economic status such as lower levels of educational attainment and higher rates of unemployment compared to non-garden tracts. These results are encouraging because they indicate that residents perhaps *most* in need of healthy food are often within close proximity to urban gardening activity. Unfortunately, an analysis of the spatial distribution of food deserts and

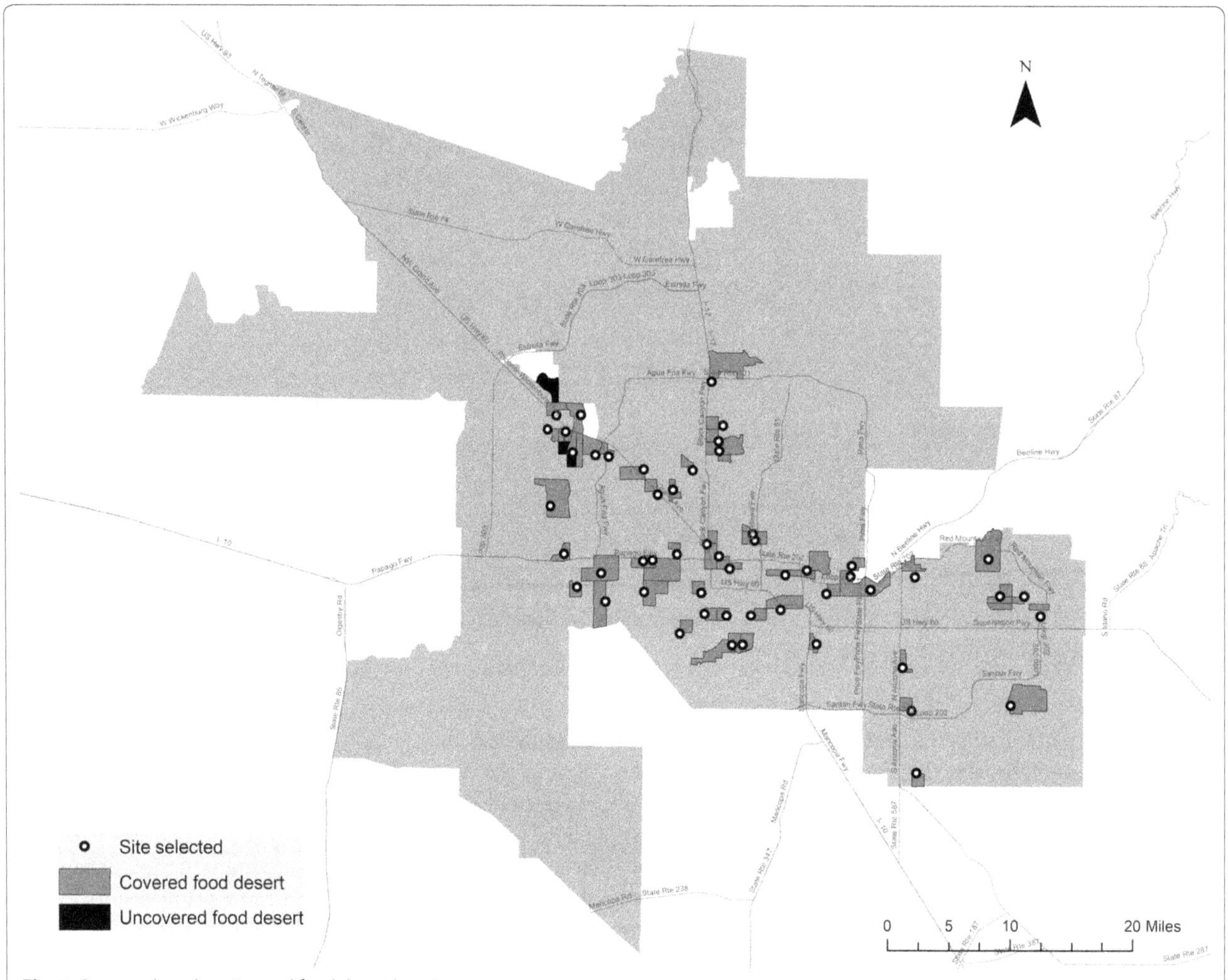

Fig. 5 Proposed garden sites and food desert locations

urban gardens reveals that the distribution of urban gardens at the time of this analysis covered less than 10% of food desert residents, which highlights that an alternative distribution of urban gardening activity would improve access to these sources of fresh fruits and vegetables. Spatial optimization models are used to suggest alternative locations of urban gardens using vacant land. These model results suggest an alternative arrangement of 53 gardens that would provide coverage of 96.4% of the food desert population.

That said, it is important to note some limitations of this analysis. First, there are additional considerations beyond the availability of land and lack of food access that will need to be investigated further in the proposed garden sites. One of these considerations is the quality of soil, which prior work has noted is a potential issue for urban gardening activity [77, 78]. Thus, it is recommended that the soil quality in the proposed sites be tested for contaminants before planting commences.

A second consideration is the potential volume of food that could be produced at garden sites. Prior studies have noted that the food production capacity of urban gardens may be insufficient to provide food in the necessary quantities needed [51]. However, other studies have noted that coordinated planning efforts to foster urban gardening activity can produce a large proportion of local food needs [79]. To account for this concern, the gardens sited in this analysis ensure that at least 5000 ft^2 are used for gardening activity. However, additional steps will need to be taken from a garden management perspective to ensure proper crop rotation and to ensure that the volume of fruits and vegetables grown is as such, that it may serve as a good supply of healthy foods for garden participants and the surrounding community. Third, once established, a concentrated and enduring effort to maintain urban gardens sites is needed to preserve these spaces. Gardens are a notoriously transient urban activity [49] and preservation plans are needed so as not to upend activity once it is commenced. This was the case with a large urban garden started as part of the Phoenix Renews project, which was shut down due to financial issues with the land on which the garden was placed [64]. Fourth, although citing gardens can reduce the physical distance to food, it may not reduce the temporal distance. Low-income people are more likely to be multiple job holders and may lack the time and also the knowledge to cook fresh vegetables. Finally, it is important to note that the mere provision of *access* to fresh fruits and vegetables is not enough to resolve dietary problems and the health issues stemming from poor diets. Studies of the built environment and health have uncovered a range of factors that influence obesity from land-use mix, crime, type of food outlets present, and urban design that is pedestrian oriented [80]. Thus, increasing access to urban gardens is just the first step to improving healthy food consumption for people. Access needs to be coupled with education efforts about the health value of fruits and vegetables grown in the gardens, as well as promotion of the gardens themselves to encourage participation by area residents. The pricing of any products sold should also be as such, that they are affordable to folks in a wide-variety of income strata. Recipes can also be provided that would educate purchasers of products about the preparation of fruits and vegetables to improve health outcomes.

Conclusion

As rapid urbanization continues globally so too are issues of food access and vacant land likely to become more prevalent. To combat these related issues, more sophisticated planning strategies are needed to improve food access for residents. Although enhancing access is just the first step in improving healthy food consumption, urban gardens represent an inexpensive way to provide food to nearby residents. As demonstrated in this paper, spatial optimization models are an analytical tool that can be used to strategically locate these food sources on unused urban land, thereby mitigating two problems evident in rapidly expanding cities around the world.

Additional files

Additional file 1. Past and Present Phoenix Garden Locations. Point shapefile of the garden data used in this analysis.

Additional file 2. Results of ANOVA tests for no garden, garden-adjacent, and garden-containing tracts. Three tables showing results of ANOVA analysis for each of the garden types and each of the variables of interest. Table includes the mean, standard deviation, and statistical significance for each variable/tract-type combination.

Additional file 3. Proposed Phoenix garden locations. Point shapefile of garden data generated from the spatial optimization analysis.

Abbreviations

ACGA: American Community Garden Association; ACS: American Community Survey; ANOVA: analysis of variance; GIS: geographic information systems; ESRI: Environmental Systems Research Institute; MAG: Maricopa Association of Governments; MCCE: Maricopa County Cooperative Extension; NHGIS: National Historic Geographic Information System; RUCA: Rural–Urban Commuting Area; USDA: United States Department of Agriculture; WHO: World Health Organization.

Authors' contributions

EM collected and analyzed the garden and related secondary data for the neighborhood context analysis, and was a major contributor in the writing of the manuscript. DT conducted the spatial optimization analysis and wrote the related methods and results for this portion of the paper. KC helped compile and analyze the garden and related secondary data for the neighborhood context analysis, and was a contributor in the writing of the manuscript. EM, DT, and KC all contributed to revisions to the manuscript. All authors read and approved the final manuscript.

Author details

[1] Department of Geography, Environment and Spatial Sciences, Michigan State University, Geography Building, 673 Auditorium Rd, Room 202, East Lansing, MI 48824, USA. [2] School of Geographical Sciences and Urban Planning, Arizona State University, Tempe, AZ 85281, USA.

Acknowledgements

Thank you to Matei Georgescu at the School of Geographical Sciences and Urban Planning, Arizona State University for support of this work.

Competing interests

The authors declare that they have no competing interests.

Availability of data and materials

The garden data used in this analysis is included in this published article as a supplementary information file with the name Additional file 1. The proposed garden data generated during this study is included in this published article as a supplementary information file with the name Additional file 3. The food desert dataset analyzed for this study is available from the United States Department of Agriculture (USDA) Food Access Research Atlas: https://www.ers.usda.gov/data-products/food-access-research-atlas/download-the-data/. The demographic and socio-economic data analyzed for this study is available from the National Historic Geographic Information System (NHGIS): https://www.nhgis.org/. The land use data analyzed for this study is available upon request from the Maricopa Association of Governments (MAG): http://www.azmag.gov/Information_Services/default.asp. The Rural–Urban Commuting Area (RUCA) codes used in this study may be downloaded from the United States Department of Agriculture (USDA) Economic Research Service (ERS) at: https://www.ers.usda.gov/data-products/rural–urban-commuting-area-codes/.

Funding

Work for this project was funded by National Science Foundation Grant No. 1419593 and USDA Grant No. 2015-67003-23508.

References

1. Bank W. How eight cities succeeded in rejuvenating their urban land. 2016. http://www.worldbank.org/en/news/press-release/2016/07/13/How-eight-cities-succeeded-in-rejuvenating-their-urban-land. Accessed 16 Aug 2017.
2. French M, Turkstra J, Farid M. Vacant land plots in Afghan cities: a problem and an opportunity. Urbanisation. 2016;1:79–94. doi:10.1177/2455747116671825.
3. Fazal S. Urban expansion and loss of agricultural land—a GIS based study of Saharanpur City, India. Environ Urban. 2000;12:133–49. doi:10.1630/095624700101285343.
4. Sperandelli DI, Dupas FA, Dias Pons NA. Dynamics of urban sprawl, vacant land, and green spaces on the Metropolitan Fringe of São Paulo, Brazil. J Urban Plan Dev. 2013;139:274–9. doi:10.1061/(ASCE)UP.1943-5444.0000154.
5. Foodtank. 28 Inspiring Urban Agriculture Projects. 2015. http://foodtank.com/news/2015/07/urban-farms-and-gardens-are-feeding-cities-around-the-world.
6. Bolen E, Hecht K. Neighborhood groceries: new access to healthy food in low-income communities. 2003; January:1–43. http://healthycornerstores.org/wp-content/uploads/resources/CFPAreport-NeighborhoodGroceries.pdf.
7. Saelens BE, Sallis JF, Frank LD. Environmental correlates of walking and cycling: findings from the transportation, urban design, and planning literaturesitle. Ann Behav Med. 2003;25:80–91.
8. Rundle A, Neckerman K, Freeman L. Neighborhood food environment and walkability predict obesity in New York City. Environmental. 2009. http://search.proquest.com/openview/adbaca8f16772d126705ffc2c0da8078/1?pq-origsite=gscholar&cbl=48869. Accessed 21 June 2017.
9. Larson NI, Story MT, Nelson MC. Neighborhood environments: disparities in access to healthy foods in the U.S. Am J Prev Med. 2009;36(74–81):e10. doi:10.1016/j.amepre.2008.09.025.
10. United Nations. World urbanization prospects: the 2014 revision, highlights (ST/ESA/SER.A/352). 2014. doi:10.4054/DemRes.2005.12.9.
11. Patel R. Stuffed and starved: markets, power and the hidden battle for the world food system. 2007.
12. Mayo J. The American grocery store: the business evolution of an architectural space. 1993. http://www.jstor.org/stable/pdf/1425290.pdf. Accessed 21 June 2017.
13. Grey M. The industrial food stream and its alternatives in the United States: an introduction. Hum Organ. 2000. http://www.sfaajournals.net/doi/abs/10.17730/humo.59.2.xm3235743p6618j3. Accessed 21 June 2017.
14. Morton L, Blanchard T. Starved for access: life in rural America's food deserts. Rural realities. 2007. http://eatbettermovemore.org/SA/enact/neighborhood/documents/RuralRealitiesFoodDeserts1-4.pdf. Accessed 21 June 2017.
15. Sadler RC, Gilliland JA, Arku G. An application of the edge effect in measuring accessibility to multiple food retailer types in Southwestern Ontario, Canada. Int J Health Geogr. 2011;10:34. doi:10.1186/1476-072X-10-34.
16. Armstrong D. A survey of community gardens in upstate New York: implications for health promotion and community development. Health Place. 2000;6:319–27. doi:10.1016/S1353-8292(00)00013-7.
17. Litt JS, Soobader MJ, Turbin MS, Hale JW, Buchenau M, Marshall JA. The influence of social involvement, neighborhood aesthetics, and community garden participation on fruit and vegetable consumption. Am J Public Health. 2011;101:1466–73.
18. Krusky AM, Heinze JE, Reischl TM, Aiyer SM, Franzen SP, Zimmerman MA. The effects of produce gardens on neighborhoods: a test of the greening hypothesis in a post-industrial city. Landsc Urban Plan. 2015;136:68–75. doi:10.1016/j.landurbplan.2014.12.003.
19. Van Duyn M, Pivonka E. Overview of the health benefits of fruit and vegetable consumption for the dietetics professional: selected literature. J Am Diet Assoc. 2000. http://www.sciencedirect.com/science/article/pii/S000282230000420X. Accessed 21 June 2017.
20. Ness A, Powles J. Fruit and vegetables, and cardiovascular disease: a review. Int J Epidemiol. 1997. http://ije.oxfordjournals.org/content/26/1/1.short. Accessed 21 June 2017.
21. Steinmetz K, Potter J. Vegetables, fruit, and cancer prevention: a review. J Am Diet Assoc. 1996. http://www.sciencedirect.com/science/article/pii/S0002822396002738. Accessed 21 June 2017.
22. Serdula M, Byers T, Mokdad A, Simoes E. The association between fruit and vegetable intake and chronic disease risk factors. 1996. http://journals.lww.com/epidem/Abstract/1996/03000/The_Association_between_Fruit_and_Vegetable_Intake.10.aspx. Accessed 21 June 2017.
23. Rose D, Richards R. Food store access and household fruit and vegetable use among participants in the US Food Stamp Program. Public Health Nutr. 2004;7:1081–8. doi:10.1079/PHN2004648.
24. Luan H, Law J, Quick M. Identifying food deserts and swamps based on relative healthy food access: a spatio-temporal Bayesian approach. Int J Health Geogr. 2015;14:37. doi:10.1186/s12942-015-0030-8.
25. Leete L, Bania N, Sparks-Ibanga A. Congruence and coverage. J Plan Educ Res. 2012;32:204–18. doi:10.1177/0739456X11427145.
26. Walker RE, Keane CR, Burke JG. Disparities and access to healthy food in the United States: a review of food deserts literature. Health Place. 2010;16:876–84. doi:10.1016/j.healthplace.2010.04.013.
27. Reisig V, Hobbiss A. Food deserts and how to tackle them: a study of one city's approach. Health Educ J. 2000. http://journals.sagepub.com/doi/abs/10.1177/001789690005900203. Accessed 21 June 2017.
28. Cummins S, Macintyre S. A systematic study of an urban foodscape: the price and availability of food in greater Glasgow. Urban Stud. 2002. http://journals.sagepub.com/doi/abs/10.1080/0042098022000011399. Accessed 21 June 2017.
29. Hendrickson D, Smith C, Eikenberry N. Fruit and vegetable access in four low-income food deserts communities in Minnesota. Agric Hum Values. 2006;23:371–83.
30. Larsen K, Gilliland J. Mapping the evolution of "food deserts" in a Canadian city: Supermarket accessibility in London, Ontario, 1961–2005. Int J Health Geogr. 2008;7:16. doi:10.1186/1476-072X-7-16.
31. Flynt A, Daepp MIG. Diet-related chronic disease in the northeastern United States: a model-based clustering approach. Int J Health Geogr. 2015;14:25. doi:10.1186/s12942-015-0017-5.
32. Smith C, Morton L. Rural food deserts: low-income perspectives on food access in Minnesota and Iowa. J Nutr Educ Behav. 2009. http://www.sciencedirect.com/science/article/pii/S1499404608007562. Accessed 21 June 2017.
33. Sharkey JR, Horel S, Dean WR. Neighborhood deprivation, vehicle ownership, and potential spatial access to a variety of fruits and vegetables in a large rural area in Texas. Int J Health Geogr. 2010;9:26. doi:10.1186/1476-072X-9-26.
34. Chen X, Clark J. Interactive three-dimensional geovisualization of space–time access to food. Appl Geogr. 2013. http://www.sciencedirect.com/science/article/pii/S0143622813001367. Accessed 21 June 2017.
35. Farber S, Morang MZ, Widener MJ. Temporal variability in transit-based accessibility to supermarkets. Appl Geogr. 2014;53:149–59.
36. Gordon C, Purciel-Hill M, Ghai NR, Kaufman L, Graham R, Van Wye G. Measuring food deserts in New York City's low-income neighborhoods. Health Place. 2011;17:696–700. doi:10.1016/j.healthplace.2010.12.012.
37. Bao KY, Tong D. The effects of spatial scale and aggregation on food access assessment: a case study of Tucson, Arizona. Prof Geogr. 2016;124(March):1–11. doi:10.1080/00330124.2016.1252271.
38. Blanchard T, Lyson T. Food availability and food deserts in the nonmetropolitan south. Mississippi, MS: South Rural Development Center; 2006.
39. (USDA) USD of A. USDA Food Access Research Atlas. 2017. https://www.ers.usda.gov/dataproducts/%0Afoodaccessresearchatlas/%0Adocumentation/. Accessed 15 June 2017.
40. Zhang M, Debarchana G. Spatial supermarket redlining and neighborhood vulnerability: a case study of Hartford, Connecticut. Trans GIS. 2016;20:79–100.
41. Raja S, Changxing M, Yadav P. Beyond food deserts: measuring and mapping racial disparities in neighborhood food environments. J Plan Educ Res. 2008;27:469–82. doi:10.1177/0739456X08317461.
42. Bao KY, Tong D. The effects of spatial scale and aggregation on food access assessment: a case study of Tucson, Arizona. Prof Geogr. 2017;69:337–47. doi:10.1080/00330124.2016.1252271.
43. Apparicio P, Cloutier M. The case of Montreal's missing food deserts: evaluation of accessibility to food supermarkets. International. 2007. https://ij-healthgeographics.biomedcentral.com/articles/10.1186/1476-072X-6-4. Accessed 21 June 2017.
44. Short A, Guthman J, Raskin S. Food deserts, oases, or mirages? J Plan Educ Res. 2007;26:352–64. doi:10.1177/0739456X06297795.
45. Algert SJ, Agrawal A, Lewis DS. Disparities in access to fresh pro-

duce in low-income neighborhoods in Los Angeles. Am J Prev Med. 2006;30:365–70.

46. Salois MJ. Obesity and diabetes, the built environment, and the "local" food economy in the United States, 2007. Econ Hum Biol. 2012;10:35–42. doi:10.1016/j.ehb.2011.04.001.

47. McClintock N. Institute for the study of societal issues from industrial garden to food desert : unearthing the root structure of urban agriculture in Oakland, California. Geography. 2008;5.

48. Birky J. The modern community garden movement in the United States: Its roots, its current condition and its prospects for the future. Grad Theses Diss. 2009;1–133. http://scholarcommons.usf.edu/etd/1860.

49. Lawson L. City bountiful. A century community. Gard Am. 2005. http://www.ucpress.edu/excerpt.php?isbn=9780520243439. Accessed 22 June 2017.

50. Hansen J. The progressive era. Social Welfare History. 2011. http://social-welfare.library.vcu.edu/eras/civil-war-reconstruction/progressive-era/.

51. Wang H, Qiu F, Swallow B. Can community gardens and farmers' markets relieve food desert problems? A study of Edmonton, Canada. Appl Geogr. 2014;55:127–37. doi:10.1016/j.apgeog.2014.09.010.

52. Kremer P, DeLiberty TL. Local food practices and growing potential: mapping the case of Philadelphia. Appl Geogr. 2011;31:1252–61. doi:10.1016/j.apgeog.2011.01.007.

53. Taylor JR, Lovell ST. Mapping public and private spaces of urban agriculture in Chicago through the analysis of high-resolution aerial images in Google Earth. Landsc Urban Plan. 2012;108:57–70. doi:10.1016/j.landurbplan.2012.08.001.

54. Thapa R, Murayama Y. Land evaluation for peri-urban agriculture using analytical hierarchical process and geographic information system techniques: a case study of Hanoi. Land use policy. 2008. http://www.sciencedirect.com/science/article/pii/S0264837707000658. Accessed 22 June 2017.

55. Erickson DL, Lovell ST, Méndez VE. Identifying, quantifying and classifying agricultural opportunities for land use planning. Landsc Urban Plan. 2013;118:29–39. doi:10.1016/j.landurbplan.2013.05.004.

56. Mendes W, Balmer K, Kaethler T, Rhoads A. Using land inventories to plan for urban agriculture: experiences from Portland and Vancouver. J Am Plan Assoc. 2008;74:435–49. doi:10.1080/01944360802354923.

57. Metcalf SS, Widener MJ. Growing Buffalo's capacity for local food: a systems framework for sustainable agriculture. Appl Geogr. 2011;31:1242–51. doi:10.1016/j.apgeog.2011.01.008.

58. Sadler RC. Integrating expert knowledge in a GIS to optimize siting decisions for small-scale healthy food retail interventions. Int J Health Geogr. 2016;15:19. doi:10.1186/s12942-016-0048-6.

59. Heim C. Leapfrogging, urban sprawl, and growth management: Phoenix, 1950–2000. Am J Econ Sociol. 2001. http://onlinelibrary.wiley.com/doi/10.1111/1536-7150.00063/full. Accessed 22 June 2017.

60. Ross A. Bird on fire: Lessons from the world's least sustainable city. 2011. https://books.google.com/books?hl=en&lr=&id=fVYyIpHYCKYC&oi=fnd&pg=PP1&dq=bird+on+fire&ots=_Zhn_lbPPd&sig=uJV3L3SJBNWVhkM_2e9_huo5H6Q. Accessed 22 June 2017.

61. Scott E. Phoenix has plans for its many vacant lots. The Arizona Republic. 2012. http://archive.azcentral.com/community/phoenix/articles/20121115phoenix-has-plans-its-many-vacant-lots.html.

62. Gardiner D. "Bad neighbor": Phoenix struggles to manage its vacant city-owned lots. The Arizona Republic. 2016. http://www.azcentral.com/story/news/local/phoenix/2016/11/24/phoenix-struggles-manage-city-real-estate/86875408/.

63. Reagor C. Land, land everywhere in Phoenix but not a lot to build on. The Arizona Republic. 2016. http://www.azcentral.com/story/money/real-estate/catherine-reagor/2016/07/07/land-land-everywhere-phoenix-but-not-lot-build/86773988/.

64. Gingold N. Phoenix community garden loses land to U.S. Department of the Interior. KJZZ 91.5. 2017. http://kjzz.org/content/431470/phoenix-community-garden-loses-land-us-department-interior.

65. USDA. Food desert locator. 2017. https://www.fns.usda.gov/tags/food-desert-locator.

66. Tong D, Murray AT. Location analysis: developments on the Horizon. Reg Res Front. 2017;2:193–208. doi:10.1007/978-3-319-50590-9_12.

67. Toregas C, Swain R, ReVelle C. The location of emergency service facilities. Operations. 1971. http://pubsonline.informs.org/doi/abs/10.1287/opre.19.6.1363. Accessed 22 June 2017.

68. Current J, O'Kelly M. Locating emergency warning sirens. Decis Sci. 1992. http://onlinelibrary.wiley.com/doi/10.1111/j.1540-5915.1992.tb00385.x/full. Accessed 10 Sept 2017.

69. Heckman L, Taylor H. School rezoning to achieve racial balance: a linear programming approach. Socioecon Plann Sci. 1969. http://www.sciencedirect.com/science/article/pii/0038012169900044. Accessed 10 Sept 2017.

70. Schoepfle O, Church R. A new network representation of a "classic" school districting problem. Socioecon Plann Sci. 1991. http://www.sciencedirect.com/science/article/pii/003801219190017L. Accessed 10 Sept 2017.

71. Shillington L, Tong D. Maximizing wireless mesh network coverage. Int Reg Sci. 2011. http://journals.sagepub.com/doi/abs/10.1177/0160017610396011. Accessed 10 Sept 2017.

72. Church Velle. The maximal covering location problem. Pap Reg Sci. 1974;32:101–18.

73. Anselin L. Local indicators of spatial association—LISA. Geogr Anal. 1995. http://onlinelibrary.wiley.com/doi/10.1111/j.1538-4632.1995.tb00338.x/full. Accessed 22 June 2017.

74. Denver Urban Gardens. Growing community gardens: a Denver urban gardens' best practices handbook for creating and sustaining community gardens. 2012. http://www.nccgp.org/images/uploads/resource_files/Best_Practices_for_Community_Gardens_-_Denver_Urban_Gardens.pdf.

75. Cassady D, Jetter K, Culp J. Is price a barrier to eating more fruits and vegetables for low-income families? J Am Diet Assoc. 2007. http://www.sciencedirect.com/science/article/pii/S0002822307016252. Accessed 21 June 2017.

76. Cummins S, Macintyre S. Food environments and obesity—neighbourhood or nation? Int J Epidemiol. 2006. http://ije.oxfordjournals.org/content/35/1/100.short. Accessed 21 June 2017.

77. Clark H, Brabander D. Sources, sinks, and exposure pathways of lead in urban garden soil. J Environ. 2006. https://dl.sciencesocieties.org/publications/jeq/abstracts/35/6/2066. Accessed 22 June 2017.

78. Finster M, Gray K, Binns H. Lead levels of edibles grown in contaminated residential soils: a field survey. Sci Total Environ. 2004. http://www.sciencedirect.com/science/article/pii/S0048969703004777. Accessed 22 June 2017.

79. Grewal SS, Grewal PS. Can cities become self-reliant in food? Cities. 2012;29:1–11. doi:10.1016/j.cities.2011.06.003.

80. Booth KM, Pinkston MM, Poston WSC. Obesity and the built environment. J Am Diet Assoc. 2005;105(5 Suppl):S110–7.

81. Bureau USC. Geographic terms and concepts—census tract. 2012. https://www.census.gov/geo/reference/gtc/gtc_ct.html. Accessed 15 June 2017.

82. Clarke G, Eyre H, Guy C. Deriving indicators of access to food retail provision in British cities: studies of Cardiff, Leeds and Bradford. Urban Stud. 2002. http://journals.sagepub.com/doi/abs/10.1080/0042098022000011353. Accessed 21 June 2017.

83. Acheson D, Barker D. Independent inquiry into inequalities in health: report. 1998. http://journals.sagepub.com/doi/pdf/10.1177/14664240081280030701. Accessed 21 June 2017.

84. Shaw HJ. Food deserts: towards the development of a classification. Geography. 2006;88:231–47.

85. Whelan A, Wrigley N, Warm D, Cannings E. Life in a 'food desert'. Urban Stud. 2002. http://journals.sagepub.com/doi/abs/10.1080/00420980220000011371. Accessed 21 June 2017.

5

Measurement of the potential geographic accessibility from call to definitive care for patient with acute stroke

J. Freyssenge[1,2,3]* [ORCID], F. Renard[3], A. M. Schott[1,4], L. Derex[1,5], N. Nighoghossian[5,6,7,8], K. Tazarourte[1,9] and C. El Khoury[1,2]

Abstract

Background: The World Health Organization refers to stroke, the second most frequent cause of death in the world, in terms of pandemic. Present treatments are only effective within precise time windows. Only 10% of thrombolysis patients are eligible. Late assessment of the patient resulting from admission and lack of knowledge of the symptoms is the main explanation of lack of eligibility.

Methods: The aim is the measurement of the time of access to treatment facilities for stroke victims, using ambulances (firemen ambulances or EMS ambulances) and private car. The method proposed analyses the potential geographic accessibility of stroke care infrastructure in different scenarios. The study allows better considering of the issues inherent to an area: difficult weather conditions, traffic congestion and failure to respect the distance limits of emergency transport.

Results: Depending on the scenario, access times vary considerably within the same commune. For example, between the first and the second scenario for cities in the north of Rhône county, there is a 10 min difference to the nearest Primary Stroke Center (PSC). For the first scenario, 90% of the population is 20 min away of the PSC and 96% for the second scenario. Likewise, depending on the modal vector (fire brigade or emergency medical service), overall accessibility from the emergency call to admission to a Comprehensive Stroke Center (CSC) can vary by as much as 15 min.

Conclusions: The setting up of the various scenarios and modal comparison based on the calculation of overall accessibility makes this a new method for calculating potential access to care facilities. It is important to take into account the specific pathological features and the availability of care facilities for modelling. This method is innovative and recommendable for measuring accessibility in the field of health care. This study makes possible to highlight the patients' extension of care delays. Thus, this can impact the improvement of patient care and rethink the healthcare organization. Stroke is addressed here but it is applicable to other pathologies.

Keywords: Stroke, Geographic accessibility, Road network, Medical transport, Health services

Background

Stroke is the main cause of non-traumatic disability and the second major cause of death in the world. WHO (World Health Organization) refers to stroke in terms of pandemic. Indeed, stroke caused 6.7 million deaths in 2012 [1]. Today, the pathology affects one person each second in the world. In 2015, a case of stroke occurred every 4 min in France, with 130,000 full hospitalisations [2]. The financial cost of stroke is high, with an annual 8.4 billion euros of sanitary and medical and social expenditure and an average €9642 per year for patients who have suffered stroke causing invalidity (about 14% more than

*Correspondence: j.freyssenge@resuval.fr
[1] Univ. Lyon, University Claude Bernard Lyon 1, HESPER EA 7425, 69008 Lyon, France
Full list of author information is available at the end of the article

for a long-term patient with Alzheimer's disease), covered by state medical insurance [3].

Stroke is a pathology bound to the notion of time. The effectiveness of treatment today is limited to precise temporal windows. For eligible patients, thrombolysis must be performed within 4 h 30 min of the appearance of the symptoms and thrombectomy within 6 h. Only 10% of patients are eligible for thrombolysis. This small proportion would seem to be the result of the late presentation of the patient and poor knowledge of the symptoms [4]. On the principle of 'time is brain', the aim of this paper is therefore to measure the access times to treatment facilities for stroke patients. This measurement is assessed using innovative methodology that models access time from the existing road network and using various means of transport.

Assessment of geographic accessibility is essential in many kinds of pathology. With the development and perfecting of Geographic Information Systems (GIS) in recent years, attempts have been made in a number of studies to model this accessibility as the use of a GIS to assess access times has been validated [5, 6]. Two studies have been essential for the development of this approach. The first [6] aimed to demonstrate the advantages of a GIS. Nadine Schuurman et al. [7] mention the 'array of spatial analysis methods' offered by GIS, providing 'an efficient and flexible way' to examine models of geographic access to health services. The study by Apparicio et al. [8] has also been a solid base for the use of GIS in assessing geographic access to a pathology. Indeed, in this case, the question is that of understanding the use of GIS to calculate accessibility that matches the phenomenon and the area observed as best as possible and that limits clumping errors. From 1980, a large number of articles have been published on the geographical accessibility topic, and this number is growing since the 2000s [9]. In our study, the topic of spatial accessibility is developed, defined like the fusion between accessibility dimension (distance or time between patient and service points) and availability dimension (number of service points from which a patient can choose) by Mark Guagliardo [10]. The measure of spatial accessibility can be classified in four categories: provider-to-population ratios, distance to the nearest provider, average distance to a set of providers, gravitational models of provider influence [10]. In this study, the travel impedance to nearest provider is studied. The travel impedance to nearest provider considers the accessibility but not the availability. Some other methods of spatial accessibility measures take into account these two dimensions [6, 10–12]: the two step floating catchment area method '2SFCA' [13, 14], gravity model [15] and the Kernel density model [10].

In the case of travel impedance to nearest provider [11, 12] a first work on modelling geographic access to emergency departments was conducted in 2009 in the United States [16]. The paper was a precursor as accessibility was addressed in terms of travelling time from the road network at different time steps, making possible the analysis of regional availability of emergency care. However, many non-geographic factors such as traffic congestion or difficult weather conditions (snow, fog, heavy rain, etc.) that disturb traffic were not taken into account and this feature seems to be an important limit to the study. One of the most complete studies so far towards accessibility is that of Alford-Teaster et al. [17] on mammography access. The use of care facilities is examined along with geographic accessibility. The study was performed from the angle of various factors such as demographic and economic criteria and land use. However, movements of patients in vehicles other their own are not shown in the study. Two studies are particularly interesting regarding to stroke. The first, by Scott et al. [18], showed the advantages of GIS for calculating time steps of journeys established according to the identification of symptoms for access to thrombolysis and using the positions of hospitals in Canada with a Stroke Unit. This study is nearly 20 years old. GIS techniques have been improved and perfected and the same modelling would be more representative of areas and the road network and hence more pertinent today. Concerning stroke care, the study of Adeoye et al. [19] seems to be the most complete study on accessibility. It describes access of the US population to hospital stroke care facilities on the basis of transport by medicalised ambulance in every case.

A review of the literature on the accessibility of stroke care facilities shows that no study of this kind had been performed in France. It was therefore essential to perform such analysis to learn more about territorial accessibility in the Rhône area. Furthermore, the limits of previous studies were taken into account—factors that are not inherently geographic such as traffic difficulties and the modelling of different types of transport and transporter. This consideration also made it possible to use different accessibility scenarios to adapt the study to territorial issues.

The aim of this study was to develop a measure method of accessibility according to the localization of patients and the different means of care.

Methods
Study area and data sources
Our study area is the Rhône administrative county in France (Fig. 1). The county covers an area of 3249 km² with a population of 1,798,511 in 2014 (source: *Institut national de la statistique et des études*

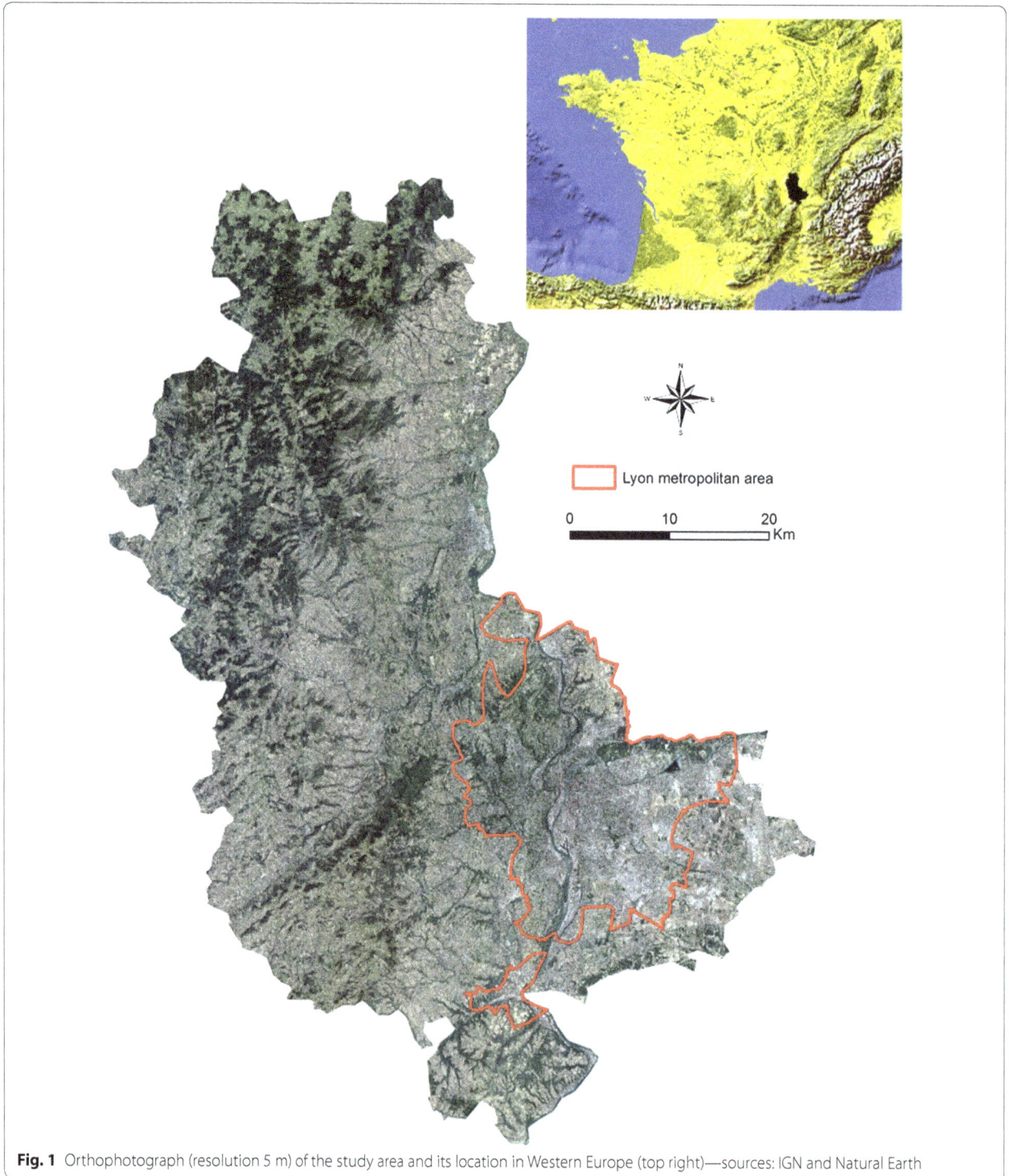

Fig. 1 Orthophotograph (resolution 5 m) of the study area and its location in Western Europe (top right)—sources: IGN and Natural Earth

économiques, Insee), i.e. 543 persons per square kilometre. Persons over 65, known to have a greater risk of stroke [20, 21], form 15.5% of the total population. A tendency for ageing is observed in the county, as is seen in all developed countries [22] as these have completed their demographic transition. Thus the number of over-60 s increased by 12% from 2007 to 2012 whereas the population as a whole increased by only 5%. The Rhône-Alpes region accounted for 9.7% of the French Gross Domestic Product (GDP), making it the second region in France and the seventh in Europe in terms of economic weight [23]. The driving force of the area is the metropolis of Lyon (Lyons), the second largest urban area of France with a population of 1.3 million.

The choice of road network is primordial for modelling transport operations. Description of accessibility using Euclidian distances [24] is a first approach but remains fairly limited. Geographic Information Systems have evolved and became essential to model access according to the road network. In previous French studies [25, 26], measurement of accessibility had used the *Route500* road database of the *Institut national de l'information géographique et forestière* (IGN). This database shows the main 500,000 kilometres of French roads: motorways, national main roads and departmental roads but passes over many residential and urban sections. Therefore, we have chosen to use the IGN *BDCarto* database, with more than a million kilometres of roads—the entire French road network—to get a more complete picture of the territory.

Pre-hospital emergency system

The ability of a care system to handle acute complications of medical or traumatic pathologies depends on many geographic and spatial criteria, making it a key public health issue. The times needed for access to treatment are a major factor in the care system. Two main types of vital emergency care system coexist in developed countries. The 'Anglo-Saxon' system relies on management of prehospital emergency by paramedics in order to transfer the patient to the nearest hospital. In this context, the goal is the fastest transport to medical facility. This system is mostly that of United States, Canada and United Kingdom where most of intensive care is performed at the hospital. The other system relies on emergency physicians involved at the scene of injury. This Emergency Medical Service (EMS) system is effective in France, Greece, Germany, Canada or Austria for example [27]. The 'French' system is based on sending to the patient a medical team called a *Unité Mobile Hospitalière*, UMH (a 'Mobile Hospital Unit') before entry to a hospital. The mobile unit assesses the seriousness of the case, makes a diagnosis, performs the necessary emergency and therapeutic support and then transfers the patient to a suitable hospital with facilities available—which is not necessarily the nearest one.

In France, the UMHs are part of *Structures Mobile d'Urgence et de Réanimation*, SMUR (Mobile Intensive Care Unit) that are located at public hospitals. Each SMUR is in charge of operational coverage of a defined population area. The segmentation of SMUR sectors depends on administrative boundaries without considering care access times for the population.

The *Service d'Aide Médicale Urgente* or SAMU (Medical Dispatch Call Center) is in charge of the reception and the triage of calls for each SMUR area. It is responsible for all prehospital medical or traumatic emergencies 24 h a day and 7 days a week, using the 15 call. Each centre is equipped with advanced telephone equipment and numerous information systems (geolocalisation, computerised filing, operational listing of resources). The SAMU centres are manned by medical staff, triage emergency doctors, general practitioners and non-medical staff (medical triage assistants).

The work of SAMU units is specified by decree and can be summarised in five broad categories:

- Decide and implement the most suitable response to the call as rapidly as possible,
- Check the availability of the public or private hospitalisation facilities appropriate for the condition of the patient, and ensure that arrangements were made for the arrival of the latter,
- If necessary, organise transport to a public or private hospital, using a public service (the fire brigade) or a private ambulance company,
- Oversee the admission of the patient, involving coordination of on-site care by the SMUR team and the hospital admission service,
- Provide support in the search for a specialised technical facility for non-academic hospitals.

The EMS system in France is not only based on UMH care. In fact, UMHs are the second level of EMS system. The first level is composed of basic life support (BLS) fire department ambulances, based at fire stations [19].

In Rhône county, it is not possible for patient to go directly to the Comprehensive Stroke Center (CSC), with private car. The patients are constantly transported by ambulances (SAMU or firemen ambulance). For stroke care there is a dedicated procedure from the call to EMS to the admission in CSC who not includes transport by private car. In most cases, stroke patients are transported to hospital by firemen because they don't need medical transport.

Data analysis

All the cartographic analyses shown in this work were produced using the program ArcMap *10.4.1* [28]. Measurements of accessibility were performed on the territory concerned by the study (the Rhône county) and neighbouring counties. Incorporating the road network in these areas in the model makes it possible to show the border effects associated with neighbouring counties population flows. The logic of movements is therefore evaluated here. Once the study area had been clearly established, it was essential to determine the speed limits allocated to each section according to the *Code de la Route* (Highway Code). As the *BDCarto* database does not include this information, the collaborative database *OpenStreetMap* [29] was used. However, information was lacking for 13% of the segments once the speed limits of the segments had been completed using this database. Therefore, thanks to CORINE Land Cover [30], a European georeferenced vectorial database showing land use, the speed limits were completed where they were lacking in the 13% of sectors. A speed limit of 50 kph (31 mph) was applied in urban zones and 90 kph (56 mph) in rural zones. Noting the speed limit in each section thus means that accessibility can be calculated in terms of time and not just in terms of distance.

Modelling according to accessibility scenarios

Various kinds of modelling were conducted with the varying of speed limits to take into account all the territorial issues involved in the Rhône county. The *Network Analyst* extension of *ArcMap 10.4.1* was used for these scenarios [7, 8, 19]. Four scenarios are shown in this study. They depend on traffic conditions and type of transport (Table 1).

The first scenario is the case of patient transportation by private car, the driver respects the speed limitations. The postulate is the movement of patients by their own means (their own vehicle or with help of a friend or relation) to the closest treatment facility. If the driver of private car decides not to respect the speed limitations, the other scenarios can be applied.

Scenario 2 is for driving in an emergency situation. The following hypothesis is used when modelling tends to show access to stroke care facilities from all points in the network: for private car, a third part transports the patient and takes the decision not to respect the speed limits. Petzäll et al. [31] measured an increase by 21.5 kph (13.3 mph) for emergency transportation by ambulances for cardiovascular disorders, 19.8 kph (12.3 mph) in urban area, 23.2 kph (14.4 mph) in rural area and 21.1 kph (13.1 mph) for extensive need of care, for a study based on the Swedish road network. Furthermore, an analysis based on SAMU interventions has been realized. From 2012 to 2016, the SMUR of Lyon has realized 646 interventions for stroke patients, prehospital medical management of stroke is indicated in case of a coma and concerns about 5% of strokes. From this reported data, the SMUR moves with an average speed of 21.46 kph (13.33 mph) faster than a private care with similar driving conditions. This average speed transport has been calculated from the precise location of SMUR departure center to the centroid of destination city (the precise location of patient care is not reported). According to these statements, the speed limits have been increased by 20 kph (12 mph) for scenario 2.

Scenario 2' is a complementary scenario which models the accessibility depending on the kind of area. In fact, on the basis of variation times between urban and rural areas [16, 31–33], the speed limitations are always increased by 20 kph (12 mph) in rural areas and decreased by 10 kph (6.2 mph) in urban areas, based on the Petzäll et al. [31] who has measured a speed difference of 30 kph (18.6 mph) between rural and urban areas.

In Scenario 3, with lower speeds due to severe weather conditions, we consider that the driver takes the decision to reduce his speed by 20 kph (12 mph) and thus respect the R413-2 article of French Highway Code recommendations if weather conditions are difficult [34].

The fourth scenario is an adaptation of scenario 2 and analysis of SAMU interventions during traffic jam hours.

Table 1 Characteristics of the different scenarios used (French law limits speeds to 130 kph (81 mph) or 110 kph (68 mph) on motorways, 90 kph (56 mph) in rural and periurban areas and 50 kph (31 mph) in built-up areas. However, local special features may be applied according to the context

Scenario	Modelling	Speed	Justification of speed adaptations
Scenario 1	Initial database	Respect of national speed limits	Private car submitted to French Highway Code respect
Scenario 2	Emergency transport	20 kph (12 mph) above the limit throughout the road network	Analysis based on Rhône's SAMU stroke interventions between 2012 and 2016, and Petzäll et al. [31] study
Scenario 2'	Emergency transport in urban and rural areas	20 kph (12 mph) higher in rural areas and 10 kph (6.2 mph) lower in urban areas	Complementary scenario for sensitivity analysis, based on literature review (Petzäll et al. [31]) and SAMU interventions analysis
Scenario 3	Difficult weather conditions (rain, fog, snow)	20 kph (12 mph) lower than the limit throughout the road network	Respect of the R413-2 article French Highway Code when there is severe weather conditions
Scenario 4	Emergency transport with traffic jams in the Lyons city area	20 kph (12 mph) lower in the Lyons metropolitan network (59 communes), 20 kph (12 mph) higher in the rest of the network	Petzäll et al. [31] study and SAMU interventions analysis for 20 kph higher and SAMU interventions analysis during traffic jam for 20 kph lower

Cartographic representation

A series of polygons was calculated for the zones covered (isochrones) representing the distance that can be attained from each stroke treatment facility in a particular length of time. The first stage thus consists of listing and geolocalising each stroke treatment infrastructure. Thus, public hospital emergency departments, Primary Stroke Center (PSC) and Comprehensive Stroke Center (CSC) [35] in the Rhône and neighbouring counties were geolocalised using their precise postal addresses (Table 2).

Preliminary measurement of accessibility to facilities from all points in the network with 10, 20, 30, 45 and 60-min access time was thus calculated. These time steps were chosen after bibliographic analysis [7, 16–19, 36, 37]. Each scenario was applied to this modelling.

Although it is pertinent to characterise the area according to the time required for travel from any point in the network to the treatment facility, it is even more interesting to model overall admission time. Treatment of stroke requires the best possible upstream taking in hand of the patient [4, 38]. This means that it is necessary to know the pattern of the territory according to the type of transport and also the positions of stroke treatment facilities. In our case, the development of thrombectomy and recent studies have shown its advantages for patients [39–41] and modelling overall patient reception was performed using the location of the CSC. With this model it is possible to characterize the territory by care delays from the emergency call to the admission in nearest CSC. It is a global approach of care because all the times of pre-hospital emergency care for stroke patients are taken into account. The second phase of our study was therefore

aimed at georeferencing each fire station in the Rhône and neighbouring counties, together with each SMUR team, using their precise addresses. After this georeferencing, supply zones were calculated for these facilities and then for each CSC to finally show total admission time—i.e. the estimated times from SMUR centres or fire stations to all the points in the network and then from any point to the CSC (Fig. 2). In this model, private car is not considered because it is not possible for patient to go directly to the CSC by his own. It was interesting to take intervention and triage times into account to better estimate the time. Thus, after a review of the literature, average time for ambulance dispatch, time spent at the scene and transport to a Comprehensive Stroke Center and intervention at the site of occurrence determined by Adeoye [19] were chosen (Fig. 2). The final times were calculated using the United States EMS (Emergency Medical Service) register for stroke cases alone.

This overall approach was represented on the basis of IRIS area units (*Ilots Regroupés pour l'Information Statistique*, small zones grouped for statistical information), the smallest administrative division of Insee (*Institut National de la Statistique et des Etudes Economiques*) and that respect demographic (populations of 2000) and geographic criteria [42]. This representation gives an accurate view and characterisation of areas according to access time to an CSC. For thrombectomy, discussions are in progress with regard to direct admission to CSC (Mothership) or a first stop at PSC ('Drip 'n Ship') [35]. In this study accessibility has been modelled using the Mothership pattern.

Results

Potential accessibility to care facilities in the Rhône county

The various scenarios (Table 1) combined with the diversity of infrastructure density in the area reveal marked differences in accessibility.

Logically, for each scenario, as there are more emergency services that PSCs, and are much more numerous than CSCs, access times to the latter are shorter. Certain zones in the area are under-privileged, whatever the scenario considered. Indeed, towns in the northern part of the Rhône such as Monsols, Aigueperse and Proprières are at least 30 min from the closest emergency department when speed limits are respected (Fig. 3a). The north of the county is again more than 30 min from an PSC facility. The area concerned is sometimes larger in this case and a zone with travelling times of more than 30 min is seen in a large south-western part: this is the case of the towns Bessenay and Duerne (Fig. 3b). For CSC, more than half of the county is more than 30 min from a facility and the journey from the commune of Aigueperse takes more than 60 min (Fig. 3c).

Table 2 Distribution of patient admission infrastructure

Infrastructure	County	Staff
Emergency department	Rhône (69)	7
	Ain (01)	3
	Saône-et-Loire (71)	6
	Isère (38)	7
	Loire (42)	6
PSC	Rhône (69)	2
	Ain (01)	1
	Saône-et-Loire (71)	1
	Isère (38)	2
	Loire (42)	2
CSC	Rhône (69)	1
	Ain (01)	0
	Saône-et-Loire (71)	0
	Isère (38)	1
	Loire (42)	1

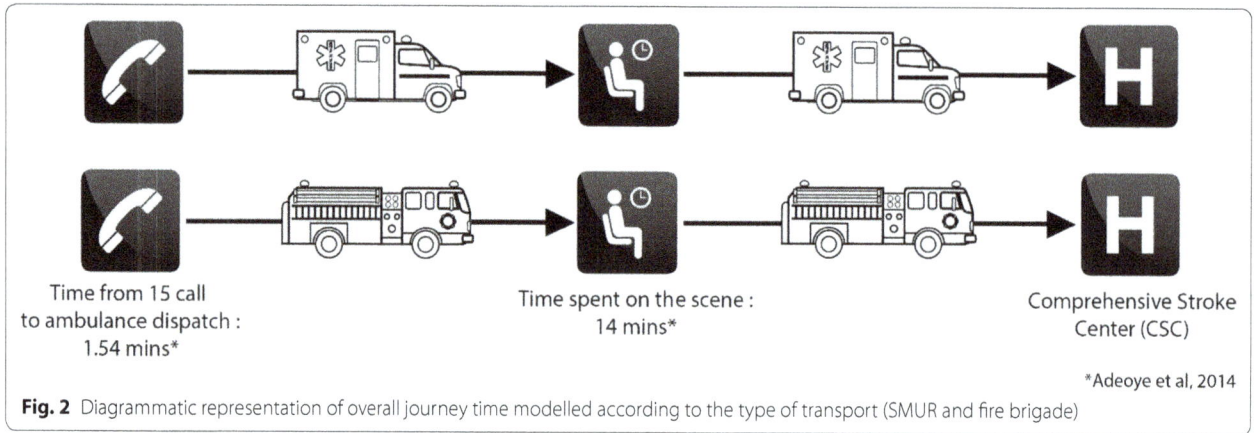

Fig. 2 Diagrammatic representation of overall journey time modelled according to the type of transport (SMUR and fire brigade)

Time from 15 call
to ambulance dispatch :
1.54 mins*

Time spent on the scene :
14 mins*

Comprehensive Stroke
Center (CSC)

*Adeoye et al, 2014

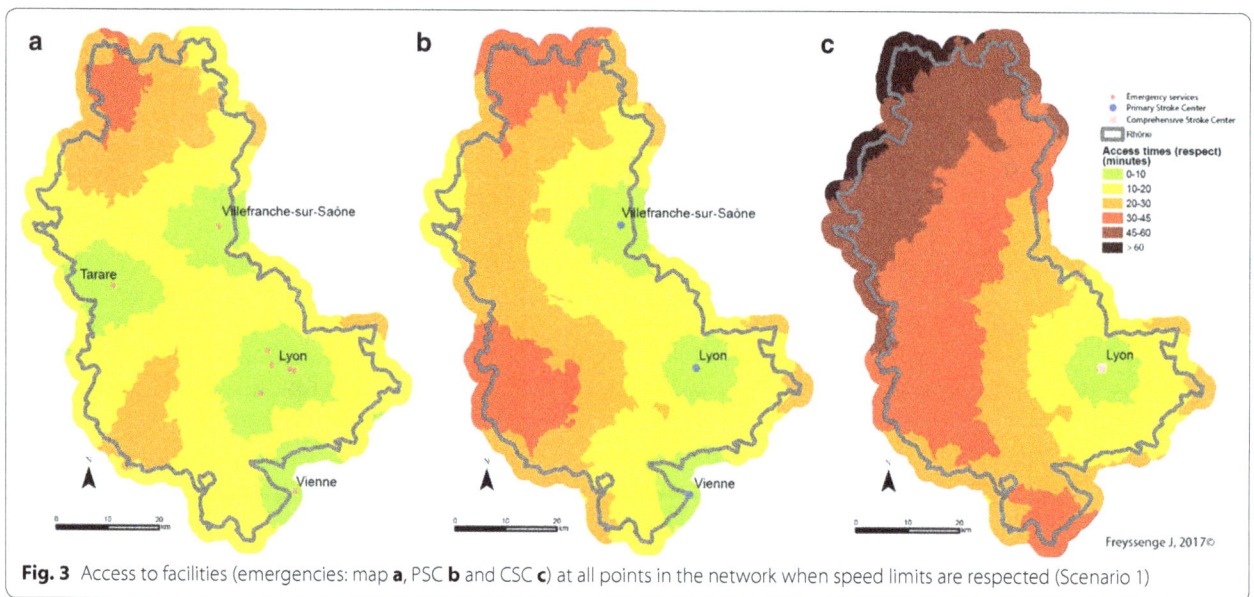

Fig. 3 Access to facilities (emergencies: map **a**, PSC **b** and CSC **c**) at all points in the network when speed limits are respected (Scenario 1)

When speed limits are not respected with an additional 20 kph for each section (Scenario 2), the entire territory is less than 30 min from the closest emergency department. Similarly, for PSC, with the exception of a very small part of the area (the northern and western extremes), communes in the Rhône county have access in less than 30 min. However, the north-western third of the Rhone area is more than 30 min from the nearest CSC (Fig. 4). There are no major variations with scenario 2', the service area for PSC and CSC is less extended in urban areas but it is not really significative (Fig. 5).

The third scenario consists of travelling 20 kph (12 mph) slower than the speed limits because of difficult weather conditions (fog, ice or snow for example). Access time is naturally longer in this case. The northern part of the Rhône—the Beaujolais area in particular—is harder hit once again. This section is more than 30 min from the nearest emergency department. The western and

northern parts of the county are thus more than 30 min from a facility and even more than 45 min from a facility when potential access times to the closest PSC units are measured. Few CSC facilities are available in the Rhône and neighbouring counties and potential access time is very varied. Indeed, some areas are distinctly under-privileged. Access to thrombectomy for the populations of the communes concerned is thus affected. Here again, the north-western part of the county has markedly fewer facilities and access times exceed 60 min (Fig. 6).

The final scenario showing road congestion does not seem to cause significant changes in access times to the various facilities times except in Greater Lyons. However, as the communes in the metropolis of Lyons are not concerned by major lack of access, traffic jams do not seem to be an obstacle to care (Fig. 7).

The proportion of population with access to facilities in a given time varies considerably. When speed limits

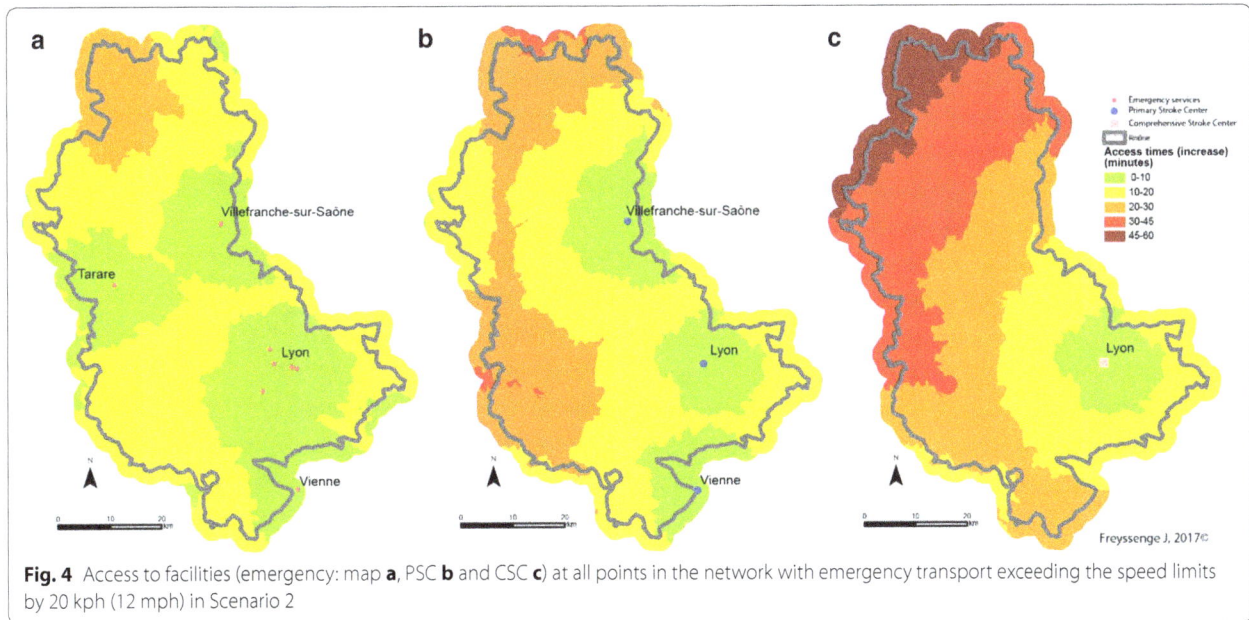

Fig. 4 Access to facilities (emergency: map **a**, PSC **b** and CSC **c**) at all points in the network with emergency transport exceeding the speed limits by 20 kph (12 mph) in Scenario 2

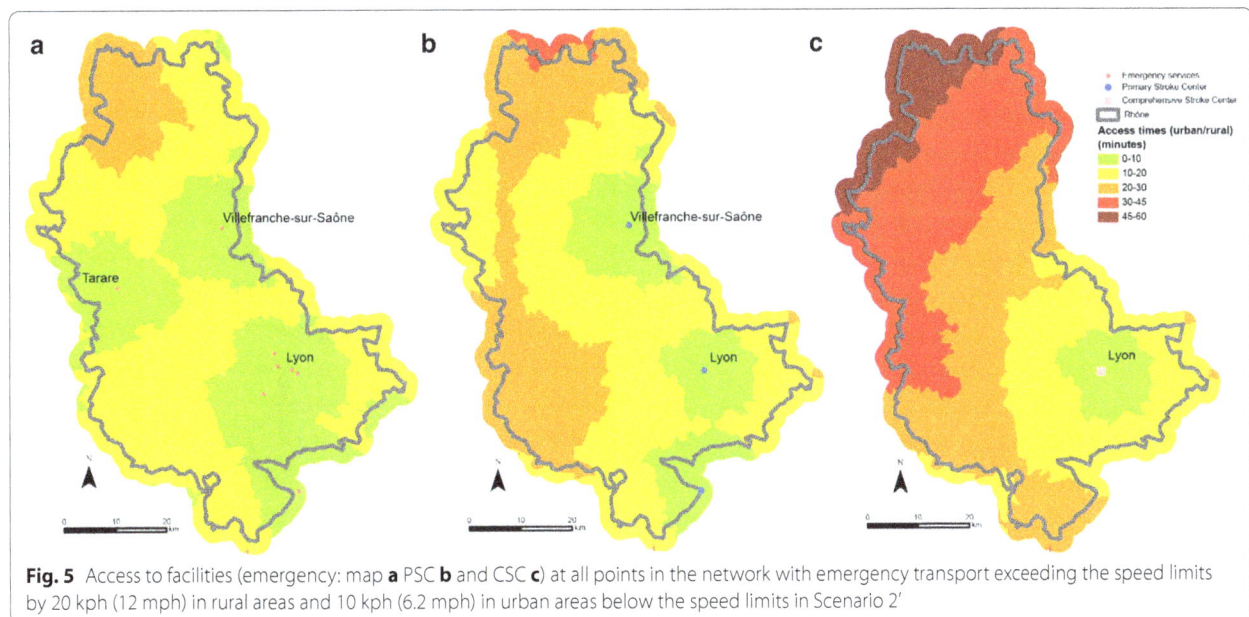

Fig. 5 Access to facilities (emergency: map **a** PSC **b** and CSC **c**) at all points in the network with emergency transport exceeding the speed limits by 20 kph (12 mph) in rural areas and 10 kph (6.2 mph) in urban areas below the speed limits in Scenario 2'

are respected (Scenario 1), 98% have 20-min access time to the nearest emergency department (Fig. 8), 90% has 20-min access time to an PSC facility (Fig. 9) and 75% has 20-min access time to an CSC facility (Fig. 10). Thus, virtually a quarter of the population of Rhône county does not have access to CSC in less than 20 min whereas this access time is practically 100% for emergency services. This raises the question of the eligibility of patients for treatment of stroke as we know that patients have little

awareness of the symptoms and are often long to call the emergency number (15) or to go to an emergency department. For example, poor accessibility of CSC plays an important role for patients who arrive too late for thrombectomy.

However, access to facilities from all points in the network is evaluated here. For a real assessment of access to facilities, it seems more interesting to perform an

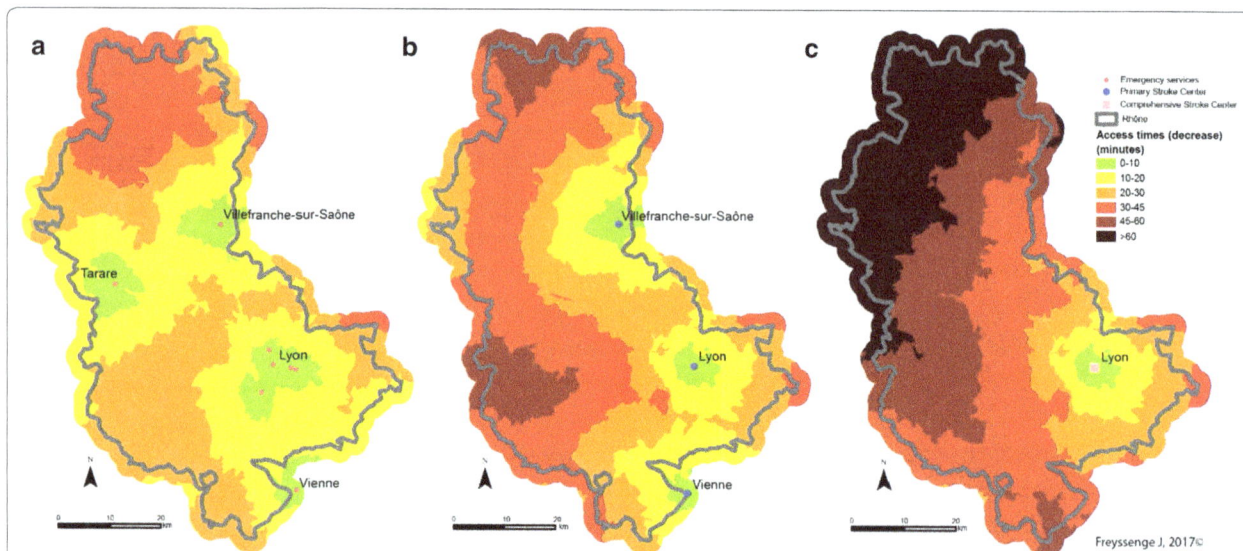

Fig. 6 Access to facilities (emergency: map **a** PSC **b** and CSC **c**) at all points in the network with adverse weather conditions (reduction of regulation speed by 20 kph (12 mph) Scenario 3)

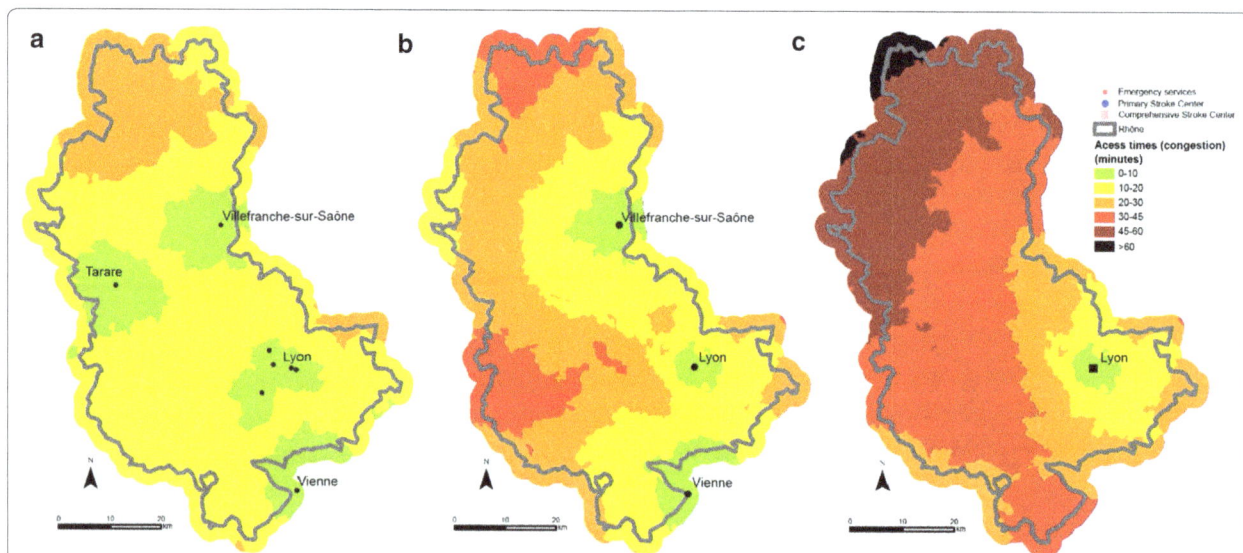

Fig. 7 Access to facilities (emergency: map **a** PSC **b** and CSC **c**) at all points in the network during traffic congestion in the Lyons urban area (Scenario 4)

examination of the full admission of patients from emergency call to arrival in an CSC facility.

Potential accessibility according to the type of patient intake procedure: complete approach from emergency call to the nearest CSC

Analysing accessibility at all points in the network of each stroke patient admission facility is an approach that has already been studied [16, 18, 19, 24], but with no allowance for different traffic scenarios. The analysis described here is innovative as—for the first time—it covers overall admission time starting with the emergency call and depending on the type of transport and traffic conditions. A great majority of stroke patients are transported by the fire brigade [4]. There are more fire stations than SMUR emergency units in the territory concerned. From the purely theoretical point of view and assuming that all fire stations and SMUR units are available,

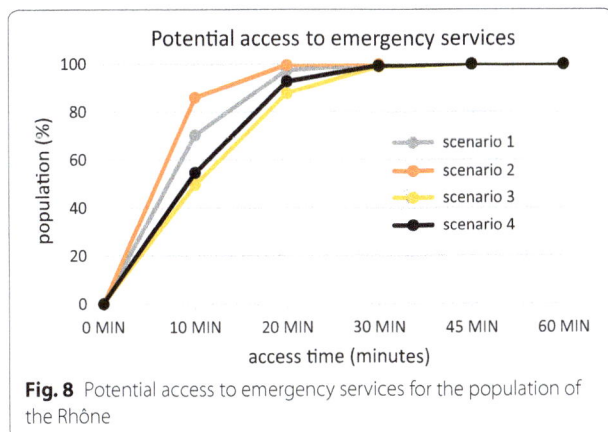

Fig. 8 Potential access to emergency services for the population of the Rhône

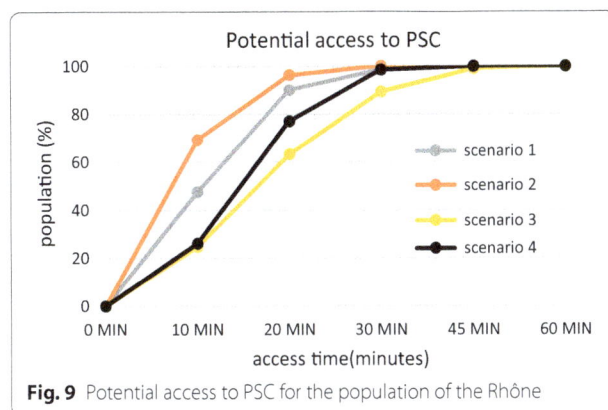

Fig. 9 Potential access to PSC for the population of the Rhône

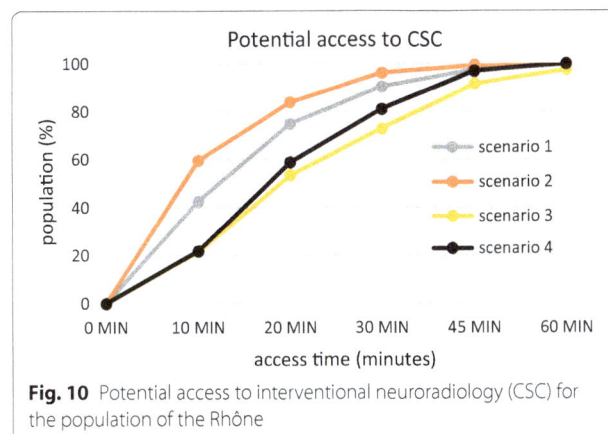

Fig. 10 Potential access to interventional neuroradiology (CSC) for the population of the Rhône

accessibility has been compared according to the mode of transport.

It is reminded that fire brigade access capability is greater than that of the SMUR medical teams. This greater density explains why potential access to patients by firemen and the admission of the formers to care facilities is greater than that of the SAMU, whatever the

scenario. Thus the median access time by fire brigades is the best, as it is the average time. When speed limits are respected, median time for the firemen is 40.9 min and average time is 45.7 min from access to admission to the closest CSC facility, in comparison with a median of 45.9 min and an average of 55.9 min for the SAMU.

As regards the territory, the towns at the northern extremity of the county display the most marked deficit in case of transport by the SMUR rather than the fire brigade, should every fire station be available. Thus stroke victims in the town of Monsols are between 1 h 45 min and 2 h 10 min from the CSC when transported by the SAMU and between 1 h 10 min and 1 h 30 min with the fire brigade—a gain of between 15 min and 1 h when speed limits are respected (Fig. 11). Admission times to CSC care are greatest in these areas that are the farthest from SMUR centres.

The pattern is the same when speed limits are raised (Fig. 12) or lowered (Fig. 13). However, several features of individual scenarios should be noted.

Increasing the limits by 20 kph (12 mph) highlights the influence of the Lyons metropolis on the territory. The density of facilities—fire stations, SMUR units and CSC—here accounts for the marked influence of the Lyons urban area. Here, whatever the type of transport, patients are less than 45 min from admission to an CSC facility. In addition, in most of the territory increasing the speed limits by 20 kph can result in the patient gaining 15 min in CSC admission.

Finally, the main observation about reducing speed limits by 20 kph concerns the question of the eligibility of the patient for treatment. Travelling time in the northern most part of the Rhône county is 2 h with the firemen and possibly more with the SMUR. Without allowing for inter-hospital time but only times between the onset of symptoms and the 15 (emergency) call at between 15 min and 5 h [43], most of the patients in these areas are no longer eligible for thrombectomy.

Discussion

The prime interest of the study is to model various scenarios based on different transport speeds. These multiple speeds are based on a review of the literature and on SAMU interventions.

This study has some practical implications. The different kind of transport are described and modelled. This modelling relies on transport times based on measured times that allows the comparison, for equivalent care conditions, between three kinds of transportation: private car and ambulances (firemen ambulance or SAMU ambulance) triggered by SAMU.

Classically, the accessibility is measured from patient's care place to the nearest facility. This problematic has

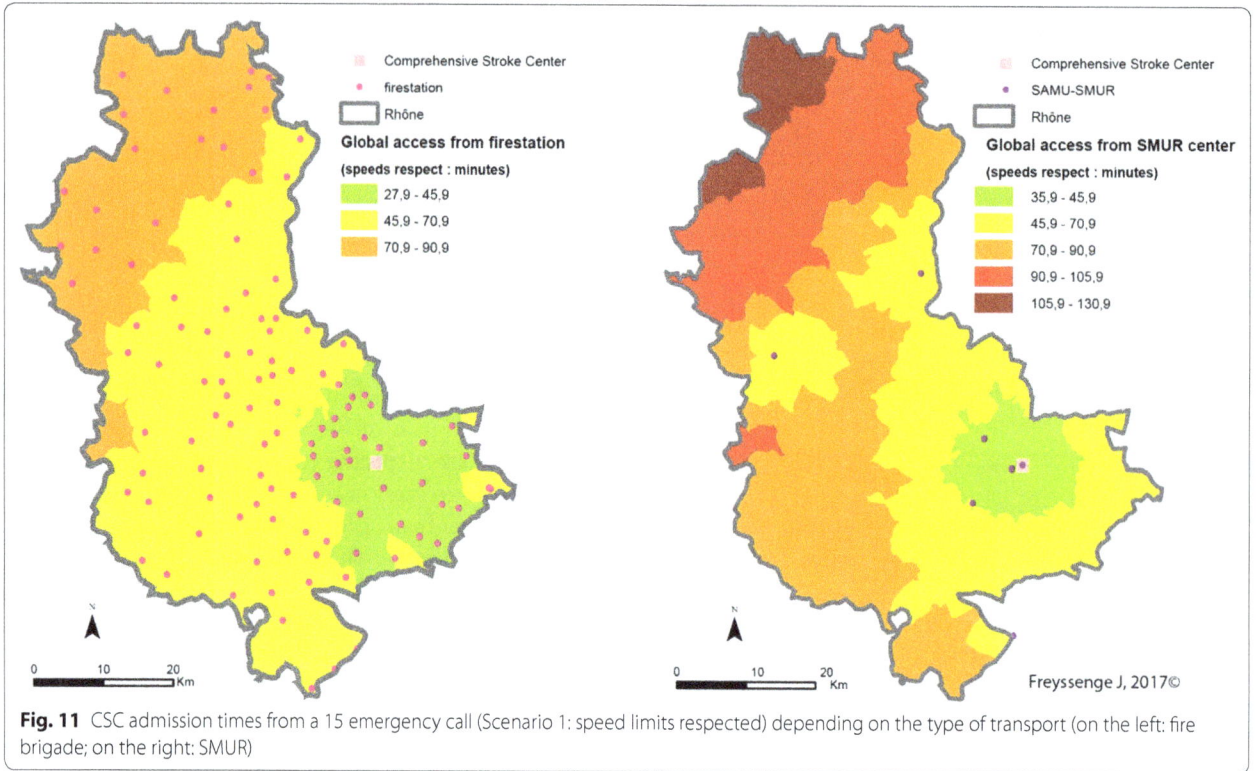

Fig. 11 CSC admission times from a 15 emergency call (Scenario 1: speed limits respected) depending on the type of transport (on the left: fire brigade; on the right: SMUR)

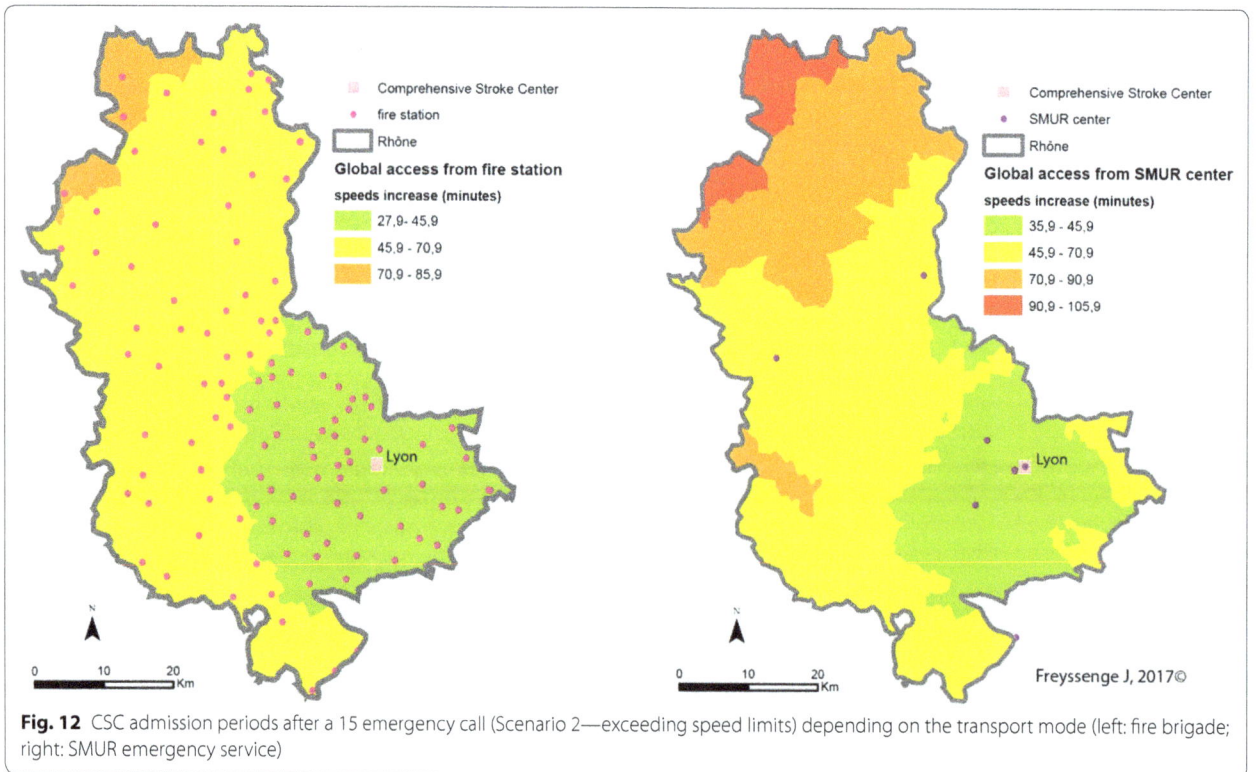

Fig. 12 CSC admission periods after a 15 emergency call (Scenario 2—exceeding speed limits) depending on the transport mode (left: fire brigade; right: SMUR emergency service)

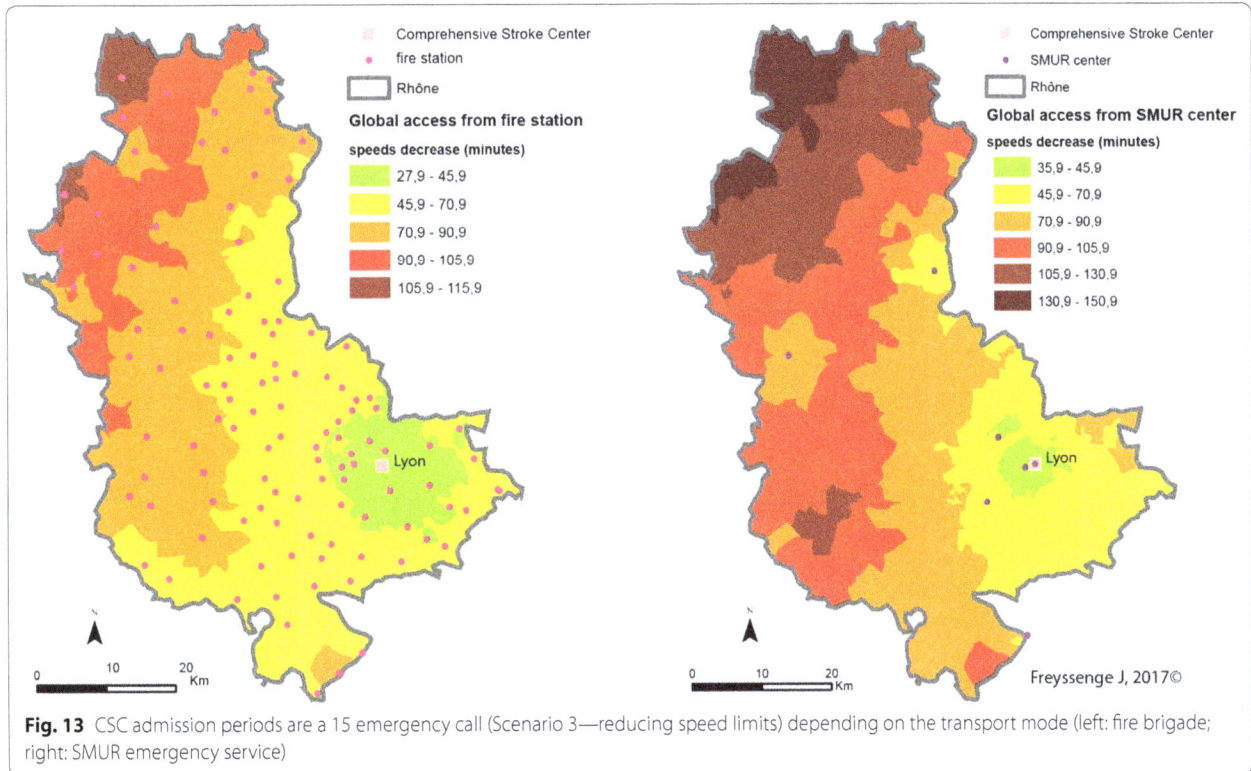

Fig. 13 CSC admission periods are a 15 emergency call (Scenario 3—reducing speed limits) depending on the transport mode (left: fire brigade; right: SMUR emergency service)

been analysed in this study, but the model has been more developed. Like it is observed in real case of care, the patient cannot go to the facility with his own mean. In a real context, the patient depends on modal transport and the access times linked to his care are from the trigger of transport care to his admission in a facility. The model presented gives a response to these care conditions.

Another practical implication is the emergence of territorial disparities. The measurement of access times to stroke patients allows to bring to light areas where we observe an extension of access delays to treatment.

As the method has been set out clearly, the finesses of modelling should now be improved. For example, 'travel impactors' [7] were not taken into account. These are in particular traffic lights and signs that lower the average speed of the vehicles carrying patients. The question of taking these impactors into account is raised especially for the modelling of patients travelling in their own vehicles.

Another limit but that is also a strong point of the study is the method used to know the maximum permitted speed in each section. *Route500*, the *Institut Géographique National* database commonly used in France for the various studies of this kind makes possible to use the Odomatrix program [44] to calculate travel time. Route 500 contains only 500,000 kilometres of the French road network. Furthermore, the maximum

authorised speeds in each section are obtained for the category of each section of road (motorway, main road, regional link, local service) and the geographic environment traversed (urban, rural), which might not be truly representative. Indeed, numerous local features can be related to the setting of a speed limit. It was therefore chosen here to use the *BDCarto* database for its considerable exhaustiveness as it covers more than 1 million kilometres of road network. Although the use of this database is essential for the best possible analysis of the territory and to be as close to reality as possible, no speed limits are attributed to the sections. It was therefore necessary to use a participative facility—*Open Street Map* in this case—to model access times. This type of information can be one of the limits of the study. It is therefore planned to acquire a professional database such as Garmin® or TomTom® to gain accuracy in modelling.

The various modelling takes into account the accessibility of the territory at all points in the road network. The improvement of modelling would require integration of the time taken by emergency teams from the road network to the patient's door. The question of accessibility is raised in particular for large housing block areas and residential zones where access to the patient's door from the road network may require time in the light of the complex configuration of buildings and in particular blocks with no lifts.

Another note is about the required average time at the time regulation for decision-making and intervention average time. In the study, we use the set times by Adeoye et al. [19], from the US Emergency Medical Service (EMS) register. From one country to another, and from one region to another, emergency medical services organization varies greatly [45]. It's therefore essential to estimate this times thanks to the SAMU registry. Thus, the models realized will be as close as possible to real life.

The modes of transport, firemen vs EMS, were compared is this study. This comparison was done to validate the method. In fact, in most cases, stroke patients are transported to hospital by firemen because they don't need medical transport. Given the proportion of interventions, this comparison doesn't have a high interest. Furthermore, the fire stations representation, which reflects the faster response of firemen, must be put into perspective. In fact, the future models should highlight the fire stations capacity to intervene. Apart from the highly-urbanized areas like Lyon and his urban agglomeration, firemen in rural fire stations are mostly volunteers. For this reason, if the nearest fire station doesn't have the sufficient number of firemen, they can't intervene and manage stroke patient which would extend access delays. The modelling of fire station ability to intervene will be feasible by representing their capacity according to the moment of the day, day/night in particular.

Conclusions

This study is innovative and allows a characterization of the territory in term of potential accessibility by network and localization of every mode of transport, in term of patient location. In this case, the comparison between EMS (SMUR) and firemen transport will be improved, yet the study shows the capacities of GIS. Only access delays for a patient to healthcare structure are evaluated, the medical aspect linked to the patient psychological state at the moment of his management is not studied.

These different models are a method of decision making for healthcare organization. The use of our method and models as a complementary tool for regulation could be the subject of future studies.

Furthermore, this study is also innovative because the transport care is estimated as a whole, from 15 call to admission in CSC. With this kind of model, it's easier to estimate the patient eligibility to thrombolysis and thrombectomy, with assumption of quickly recognizing of signs by the patient or people in his environment.

Abbreviations
EMS: Emergency medical service; SAMU: Service d'Aide Médicale Urgente; SDIS: Service Départemental d'Incendie et de Secours; GDP: Gross domestic product; GIS: Geographic information systems; IGN: Institut National de l'information Géographique et forestière; Insee: Institut National de la Statistique et des Etudes Economiques; IRIS: Ilots Regroupés pour l'Information Statistique; SMUR: Structure Mobile d'Urgence et de Réanimation; PSC: Primary Stroke Center; CSC: Comprehensive Stroke Center; UMH: Unité Mobile Hospitalière; WHO: World Health Organization.

Authors' contributions
JF, FR and KT conceived the study. KT, NN, LD, AMS and CEK participated in the design. JF carried out the GIS, statistical and mapping analyses, and drafted the manuscript. All authors read and approved the final manuscript.

Author details
[1] Univ. Lyon, University Claude Bernard Lyon 1, HESPER EA 7425, 69008 Lyon, France. [2] Emergency Department and RESCUe Network, Lucien Hussel Hospital, Vienne 38200, France. [3] UMR 5600 Environnement Ville Société CNRS, University Jean Moulin Lyon 3, 18, rue Chevreul, 69007 Lyon, France. [4] Pôle IMER, Hospices Civils de Lyon, 69003 Lyon, France. [5] Department of Stroke Medicine, Hospices Civils de Lyon, 69003 Lyon, France. [6] Department of Neuroradiology, Hospices Civils de Lyon, 69003 Lyon, France. [7] CREATIS, CNRS-UMR5220 INSERM-U1044, Lyon 69008, France. [8] INSA-Lyon, Lyon 69008, France. [9] Emergency Department, Hospices Civils de Lyon, 69003 Lyon, France.

Acknowledgements
The authors gratefully acknowledge Pr. Schott research team at Pôle IMER and RESCUe-RESUVal team for the support. We also thank Simon Barnard for his translation. The authors acknowledge the reviewers of the journal for their thoughtful comments that have led to some significant improvements on the paper.

Competing interests
The authors declare that they have no competing interests.

Funding
This work was supported by RESUVal (Réseau des Urgences de la Vallée du Rhône).

References
1. OMS | Maladies cardiovasculaires. WHO. http://www.who.int/mediacentre/factsheets/fs317/fr/. Accessed 13 Dec 2016.
2. L'accident vasculaire cérébral—Accident Vasculaire Cérébral (AVC)—Ministère des Affaires sociales et de la Santé. http://social-sante.gouv.fr/soins-et-maladies/maladies/maladies-cardiovasculaires/accident-vasculaire-cerebral-avc/article/l-accident-vasculaire-cerebral. Accessed 13 Dec 2016.
3. Fery-Lemonnier E. La prévention et la prise en charge des accidents vasculaires cérébraux en France : rapport à Madame la ministre de la santé et des sports. Ministèere de la santé et des sports; 2009. http://social-sante.gouv.fr/IMG/pdf/AVC_-_rapport_final_-_vf.pdf. Accessed 13 Dec 2016.
4. Derex L, Adeleine P, Nighoghossian N, Honnorat J, Trouillas P. Factors influencing early admission in a French stroke unit. Stroke. 2002;33:153–9.
5. Haynes R, Jones AP, Sauerzapf V, Zhao H. Validation of travel times to hospital estimated by GIS. Int J Health Geogr. 2006;5:1.
6. Higgs G. A literature review of the use of GIS-based measures of access to health care services. Health Serv Outcomes Res Methodol. 2004;5:119–39.
7. Schuurman N, Fiedler RS, Grzybowski SC, Grund D. Defining rational hos-

pital catchments for non-urban areas based on travel-time. Int J Health Geogr. 2006;5:43.

8. Apparicio P, Abdelmajid M, Riva M, Shearmur R. Comparing alternative approaches to measuring the geographical accessibility of urban health services: distance types and aggregation-error issues. Int J Health Geogr. 2008;7:7.

9. Apparicio P, Gelb J, Dubé A-S, Kingham S, Gauvin L, Robitaille É. The approaches to measuring the potential spatial access to urban health services revisited: distance types and aggregation-error issues. Int J Health Geogr. 2017. https://doi.org/10.1186/s12942-017-0105-9.

10. Guagliardo MF. Spatial accessibility of primary care: concepts, methods and challenges. Int J Health Geogr. 2004;3:3.

11. Yang D-H, Goerge R, Mullner R. Comparing GIS-based methods of measuring spatial accessibility to health services. J Med Syst. 2006;30:23–32.

12. Wang F. Measurement, optimization, and impact of health care accessibility: a methodological review. Ann Assoc Am Geogr. 2012;102:1104–12.

13. Luo W, Wang F. Measures of spatial accessibility to health care in a gis environment: synthesis and a case study in the Chicago region. Environ Plan B Plan Des. 2003;30:865–84.

14. McGrail MR. Spatial accessibility of primary health care utilising the two step floating catchment area method: an assessment of recent improvements. Int J Health Geogr. 2012;11:50.

15. Crooks VA, Schuurman N. Interpreting the results of a modified gravity model: examining access to primary health care physicians in five Canadian provinces and territories. BMC Health Serv Res. 2012;12:230.

16. Carr BG, Branas CC, Metlay JP, Sullivan AF, Camargo CA. Access to emergency care in the United States. Ann Emerg Med. 2009;54:261–9.

17. Alford-Teaster J, Lange JM, Hubbard RA, Lee CI, Haas JS, Shi X, et al. Is the closest facility the one actually used? An assessment of travel time estimation based on mammography facilities. Int J Health Geogr. 2016;15:10.

18. Scott PA, Temovsky CJ, Lawrence K, Gudaitis E, Lowell MJ. Analysis of Canadian population with potential geographic access to intravenous thrombolysis for acute ischemic stroke. Stroke. 1998;29:2304–10.

19. Adeoye O, Albright KC, Carr BG, Wolff C, Mullen MT, Abruzzo T, et al. Geographic access to acute stroke care in the United States. Stroke. 2014;45:3019–24.

20. Bohic N. Prévention des accidents vasculaires cérébraux et vieillissement: impact des inégalités sociales et territoriales de santé. Gérontol Soc. 2012;35:217.

21. de Peretti C, Chin F, Tuppin P, Béjot Y, Giroud M, Schniztler A, et al. Personnes hospitalisées pour accident vasculaire cérébral en France: tendances 2002–2008. Bull Epidemiol Hebd. 2012;10:125.

22. Joseph V, Guye O. Les personnes âgées en Rhône-Alpes : évaluation des besoins de prise en charge de la dépendance à l'horizon 2020. ORS Rhône-Alpes; 2005.

23. Sedeno A, Chambard P-J. Rhône-Alpes : une croissance de long terme soutenue par l'industrie, la métropolisation et l'économie résidentielle. Insee; 2014.

24. Ward MJ, Shutter LA, Branas CC, Adeoye O, Albright KC, Carr BG. Geographic Access to US Neurocritical Care Units Registered with the Neurocritical Care Society. Neurocrit Care. 2011;16:232–40.

25. Tazarourte K. Espace francilien et organisation des urgences vitales préhospitalières : les traumatismes crâniens graves pris en charge par les SAMU. PARIS X NANTERRE; 2012.

26. Bourgueil Y. L'évaluation économique et la recherche sur les services de santé. Paris; 2016.

27. Roudsari BS, Nathens AB, Arreola-Risa C, Cameron P, Civil I, Grigoriou G, et al. Emergency Medical Service (EMS) systems in developed and developing countries. Injury. 2007;38:1001–13.

28. Esri - GIS Mapping Software, Solutions, Services, Map Apps, and Data. http://www.esri.com/. Accessed 13 Dec 2016.

29. OpenStreetMap. OpenStreetMap. https://www.openstreetmap.org/. Accessed 13 Dec 2016.

30. Pageaud D, Carré C. La France vue par CORINE Land Cover, outil européen de suivi de l'occupation des sols. Commissariat général du développement durable: Le point sur; 2009.

31. Petzäll K, Petzäll J, Jansson J, Nordström G. Time saved with high speed driving of ambulances. Accid Anal Prev. 2011;43:818–22.

32. Branas CC, MacKenzie EJ, Williams JC, Schwab CW, Teter HM, Flanigan MC, et al. Access to trauma centers in the United States. JAMA. 2005;293:2626–33.

33. Carr BG, Caplan JM, Pryor JP, Branas CC. A meta-analysis of prehospital care times for Trauma. Prehosp Emerg Care. 2006;10:198–206.

34. Code de la route—Article R413-2.

35. Milne MSW, Holodinsky JK, Hill MD, Nygren A, Qiu C, Goyal M, et al. Drip 'n ship versus mothership for endovascular treatment. Stroke. 2017;48:791.

36. Mullen MT, Wiebe DJ, Bowman A, Wolff CS, Albright KC, Roy J, et al. Disparities in accessibility of certified primary stroke centers. Stroke. 2014;45:3381–8.

37. Ripley DCC, Kwong PL, Vogel WB, Kurichi JE, Bates BE, Davenport C. How does geographic access affect in-hospital mortality for veterans with acute ischemic stroke? Med Care. 2015;53:501–9.

38. Saver JL. Time Is Brain—Quantified. Stroke. 2006;37:263–6.

39. Goyal M, Jadhav AP, Bonafe A, Diener H, Mendes Pereira V, Levy E, et al. Analysis of workflow and time to treatment and the effects on outcome in endovascular treatment of acute ischemic stroke: results from the SWIFT PRIME randomized controlled trial. Radiology. 2016;279:888–97.

40. Berkhemer OA, Fransen PSS, Beumer D, van den Berg LA, Lingsma HF, Yoo AJ, et al. A randomized trial of intraarterial treatment for acute ischemic stroke. N Engl J Med. 2015;372:11–20.

41. Palaniswami M, Yan B. Mechanical thrombectomy is now the gold standard for acute ischemic stroke: implications for routine clinical practice. Interv Neurol. 2015;4:18–29.

42. Définition—IRIS | Insee. https://www.insee.fr/fr/metadonnees/definition/c1523. Accessed 28 Dec 2016.

43. Desseigne N, Akharzouz D, Varvat J, Cheynet M, Pouzet V, Marjollet O, et al. Quels sont les facteurs influençant les délais d'admission des patients arrivant aux urgences pour une suspicion d'accident vasculaire cérébral. Presse Méd. 2012;41:e559–67.

44. Hilal M. Odomatrix : Calcul de distances routières intercommunales. INRA; 2008. https://www6.inra.fr/cahier_des_techniques/content/download/3280/31761/version/1/file/41_Hilal_Odomatrix.pdf. Accessed 13 Dec 2016.

45. Fassbender K, Balucani C, Walter S, Levine SR, Haass A, Grotta J. Streamlining of prehospital stroke management: the golden hour. Lancet Neurol. 2013;12:585–96.

6

Ovarian cancer: density equalizing mapping of the global research architecture

Dörthe Brüggmann[1,2]*, Katharina Pulch[2], Doris Klingelhöfer[2], Celeste Leigh Pearce[3] and David A. Groneberg[2]

Abstract

Background: Despite its impact on female health worldwide, no efforts have been made to depict the global architecture of ovarian cancer research and to understand the trends in the related literature. Hence, it was the objective of this study to assess the global scientific performance chronologically, geographically and in regards to economic benchmarks using bibliometric tools and density equalizing map projections.

Methods: The NewQIS platform was employed to identify all ovarian cancer related articles published in the Web of Science since 1900. The items were analyzed regarding quantitative aspects (e.g. publication date, country of origin) and parameters describing the recognition of the work by the scientific community (e.g. citation rates).

Results: 23,378 articles on ovarian cancer were analyzed. The USA had the highest activity of ovarian cancer research with a total of n = 9312 ovarian cancer-specific publications, followed by the UK (n = 1900), China (n = 1813), Germany (n = 1717) and Japan (n = 1673). Ovarian cancer-specific country h-index also showed a leading position of the USA with an h-index (HI) of 207, followed by the UK (HI = 122), Canada (HI = 99), Italy (HI = 97), Germany (HI = 84), and Japan (HI = 81). In the socio-economic analysis, the USA were ranked first with an average of 175.6 ovarian cancer-related publications per GDP per capita in 1000 US-$, followed by Italy with an index level of 46.85, the UK with 45.48, and Japan with 43.3. Overall, the USA and Western European nations, China and Japan constituted the scientific power players publishing the majority of highly cited ovarian cancer-related articles and dominated international collaborative efforts. African, Asian and South American countries played almost no visible role in the scientific community.

Conclusions: The quantity and scientific recognition of publications related to ovarian cancer are continuously increasing. The research endeavors in the field are concentrated in high-income countries with no involvement of lower-resource nations. Hence, worldwide collaborative efforts with the aim to exchange epidemiologic data, resources and knowledge have to be strengthened in the future to successfully alleviate the global burden related to ovarian cancer.

Keywords: Ovarian carcinoma, Density equalizing mapping, Socio-economic analysis

Background

Ovarian cancer is the most lethal gynecological tumor in high income-countries; it represents the seventh-most common female cancer worldwide [1, 2]. In the United States, approximately 22,000 new ovarian cancer cases are diagnosed annually, 14,200 related deaths occur each

year [3]. The majority of invasive ovarian malignancies originate from epithelial cells. Each histotype—high-grade serous, low-grade serous, mucinous, clear cell and endometrioid—exhibits distinct clinical and pathological characteristics [4].

During the last three decades, multiple breakthrough discoveries have been reported in the field: for the last 10 years it has been accepted that two types of epithelial ovarian cancers exist [1, 5]. Type I tumors include low-grade serous, endometrioid and clear cell histologies [6, 7]. The association of Type I cancers with endometriosis

*Correspondence: doerthe.brueggmann@med.usc.edu
[2] Department of Female Health and Preventive Medicine, Institute of Occupational Medicine, Social Medicine and Environmental Medicine, Goethe-University, Theodor-Stern Kai 7, 60590 Frankfurt, Germany
Full list of author information is available at the end of the article

was found in 2012. This benign condition increases the risk of low-grade serous and endometrioid cancers by approximately twofold, for clear cell subtypes by three-fold [1, 8]. Also, *ARID1A* gene mutations were described for endometriosis-associated endometrioid and clear cell cancers [9]. Type II high-grade serous carcinomas are the most common ovarian malignancies. In 2006, Medeiros et al. presumed their origin from the fimbriae of the fallopian tube [10]. In the last years, the identification of relevant somatic and germline mutations gained relevance as a first step towards screening strategies and novel targeted therapies: *KRAS, BRAF, ERBB2, CTNNB1, PTEN, PIK3CA, ARID1A, PPP2R1A*, and *BCL2* mutations were found in Type I carcinomas. 96% of high-grade serous Type II tumors had *TP53* mutations [1, 5, 11]. In 1994 and 1995, *BRCA 1/2* mutations were described in hereditary Type II cancers; since then they have gained importance for clinical risk prediction and patient counseling [12, 13].

The volume of scientific literature in oncology increased rapidly during the last 50 years [14]. Systematic evaluation of research output is necessary to guide individual reading, to plan research activities according to shortcomings and to quantify individual and collaborative productivity on national and international level. These assessments play an integral role in career decisions, allocation of grant funding and prioritizing research resources [14]. Scientometric methods provide the standardized analysis of journal articles in reference to their content and citations describing developments in origin and dissemination of published data. Specific to ovarian cancer, no systematic evaluation of the global scientific output is available to date, and no efforts have been made to understand trends in the related literature. Therefore, the topic of ovarian cancer was elected by the New Quality and Quantity Indices in Science (New-QIS) project [15] for a scientometric in-depth analysis. The study objectives included (1) the assessment of the worldwide publication output regarding quantitative aspects, parameters describing the recognition within the scientific community (e.g. citation rates) and research networks as well as (2) the evaluation of the country-specific productivity related to socio-economic variables. Also, we identified the leading journals publishing in the field and the most recognized articles since 1900.

Methods
NewQIS study
We employed the established NewQIS platform [15, 16] to conduct this study. The NewQIS platform was developed in 2009 as a multidisciplinary project involving scientists from different backgrounds such as engineering, computer sciences and medicine and numerous studies

were published so far using the platform [17–32]. It constitutes a novel tool that was designed for the objective, precise and reliable scientometric analyses of research productivity based on validated protocols. Benefits of the platform include the efficient and standardized investigation of the scientific progress chronologically and geographically, the visualization of the results in expressive global maps via density equalizing map projections (DEMP), as well as unique evaluation tools deciphering national and international scientific relations and gender distribution among authors.

Data source
We used an index database of the Web of Science (WoS core collection, Thomson Scientific) and analyzed the total research productivity by quantification of ovarian cancer-specific publications. Parameters describing the articles' recognition by the scientific community were assessed based on the number of related citations, i.e. h-indices and citation rates.

The WoS was selected as data source because of its unique Citation Report function allowing the extraction of citation performance parameters [33]. We refrained from extracting data from other platforms such as Google Scholar or Scopus due to the lack of data congruence in these three databases hampering triangulating, comparing and integrating data related to ovarian cancer research since 1900 [34].

Search strategy
We conducted a "title" search for the time period of 1900 (01-01) to 2014 (31-12). The search term ["(*ovarian OR ovary) AND (cancer OR neoplasm OR carcinoma)*"] was used. The year 2015 was excluded to avoid incomplete data acquisition at the time the study was performed. We used the filter option "document type" to restrict our search to "original articles" as described previously [15].

Data analysis and categorization
Articles were saved in a plain text format using the download application provided by the WoS. All related metadata were collected in an interim database and, analyzed according to the following criteria: originating country, language, citations, cited references, authors, journal, year published and subject categories. The subject categories represent standard categories assigned to every publication by the Journal Citation Reports (provided by the Thompson Reuters/Institute of Scientific Information) during the publication process. We computed the country-specific modified h-index (HI) and the citation rate (CR, number of all citations per total ovarian cancer publication volume). In 2005, the HI was developed by Jorge Hirsch to assess the recognition of an author's

research performance in the scientific community [35]. In our study, this proxy measure was adapted to evaluate the productivity of single countries in ovarian cancer research and therefore termed "modified HI". Also, a glossary was added in the Additional file 1 describing important terms used in this manuscript.

Density equalizing map projections (DEMP)

DEMP visualize benchmarking processes by the creation of anamorphic world maps. After the transfer of the metadata to excel charts and parameter analysis, DEMP were calculated based on the algorithms of Gastner and Newman. Therefor, the territories of countries publishing ovarian cancer research were resized in proportion to the selected criteria (i.e. the total number country-specific articles) [36].

Socio-economic analysis

In order to quantify country-specific contributions to ovarian cancer research in regards to their economic resources and manpower, we evaluated research productivity in relation (1) to the gross domestic product (GDP) per capita, (2) to the total economic power index GDP per 1000 billion US-$ and (3) to the population size. Economic facts were obtained from the *World Economic Outlook Database of the International Monetary Fund* of 2014 [37]. Only countries with a minimum of 50 ovarian cancer publications were included. We also collected the absolute numbers of ovarian cancer incidence and the crude rate (defined as the new cancer cases diagnosed in a specific year per 100,000 persons at risk) of the 25 countries that have published more than 100 ovarian cancer items during the investigated time span. The data reflect the incidence of ovarian cancer in 2012 and were obtained from http://globocan.iarc.fr/Pages/summary_table_pop_sel.aspx. Based on these numbers we calculated the ratio of country-specific articles per each new ovarian cancer case.

Analysis of ovarian cancer research collaborations

To determine research collaborations from a global viewpoint, affiliations of authors were analyzed and chart diagrams were computed as previously described [38]. We defined an article as "collaborative" if at least two authors, who work in different countries as stated in the affiliations, contributed to the work. Publications with shared authorship were counted one time only (independent of the number of authors from the same country defined in the affiliations) towards the complete count of joint publications this specific country is involved in. For example, when 10 publications were analysed of which eight were affiliated with the USA, five with the UK and three items were joint publications, these were counted as 3

out of 8 for the USA and 3 out of 5 for the UK. Also, we related the total count of collaborative items to the overall number of publications for each investigated country. For example, 2240 items were published by US-American authors in a joint effort with other countries. These were related to the overall scientific productivity of the USA represented by 9312 items (24%). 747 collaborative publications were identified for the UK; these accounted for 39% out of 1900 items. In Fig. 3, vectors represent the productivity of collaborations for each pair of countries. These are proportional in line width and shade of grey to the number of collaborations.

Results
General parameters

In 115 years, a total of 23,378 original articles were published in the WoS. The publication activities increased continuously throughout the decades: Until the 1950s we identified up to 10 articles each year; this number increased to more than 100 publications/year from 1979 onwards and doubled after 1984. In the next decade, the productivity increased to more than 500 annual items and doubled again after 2008. In 2014, 1540 articles were published (Fig. 1a). The number of participating authors per publication increased from 2.5 authors in 1972 to 8.18 authors per ovarian cancer-related article in 2014.

Country-specific analysis

A total of 99 countries participated in the publication of all articles. The majority of publication volume originated from a small number of countries: The United States of America (USA) was the most productive with 9312 ovarian cancer-specific articles. It was followed by the United Kingdom (UK, 1900 articles), China (1813 articles), Germany (1717 articles), Japan (1673 articles) and Italy (1672 articles). Hence, DEMP analysis demonstrated a distorted world map with the main focus on North America and Western Europe and a prominent China and Japan (Fig. 1b). Asian, South American and African countries occupied only minimal areas on the cartogram.

Citation analysis

The citation count of yearly published articles showed a course similar to the annual publication activity: After a very modest increase until 1974 the citations increased steadily with peaks in 1979, 1989, 1994, 1996, 2004. After 2005, we documented a steep decline in citation numbers until 2014 with the exception of a small plateau in 2008 (Fig. 2a).

Country-specific citation analysis indicated a leading position of the USA with 354,891 citations (41.2% of all citations). It was followed by the UK (71,562 citations), Canada (55,964 citations), Italy (49,422 citations),

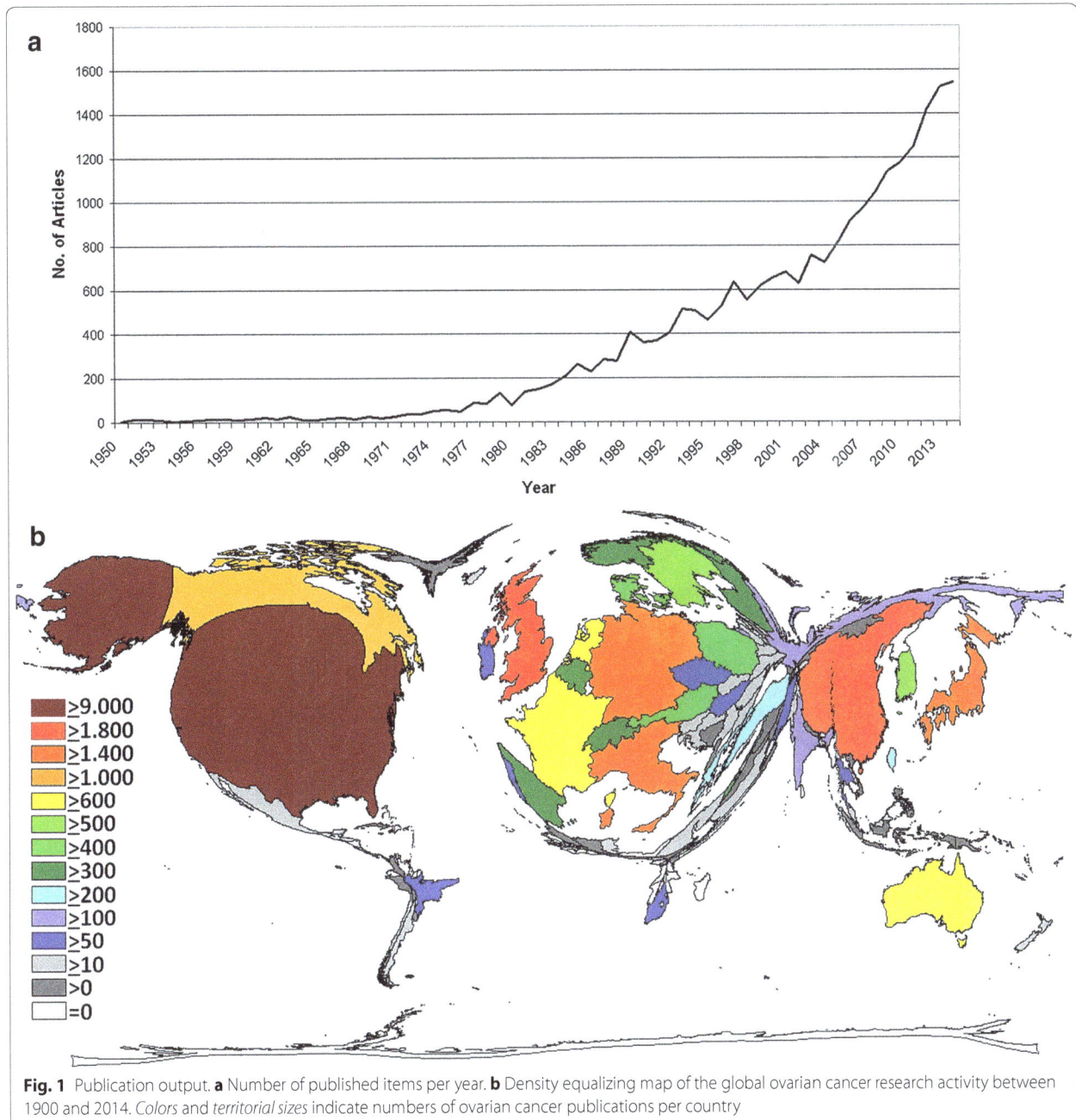

Fig. 1 Publication output. **a** Number of published items per year. **b** Density equalizing map of the global ovarian cancer research activity between 1900 and 2014. *Colors* and *territorial sizes* indicate numbers of ovarian cancer publications per country

Japan (35,995 citations), and Germany (34,278 citations) (Fig. 2b). In contrast to publication activities, China dropped from third to position 10 when citations were quantified.

The USA dominated the country-specific HI analysis (HI of 207), and was followed by the UK (HI = 122), Canada (HI = 99), Italy (HI = 97), Germany (HI = 84), and Japan (HI = 81) (Table 1). Regarding the citation rate (CR) of countries with a minimum of 30 articles published on ovarian cancer, we identified Canada (CR = 43.52) in the leading position. Then Finland (CR = 39.17), Hungary (CR = 38.81), the USA (CR = 38.11) and the UK (CR = 37.66) were followed by the Western European countries Belgium (CR = 36.92), Sweden (CR = 36.61), the Netherlands (CR = 34.03), Norway (CR = 31.8), Italy (CR = 29.56) and France (CR = 23.79). China dropped to a CR of 11.05 (Table 2).

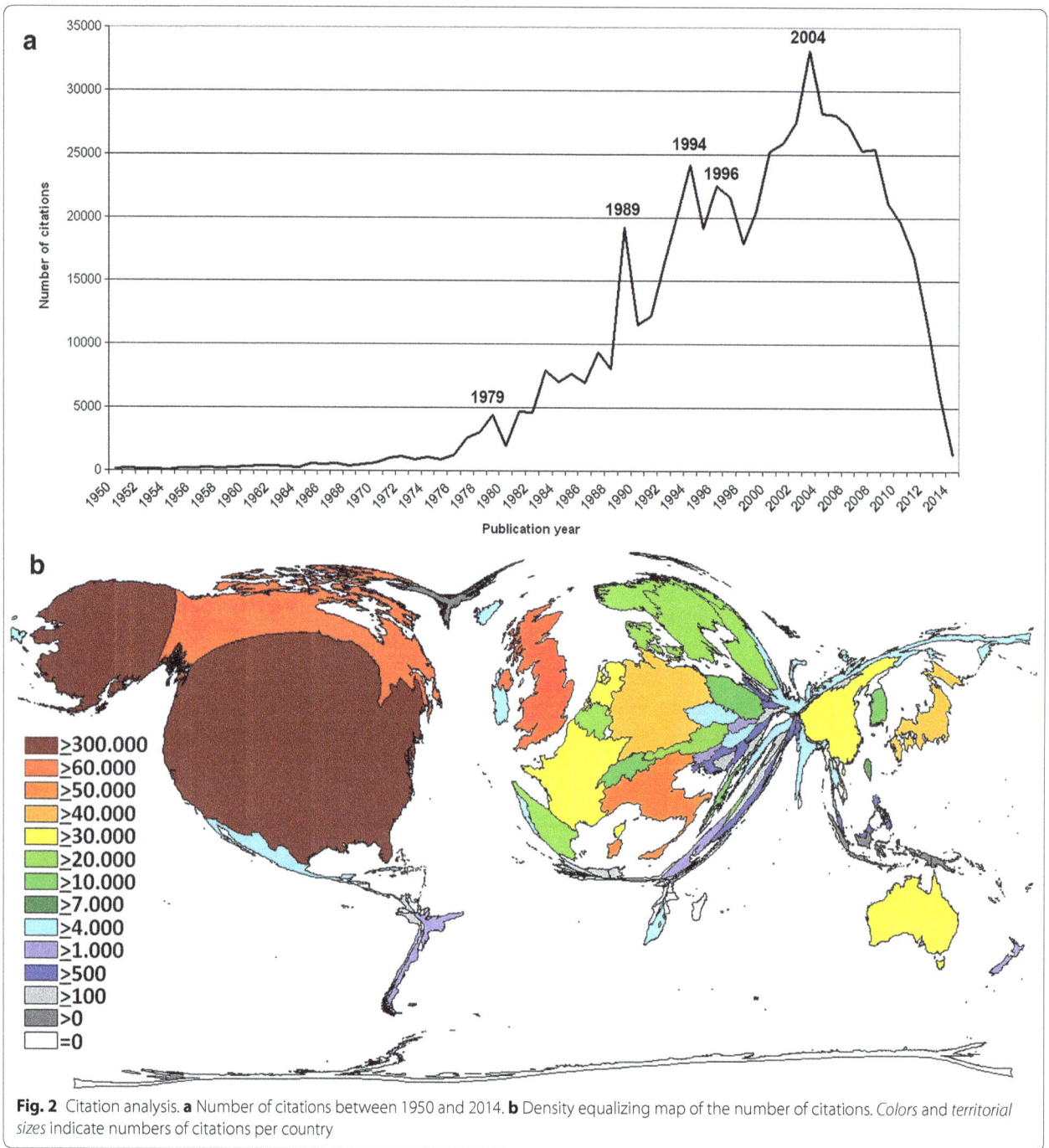

Fig. 2 Citation analysis. **a** Number of citations between 1950 and 2014. **b** Density equalizing map of the number of citations. *Colors* and *territorial sizes* indicate numbers of citations per country

Socio-economic analysis of ovarian cancer research

When the country-specific publications were related to the gross domestic product (GDP) per capita, the USA was ranked first with an average of 169.9 ovarian cancer-related publications per GDP per capita in 1000 US-$ (Q1). The USA was followed by China as the first middle-income country in the ranking (Q1: 140.5), the UK (Q1: 50.4), Italy (Q1: 48.5) and Japan (Q1: 44.3) (Table 3).

For the total economic power index GDP, Denmark was positioned at the first place with a total of 1293.2 ovarian cancer-specific articles per 1000 billion US-$ GDP (Bio US-$ GDP, Q2), followed by Israel (Q2: 1272). Amongst the high-income countries, the UK ranked at position 12 (Q2: 667.1), followed by Belgium (Q2: 629) and the USA (Q2: 534.6). China (Q2: 157) occupied the 4th rank of the middle-income countries and the 32nd position of all

Table 1 Modified h-indices

Rank	Country	h-index
1	United States	207
2	United Kingdom	122
3	Canada	99
4	Italy	97
5	Germany	84
6	Japan	81
7	Netherlands	78
8	Australia	74
9	France	70
10	Sweden	68
11	Belgium	58
12	China	57
13	Finland	55
14	Denmark	54
15	Norway	54
16	Israel	52
17	Austria	51
18	Spain	49
19	Switzerland	48
20	South Korea	45
21	Greece	42
22	Poland	40
23	Taiwan	37
24	Turkey	23
25	India	22
26	Ireland	22
27	South Africa	20
28	Hungary	20
29	Portugal	20
30	Czech Republic	19
31	Russia	18
32	Thailand	18
33	Singapore	18
34	Iceland	18
35	Brazil	16
36	New Zealand	15
37	Mexico	14
38	Slovakia	14
39	Slovenia	13
40	Chile	13
41	Croatia	12
42	Egypt	12
43	Malaysia	12
44	Iran	10
45	Saudi Arabia	10
46	Argentina	10
47	Belarus	10
48	Serbia	9
49	Romania	8

Table 1 continued

Rank	Country	h-index
50	Pakistan	8
51	Lithuania	8
52	Bulgaria	7
53	Latvia	6
54	Ukraine	4
55	Tunisia	3

The table summarizes the h-indices related to research on ovarian cancer and published by the countries investigated

countries with more than 50 ovarian cancer-specific articles (Table 3).

Denmark was positioned first when the ovarian cancer research output was related to population size. Here, 80.3 ovarian cancer-specific publications were authored per 1 million citizens. It was followed by Norway (77.9 publications/1 million citizens), Iceland (65.5 publications/1 million citizens), Finland (62.2 publications/1 million citizens) and Sweden at position 5 (54.8 publications/1 million citizens). Other productive countries were the USA (29.7 publications/1 million citizens), UK (29.8 publications/1 million citizens) and China (13.4 publications/1 million citizens).

Furthermore, Israel took the lead having published one article per newly diagnosed ovarian cancer case based on the incidence data of 2012. It was followed by Norway (0.94 articles per new ovarian cancer case), Denmark (0.83 articles per new ovarian cancer case), Sweden (0.79 articles per new ovarian cancer case), the Netherlands (0.74 articles per new ovarian cancer case) and Finland (0.74 articles per new ovarian cancer case). The USA was ranked 11th; countries such as China, Russia and India were ranked last amongst the 25 investigated nations (Table 4). A DEMP shows the absolute ovarian cancer incidence numbers of the 25 counties that have published more than 100 articles during the investigated time span (Additional file 2: Figure S1).

Publishing journals and landmark articles

1685 journals published ovarian cancer-related articles since 1900. The most prolific journal was "Gynecologic Oncology" with 2710 articles and a related citation rate (CR) of 23.91 followed by "International Journal of Gynecological Cancer" (968 articles/CR = 11.06) and "Cancer Research" (637 articles/CR = 80.81). We displayed the top 15 journals including number of articles, citations and CR (Additional file 3: Table S1, Additional file 4: Figure S2) and identified the ten most cited articles in the area of ovarian cancer research (Additional file 5: Table S2).

Table 2 Ovarian cancer-specific citation rates

Rank	Country	Citation rate
1	Canada	43.52
2	Finland	39.17
3	Hungary	38.81
4	United States	38.11
5	United Kingdom	37.66
6	Belgium	36.92
7	Sweden	36.61
8	Netherlands	34.03
9	Norway	31.80
10	Australia	30.55
11	Italy	29.56
12	Portugal	29.44
13	Switzerland	29.43
14	Spain	28.76
15	Denmark	28.53
16	Ireland	28.51
17	Mexico	27.16
18	Israel	25.96
19	Greece	24.91
20	France	23.79
21	Austria	22.58
22	Slovenia	22.47
23	South Africa	22.35
24	Japan	21.52
25	New Zealand	20.66
26	Germany	19.96
27	Poland	19.33
28	Taiwan	18.17
29	Thailand	17.85
30	Czech Republic	17.16
31	Slovakia	16.69
32	South Korea	15.30
33	Egypt	13.81
34	Singapore	13.03
35	India	12.65
36	Malaysia	12.31
37	Brazil	11.90
38	China	11.05
39	Romania	10.50
40	Saudi Arabia	9.30
41	Croatia	8.82
42	Turkey	8.59
43	Russia	7.55
44	Iran	4.34
45	Serbia	4.14

The table summarizes the citation rates related to ovarian cancer research and published by investigated countries with a minimum of 30 publications

Ovarian cancer subject area analysis

The leading subject categories of ovarian cancer research were "Oncology" with 13,649 publications cited 363,896 times, "Obstetrics & Gynecology" (6878 publications, 128,161 citations), and—following with a considerable gap—"Pathology" (1238 publications and 31,921 citations) (Additional file 6: Figure S3A). The areas "General & Internal Medicine" (35,221 citations) and "Genetics & Hereditary" (33,842 citations) showed a high CR relative to the total number of publications indicating a high impact of published work in the field.

We performed a subject area analysis for the ten most active countries in ovarian cancer research to identify their particular scientific focus: Up to 80% of all publications in nine of the ten countries were attributed to "Oncology" and "Obstetrics & Gynecology". China published a high percentage of articles in "Research and Experimental Medicine", "Biochemistry and Molecular Biology" as well as "Cell Biology". Researchers from the UK, Australia, France and Canada focused on the area of "Genetics". Japanese scientists dedicated a high percentage of their work to the subject category of "Pathology". "General and Internal Medicine" was popular among researchers from France and the UK (Additional file 6: Figure S3B).

International ovarian cancer collaborations

We identified 3697 international collaborations publishing on ovarian cancer, 74% were bilateral (2733 items) and 15.4% trilateral co-operations (568 items). Joint research efforts were clearly dominated by scientists and institutions situated in the USA. US-American authors published 24% of all publications in co-operation with other countries, and collaborated with 13 different countries in total. The most active collaborations were established between the USA and Canada (433 collaborative papers), followed by US-American co-operations with the UK (385 papers), China (300 papers), Italy (291 papers) and Germany (284 papers) (Fig. 3).

Discussion

During 115 years, a total of 23,378 original research articles were published in the WoS. The number of publications rose slowly until the seventies, when a steep and steady increase of research productivity started. This pattern is detected for most biomedical research as exemplified by studies on medical curare use or bacterial meningitis [39, 40]. From 1900 to 1950, only 139 articles related to ovarian cancer were part of the WoS database. This is attributed to the following: Overall research activities were lower since the recognition and funding

Table 3 Socio-economic analysis of ovarian cancer research of the most active countries in ovarian cancer research. *Source* for GDP (Currency in 1000 Billion US Dollars) and GDP per capita (Currency in 1000 US Dollars) in 2014 was the World Economic Outlook Database of the International Monetary Fund of 2014. (Threshold: 50 ovarian cancer-specific publications)

Country	Rank	Number of articles	GDP (in 1000 Bill. US$)	Articles/GDP (1000 Bill. US$)	Rank ratio (Articles/GDP in economic group)	GDP per capita (in US$)	Articles/GDP per capita (in 1000 US$)	Rank ratio (Articles/GDP per capita in economic group)
USA	1.	9312	17.420	534.6	HIG 14	54,800	169.9	HIG 1
China	2.	1813	10.360	175.0	MIG 4	12,900	140.5	MIG 1
UK	3.	1900	2.848	667.1	HIG 12	37,700	50.4	HIG 2
Italy	4.	1672	2.129	785.3	HIG 9	34,500	48.5	HIG 3
Japan	5.	1673	4.770	350.7	HIG 22	37,800	44.3	HIG 4
Germany	6.	1717	3.820	449.5	HIG 18	44,700	38.4	HIG 5
Canada	7.	1286	1.794	716.8	HIG 11	44,500	28.9	HIG 6
India	8.	150	2.048	73.2	MIG 6	5800	25.9	MIG 2
France	9.	878	2.902	302.5	HIG 24	40,400	21.7	HIG 7
Poland	10.	458	0.552	829.4	HIG 8	24,400	18.8	HIG 8
Australia	11.	742	1.483	500.3	HIG 16	46,000	16.1	HIG 9
Netherlands	12.	762	0.880	865.5	HIG 7	47,400	16.1	HIG 10
South Korea	13.	561	1.410	397.9	HIG 20	35,400	15.8	HIG 11
Turkey	14.	290	0.813	356.6	MIG 1	19,600	14.8	MIG 3
Sweden	15.	522	0.559	933.6	HIG 6	44,700	11.7	HIG 12
Israel	16.	388	0.305	1272.1	HIG 2	33,400	11.6	HIG 13
Greece	17.	295	0.246	1197.2	HIG 4	25,800	11.4	HIG 14
Spain	18.	370	1.400	264.3	HIG 25	33,000	11.2	HIG 15
Denmark	19.	449	0.347	1293.2	HIG 1	44,300	10.1	HIG 16
Austria	20.	450	0.436	1031.9	HIG 5	45,400	9.9	HIG 17
Finland	21.	337	0.276	1219.7	HIG 3	40,500	8.3	HIG 18
Belgium	22.	332	0.528	629.0	HIG 13	41,700	8.0	HIG 19
Russia	23.	166	2.057	80.7	HIG 28	24,800	6.7	HIG 20
Taiwan	24.	265	0.530	500.5	HIG 15	43,600	6.1	HIG 21
Norway	25.	391	0.512	764.3	HIG 10	65,900	5.9	HIG 22
South Africa	26.	71	0.341	208.1	MIG 2	12,700	5.6	MIG 4
Switzerland	27.	306	0.679	450.7	HIG 17	55,200	5.5	HIG 23
Thailand	28.	74	0.374	198.0	MIG 3	14,400	5.1	MIG 5
Brazil	29.	70	2.244	31.2	MIG 7	15,200	4.6	MIG 6
Iran	30.	62	0.403	154.0	MIG 5	16,500	3.8	MIG 7
Czech Republic	31.	74	0.206	359.9	HIG 21	28,400	2.6	HIG 24
Hungary	32.	57	0.130	439.5	HIG 19	24,300	2.3	HIG 25
Portugal	33.	54	0.228	236.6	HIG 26	26,300	2.1	HIG 26
Ireland	34.	75	0.246	305.1	HIG 23	46,800	1.6	HIG 27
Singapore	35.	70	0.308	227.3	HIG 27	81,300	0.9	HIG 28

of scientists were not predominantly determined by their productivity. In 1915, Japanese researchers could provoke cancer in an animal model for the first time. Since then pathogenetic mechanisms of cancer shifted into the scientific focus paving the way to today's understanding of the disease [41]. English was not the common scientific language at this time. Hence, a considerable amount of non-English publications issued before 1950 is not represented in our analysis.

The late 1970s was an era when ovarian cancer-associated research gained increasing popularity (Fig. 1). Then, major scientific progress happened in the field as indicated by the first highly cited publication linking ovarian cancer and incessant ovulation [42–46]. The output grew

Table 4 The table depicts the absolute incidence numbers and the crude rate (defined as the new cancer cases diagnosed in a specific year per 100,000 persons at risk) of ovarian cancer of the 25 countries having published more than 100 related items and the ratio of country-specific articles per each new ovarian cancer case

Rank	Country	Article count	Incidence in 2012	Crude rate in 2012	Article/new case in 2012
1	Israel	388	380	9.8	1.02
2	Norway	391	418	16.9	0.94
3	Denmark	449	544	19.3	0.83
4	Sweden	522	659	13.8	0.79
5	Netherlands	762	1025	12.2	0.74
6	Finland	337	457	16.6	0.74
7	Austria	450	636	14.8	0.71
8	Australia	742	1424	12.4	0.52
9	Switzerland	306	621	15.8	0.49
10	Canada	1286	2648	15.2	0.49
11	United States	9312	20,874	13.1	0.45
12	Belgium	332	840	15.3	0.40
13	Greece	295	915	15.9	0.32
14	United Kingdom	1900	6692	21	0.28
15	Italy	1672	5911	19	0.28
16	Germany	1717	6673	16.1	0.26
17	South Korea	561	2349	9.8	0.24
18	France	878	4592	14.1	0.19
19	Japan	1673	8921	13.7	0.19
20	Turkey	290	2400	6.4	0.12
21	Spain	370	3236	13.7	0.11
22	Poland	458	4456	22.5	0.10
23	China	1813	34,575	5.3	0.05
24	Russia	166	13,373	17.4	0.01
25	India	150	26,834	4.4	0.01

The data reflect the incidence of ovarian cancer in 2012

dramatically in the nineties, which coincided with more landmark findings such as the discovery of the *BRCA* genes [47]. After 2008, annual research productivity increased to more than 1000 papers when new hypotheses regarding the origin of high-grade serous subtypes [10] and the association of ovarian cancers with *ARID1A* mutations and endometriosis were proposed [8, 9]. Also, publications assessing novel treatment strategies such as pathway inhibitor (e.g. PARP inhibitors) or antibody-based therapies were mainly released in the last 7 years.

Resembling the growing volume of published papers, the absolute citation count of ovarian cancer-related publications showed a steady increase until 2005 (Fig. 2a). Landmark papers (included in Additional file 5: Table S2) contributed to peaks in the graph: In 1979, Casagrande et al. [42] proposed the link between ovarian cancer and incessant ovulation. In 1989, two highly cited papers were published, which explored the pathogenetic relevance of HER2neu receptors and the efficacy of taxol as ovarian cancer treatment [48, 49]. In 1994 and 1995, the ovarian

cancer susceptibility genes—BRCA 1 and 2—were identified. Related articles lead to citation peaks in 1994 and 1996 [12, 13]. A meta-analysis investigating the ovarian cancer risk of 8139 patients with BRCA1 and BRCA2 mutations was published in 2003 and associated with the citation peak in 2004 [50]. The decrease in citations after 2005 is linked to a delay of up to 8 years between publication and appropriate scientific recognition of an article represented by a maximum number of citations [51].

When country-specific ovarian cancer research productivity was analyzed, the leading position of the USA became evident. This finding aligns with a benchmarking study assessing the scientific output from 1961 to 2007 related to 22 organ systems. With 1,893,800 of 5,527,558 publications, the USA identified as the most productive nation [52]. The success of the USA points to its commitment to allocate major resources towards biomedical research, e.g. the NCI awarded $100.6 million ovarian cancer funding in 2003 (http://www.cancer.gov/research/progress/snapshots/ovarian). In our study, the USA was

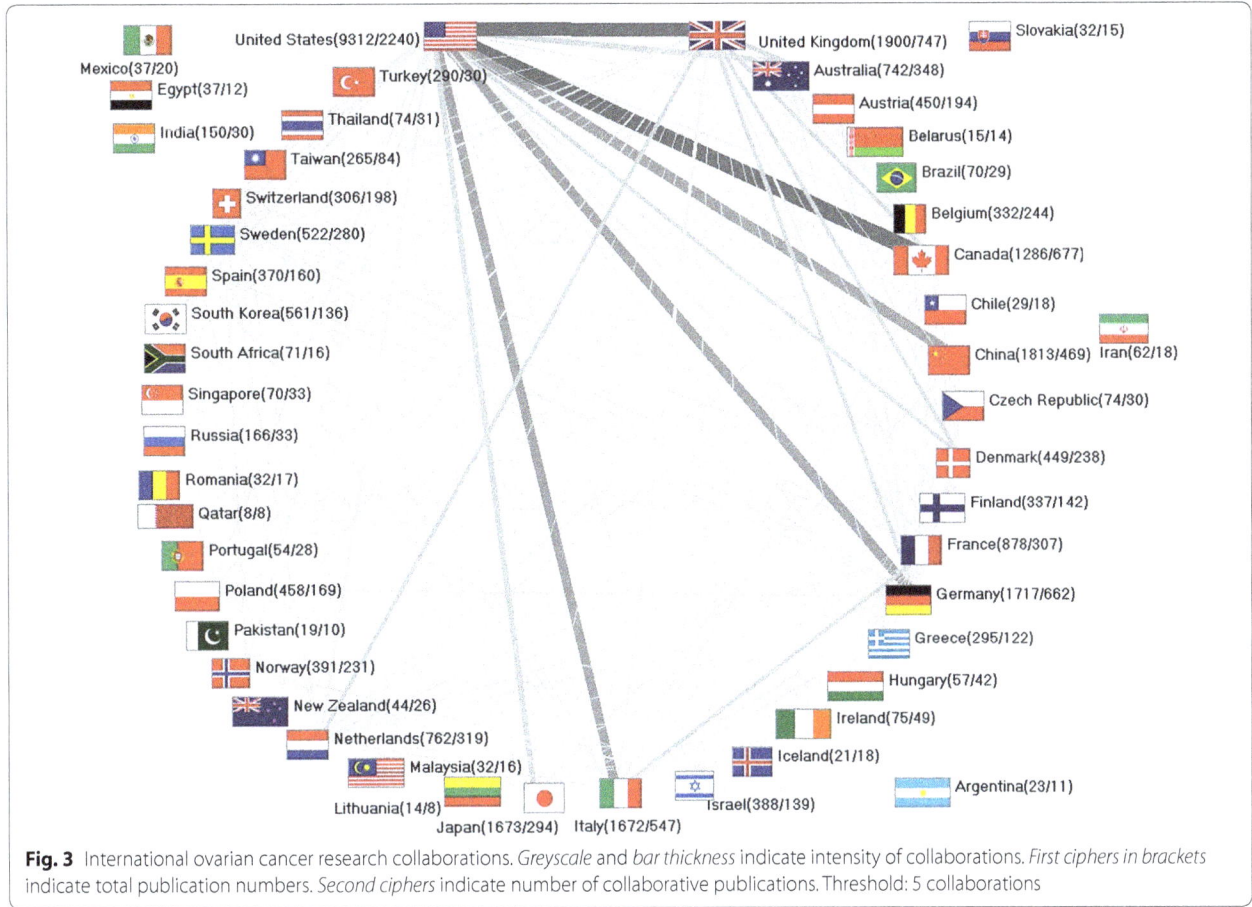

Fig. 3 International ovarian cancer research collaborations. *Greyscale* and *bar thickness* indicate intensity of collaborations. *First ciphers in brackets* indicate total publication numbers. *Second ciphers* indicate number of collaborative publications. Threshold: 5 collaborations

followed by the UK, China, Germany and Japan regarding research productivity. Glynn et al. [14] described a similar pattern for breast cancer, where the USA, the UK, Germany and Japan were also among the top five countries. China constitutes an exception: It ranked second for ovarian cancer research productivity but dropped to position 12 for breast cancer.

Citations indicate the relevance of a published item [14]. In our study, the USA, the UK and Canada dominated the ranking in term of citation counts, HI and CR. These results correspond to other studies in obstetrics and gynecology, e.g. on smoking and pregnancy. Here, the USA, the UK and Canada also achieved the highest modified HI of 128, 79 and 62 and the highest citation rates of 41.4, 8.6 and 5.3%, respectively [38]. In order to define the commitment of single countries in ovarian cancer research, we investigated scientific productivity in terms of socio-economic abilities and demonstrated two important features: First, the USA lost its leading position and other—mostly European—nations gained importance. Denmark, Norway, Iceland, Finland and Sweden ranked in the top five when article count was analyzed in relation to number of citizens. When the

total number of articles was related to the total economic power, Israel, Iceland, Denmark and Finland were leading the field. Second, when we focused on countries with a large population and high total GDPs such as China, their relative contribution to the global research output remained small compared to the USA and Europe.

Taken together, the worldwide research architecture on ovarian cancer revealed that the USA and Western European nations, China and Japan constitute the scientific power players. They publish the majority of highly cited ovarian cancer-related articles and dominate international collaborative efforts. A strong dedication of single countries to ovarian cancer research is also indicated by the prominent position of European nations—e.g. the Scandinavian countries in particular—when research productivity was related to socio-economic benchmarks. These findings coincide with other benchmarking studies [52] and with the fact that the highest incidence rates of ovarian cancer (e.g. Northern and Western Europe with incidences of 13.3 and 11.3 per 100,000 person-years as well as Northern America with an incidence of 10.7 per 100,000 person-years) are found in areas with the greatest research productivity. This association underlines that the nations, which should prioritize ovarian cancer research to alleviate the burden among its female inhabitants, actually do so. Taking the ratio of articles per every new ovarian cancer case (based on the absolute incidence data of 2012) into account, we can demonstrate a similar picture. The Scandinavian countries and the Netherlands were among the leading nations. By contrast, Canada and the USA were ranked only in the middle field with a publication output of around one article per two new ovarian cancer cases. Although China had a low incidence rate of 3.2 per 100,000 person-years reported for 2002, secular epidemiological trends project increasing numbers for the future [53]. This might explain why China supports ovarian cancer research as indicated by the strong research productivity [54].

The public health burden of ovarian cancer is significant. No considerable improvements of survival rates or decrease in morbidity and mortality have been seen over the past decades. Hence, research activity needs to be fostered, and collaborative research efforts are crucial to tackle the challenges in the field. National and international networks are equipped to do this by sharing resources, facilities and ideas leading to landmark publications [55]. In our study, the USA was the most preferred nation for collaborations based on its outstanding financial support and scientific infrastructure. We identified the most productive co-operations between the USA, Canada as well as the UK. This finding is linked to the areal proximity and cultural/language similarities, which contribute to the high productivity and quality of research produced by each of these countries. Additionally, our observation of increasing author numbers per ovarian cancer publication reflects the development of strong research networks around the globe. The Ovarian Cancer Association Consortium (OCAC) serves as an example for highly prolific global networks. Founded in 2005, this multidisciplinary, international group published more than 60 high impact papers in the areas of genetics and epidemiology.

According to the International Agency for Research on Cancer in 2012, 58% of ovarian cancer cases occurred in less developed nations [56]. Countries with the highest incidence rates of ovarian cancer were Fiji (age-standardized rate per 100,000: 14.9), Latvia (age-standardized rate per 100,000: 14.2) and Bulgaria (age-standardized rate per 100,000: 14.0) [56]. Although these countries experience a significant burden due to the disease, they were underrepresented on our map of ovarian cancer research. We did not identify one article published by Fiji. Latvia published 10 articles cited 112 times and Bulgaria issued 10 articles cited 90 times. Fiji was not part of any collaborative network. Latvia participated in only five multinational collaborations and Bulgaria in eight

bilateral collaborations. We want to point out the necessity—and almost the ethical responsibility—to include lower-resource countries with high incidence rates in scientific collaborations. Here epidemiological data, ideas and gained knowledge can be exchanged and benefit all participants.

To date, most ovarian cancer related articles were published in the subject categories of Oncology, Obstetrics/Gynecology as well as Pathology. This is not surprising. However, we found a shift in publication activity to areas such as Genetics and Internal Medicine. This development is linked to highly cited articles published by recently founded genetic-epidemiological consortia, i.e. OCAC or Ovarian Tumor Tissue Array Consortium. The increase in the subject category of Internal Medicine is explained by the growing number of high quality publications in leading journals such as the "New England Journal of Medicine", "Nature" or "Lancet", which are attributed to this category. Also, it reflects the growing interest of internal medicine physicians in the care of ovarian cancer patients.

In this study, we analyzed ovarian cancer research by assessing the country-specific publication output associated with this topic. DEMP analysis provided the visualization of computed geospatial information regarding our findings, which is a unique strength of this study. Researchers from different countries and continents can benefit from our data since they provide objective insights about the status of ovarian cancer research in their homeland or a specific country of interest. In particular, they are able to plan future research initiatives and collaborations tailored to meet the identified needs. Further, representatives of funding institution can use the presented results for the strategic allocation of resources according to obvious shortcomings. A limitation of this study is linked to the preference of the WoS to index mostly English publications. This translates into an underrepresentation of non-English items and an underestimation of the total article number, which seems to skew our findings. Since high quality research is mostly published in English journals and the WoS catalogs 90% of cited and 80% of published items related to a specific topic [57], our search identified the majority of relevant published items linked to ovarian cancer. Hence, the bias can be considered as limited. Overall, we assessed three types of bibliometric indicators gauging the publication activity on ovarian cancer: Quantitative aspects to measure the productivity of the research community, performance indicators to reflect the quality of scientific output and structural indicators to visualize the interconnectedness of research [58]. Limitations are linked to the evaluation of "qualitative" citation parameters. It is generally accepted that high citation numbers reflect outstanding scientific recognition. This relationship might be skewed due to the Matthew effect: Scientists of acknowledged standing will be cited more than little-known authors, and the citation count of their papers will increase disproportionally after their publications gained some initial popularity [59]. Also, the use of performance indicators (e.g. the citation rate) only helps gauge the quality of published research. Because citation habits and dynamics are highly variable in the investigated fields of research, all variables based on citation frequency are problematic and rather mirror the recognition of fellow scientists than truly reflect quality [59].

Conclusions

This density-equalizing mapping study represents the first concise analysis of the global ovarian cancer research architecture and illustrates the benefits of scientometrics to assess research output in a standardized way. Our study identifies historically interesting aspects in the research dynamics and relates these to landmark publications in the field. The identification of key manuscripts, subject areas as well as journals with high publication and citation rates guides individual reading and the future direction of scientific endeavors. Also, our observations highlight the outstanding importance of collaborative networks—such as OCAC—that are able to produce high quality research and apply for grant funding successfully in a joint effort. Further, lower-resource countries with a high disease burden in their population should be included in collaborative networks leading to mutual benefits due to the exchange of samples, epidemiologic data, ideas and gained knowledge.

Additional files

Additional file 1. The glossary describes important terms used in this manuscript.

Additional file 2: Figure S1. Density equalizing map of global ovarian cancer incidence numbers. Map depicts the absolute incidence numbers of ovarian cancer of the 25 countries having published more than 100 items on ovarian cancer.

Additional file 3: Table S1. Most publishing journals with number of articles, number of citations and citation rate.

Additional file 4: Figure S2. Number of articles and citation rate of the most publishing journals regarding ovarian cancer.

Additional file 5: Table S2. Most cited articles with country of origin, number of citations and journal.

Additional file 6: Figure S3. Subject area analysis of ovarian cancer research. A) Number of articles and citations per subject category. B) Relative proportions of the most assigned subject areas in most active countries.

Abbreviations

DEMP: density equalizing map projections; CR: citation rate; CIA: Central Intelligence Agency; GDP: gross domestic product; HI: Hirsch-index; NewQIS: New quality and quantity indices in science; NCI: National Cancer Institute; OCAC: Ovarian Cancer Association Consortium; UK: United Kingdom; USA: United States of America; WoS: Web of Science.

Authors' contributions

DB, KP, and DK have made substantial contributions to the conception and design of the study, acquisition of the data and interpretation. CLP and DAG have made substantial contributions to the interpretation of the data. They all have been involved in drafting and revising the manuscript. All authors read and approved the final manuscript.

Author details

[1] Department of Obstetrics and Gynecology, Keck School of Medicine of USC, Los Angeles, CA, USA. [2] Department of Female Health and Preventive Medicine, Institute of Occupational Medicine, Social Medicine and Environmental Medicine, Goethe-University, Theodor-Stern Kai 7, 60590 Frankfurt, Germany. [3] Department of Epidemiology, School of Public Health, University of Michigan, Ann Arbor, MI, USA.

Acknowledgements

We thank Cristian Scutaru for the establishment of the analysis unit and helpful comments. This study is part of a Ph.D. thesis project (KP).

Competing interests

The authors declare that they have no competing interests.

References

1. Nezhat FR, Apostol R, Nezhat C, Pejovic T. New insights in the pathophysiology of ovarian cancer and implications for screening and prevention. Am J Obstet Gynecol. 2015;213(3):262–7.
2. Prat J, Franceschi S, Denny L, Lazcano Ponce E. Cancers of the female reproductive organs. In: Stewart BW, Wild CP, editors. WHO: World Cancer Report. Geneva: WHO Press; 2014. p. 467.
3. Siegel R, Ma J, Zou Z, Jemal A. Cancer statistics, 2014. CA Cancer J Clin. 2014;64(1):9–29.
4. Gilks CB. Molecular abnormalities in ovarian cancer subtypes other than high-grade serous carcinoma. J Oncol. 2010;2010:740968.
5. Nezhat FR, Pejovic T, Reis FM, Guo SW. The link between endometriosis and ovarian cancer: clinical implications. Int J Gynecol Cancer. 2014;24(4):623–8.
6. Wang S, Qiu L, Lang JH, Shen K, Yang JX, Huang HF, Pan LY, Wu M. Clinical analysis of ovarian epithelial carcinoma with coexisting pelvic endometriosis. Am J Obstet Gynecol. 2013;208(5):413 e411–5.
7. Erickson BK, Conner MG, Landen CN Jr. The role of the fallopian tube in the origin of ovarian cancer. Am J Obstet Gynecol. 2013;209(5):409–14.
8. Pearce CL, Templeman C, Rossing MA, Lee A, Near AM, Webb PM, Nagle CM, Doherty JA, Cushing-Haugen KL, Wicklund KG, et al. Association between endometriosis and risk of histological subtypes of ovarian cancer: a pooled analysis of case–control studies. Lancet Oncol. 2012;13(4):385–94.
9. Wiegand KC, Shah SP, Al-Agha OM, Zhao Y, Tse K, Zeng T, Senz J, McConechy MK, Anglesio MS, Kalloger SE, et al. ARID1A mutations in endometriosis-associated ovarian carcinomas. New Engl J Med. 2010;363(16):1532–43.
10. Medeiros F, Muto MG, Lee Y, Elvin JA, Callahan MJ, Feltmate C, Garber JE, Cramer DW, Crum CP. The tubal fimbria is a preferred site for early adenocarcinoma in women with familial ovarian cancer syndrome. Am J Surg Pathol. 2006;30(2):230–6.
11. Kurman RJ, Shih IM. Molecular pathogenesis and extraovarian origin of epithelial ovarian cancer—shifting the paradigm. Hum Pathol. 2011;42(7):918–31.

12. Miki Y, Swensen J, Shattuck-Eidens D, Futreal PA, Harshman K, Tavtig-ian S, Liu Q, Cochran C, Bennett LM, Ding W, et al. A strong candidate for the breast and ovarian cancer susceptibility gene BRCA1. Science. 1994;266(5182):66–71.

13. Wooster R, Bignell G, Lancaster J, Swift S, Seal S, Mangion J, Collins N, Gregory S, Gumbs C, Micklem G. Identification of the breast cancer susceptibility gene BRCA2. Nature. 1995;378(6559):789–92.

14. Glynn RW, Scutaru C, Kerin MJ, Sweeney KJ. Breast cancer research output, 1945–2008: a bibliometric and density-equalizing analysis. Breast Cancer Res BCR. 2010;12(6):R108.

15. Groneberg-Kloft B, Quarcoo D, Scutaru C. Quality and quantity indices in science: use of visualization tools. EMBO Rep. 2009;10(8):800–3.

16. Groneberg-Kloft B, Fischer TC, Quarcoo D, Scutaru C. New quality and quantity indices in science (NewQIS): the study protocol of an interna-tional project. J Occup Med Toxicol (London, England). 2009;4:16.

17. Groneberg-Kloft B, Kreiter C, Welte T, Fischer A, Quarcoo D, Scutaru C. Interfield dysbalances in research input and output benchmarking: visualisation by density equalizing procedures. Int J Health Geogr. 2008;7:48.

18. Groneberg-Kloft B, Scutaru C, Dinh QT, Welte T, Chung KF, Fischer A, Quarcoo D. Inter-disease comparison of research quantity and quality: bronchial asthma and chronic obstructive pulmonary disease. J Asthma. 2009;46(2):147–52.

19. Groneberg-Kloft B, Scutaru C, Fischer A, Welte T, Kreiter C, Quarcoo D. Analysis of research output parameters: density equalizing mapping and citation trend analysis. BMC Health Serv Res. 2009;9:16.

20. Al-Mutawakel K, Scutaru C, Shami A, Sakr M, Groneberg DA, Quarcoo D. Scientometric analysis of the world-wide research efforts concerning Leishmaniasis. Parasites Vectors. 2010;3(1):14.

21. Vitzthum K, Scutaru C, Musial-Bright L, Quarcoo D, Welte T, Spallek M, Groneberg-Kloft B. Scientometric analysis and combined density-equaliz-ing mapping of environmental tobacco smoke (ETS) research. PLoS ONE. 2010;5(6):e11254.

22. Groneberg DA, Schilling U, Scutaru C, Uibel S, Zitnik S, Mueller D, Klingelhoefer D, Kloft B. Drowning—a scientometric analysis and data acquisition of a constant global problem employing density equalizing mapping and scientometric benchmarking procedures. Int J Health Geogr. 2011;10:55.

23. Bundschuh M, Groneberg DA, Klingelhoefer D, Gerber A. Yellow fever disease: density equalizing mapping and gender analysis of international research output. Parasites Vectors. 2013;6:331.

24. Fricke R, Uibel S, Klingelhoefer D, Groneberg DA. Influenza: a scientomet-ric and density-equalizing analysis. BMC Infect Dis. 2013;13:454.

25. Groneberg-Kloft B, Klingelhoefer D, Zitnik SE, Scutaru C. Traffic medicine-related research: a scientometric analysis. BMC Public Health. 2013;13:541.

26. Schmidt S, Bundschuh M, Scutaru C, Klingelhoefer D, Groneberg DA, Gerber A. Hepatitis B: global scientific development from a critical point of view. J Viral Hepat. 2014;21(11):786–93. doi:10.1111/jvh.12205.

27. Addicks JP, Uibel S, Jensen AM, Bundschuh M, Klingelhoefer D, Groneberg DA. MRSA: a density-equalizing mapping analysis of the global research architecture. Int J Environ Res Public Health. 2014;11(10):10215–25.

28. Gerber A, Klingelhoefer D, Groneberg D, Bundschuh M. Antineutro-phil cytoplasmic antibody-associated vasculitides: a scientometric approach visualizing worldwide research activity. Int J Rheum Dis. 2014;17(7):796–804.

29. Groneberg DA, Rahimian S, Bundschuh M, Schwarzer M, Gerber A, Kloft B. Telemedicine—a scientometric and density equalizing analysis. J Occup Med Toxicol (London, England). 2015;10(38):38.

30. Groneberg DA, Weber E, Gerber A, Fischer A, Klingelhoefer D, Bruegg-mann D. Density equalizing mapping of the global tuberculosis research architecture. Tuberculosis (Edinburgh, Scotland). 2015;95(4):515–22.

31. Quarcoo D, Bruggmann D, Klingelhofer D, Groneberg DA. Ebola and its global research architecture—need for an improvement. PLoS Negl Trop Dis. 2015;9(9):e0004083.

32. Bruggmann D, Richter T, Klingelhofer D, Gerber A, Bundschuh M, Jaque J, Groneberg DA. Global architecture of gestational diabetes research: density-equalizing mapping studies and gender analysis. Nutr J. 2016;15(1):36.

33. Gerber A, Klingelhoefer D, Groneberg DA, Bundschuh M. Silicosis: geo-graphic changes in research: an analysis employing density-equalizing mapping. J Occup Med Toxicol (London, England). 2014;9(1):2.

34. Falagas ME, Pitsouni EI, Malietzis GA, Pappas G. Comparison of PubMed, Scopus, web of science, and Google Scholar: strengths and weaknesses. FASEB J. 2008;22(2):338–42.

35. Hirsch JE. An index to quantify an individual's scientific research output. Proc Natl Acad Sci USA. 2005;102(46):16569–72.

36. Gastner MT, Newman ME. Diffusion-based method for producing density-equalizing maps. Proc Natl Acad Sci USA. 2004;101(20):7499–504.

37. World Economic Outlook Database. http://www.imf.org/external/pubs/ft/weo/2013/02/weodata/weorept.aspx?pr.x=75&pr.y=10&sy=2012&ey=2012&scsm=1&ssd=1&sort=country&ds=.&br=1&c=193%2C223%2C924%2C132%2C134%2C146%2C136%2C158%2C112%2C111&s=NGDPD&grp=0&a=.

38. Mund M, Kloft B, Bundschuh M, Klingelhoefer D, Groneberg DA, Gerber A. Global research on smoking and pregnancy—a scientometric and gender analysis. Int J Environ Res Public Health. 2014;11(6):5792–806.

39. Carl J, Schwarzer M, Klingelhoefer D, Ohlendorf D, Groneberg DA. Curare—a curative poison: a scientometric analysis. PLoS ONE. 2014;9(11):e112026.

40. Pleger N, Kloft B, Quarcoo D, Zitnik S, Mache S, Klingelhoefer D, Groneberg DA. Bacterial meningitis: a density-equalizing mapping analy-sis of the global research architecture. Int J Environ Res Public Health. 2014;11(10):10202–14.

41. Fujiki H. Gist of Dr. Katsusaburo Yamagiwa's papers entitled "Experimental study on the pathogenesis of epithelial tumors" (I to VI reports). Cancer Sci. 2014;105(2):143–9.

42. Casagrande JT, Louie EW, Pike MC, Roy S, Ross RK, Henderson BE. "Incessant ovulation" and ovarian cancer. Lancet (London, England). 1979;2(8135):170–3.

43. Fathalla MF. Incessant ovulation and ovarian cancer—a hypothesis re-visited. Facts Views Vis ObGyn. 2013;5(4):292–7.

44. Lowry S, Russell H, Hickey I, Atkinson R. Incessant ovulation and ovarian cancer. Lancet (London, England). 1991;337(8756):1544–5.

45. Seidman JD. The presence of mucosal iron in the fallopian tube supports the "incessant menstruation hypothesis" for ovarian carcinoma. Int J Gynecol Pathol. 2013;32(5):454–8.

46. Fathalla MF. Incessant ovulation—a factor in ovarian neoplasia? Lancet (London, England). 1971;2(7716):163.

47. Wooster R, Neuhausen SL, Mangion J, Quirk Y, Ford D, Collins N, Nguyen K, Seal S, Tran T, Averill D. Localization of a breast cancer susceptibility gene, BRCA2, to chromosome 13q12-13. Science. 1994;265(5181):2088–90.

48. Slamon DJ, Godolphin W, Jones LA, Holt JA, Wong SG, Keith DE, Levin WJ, Stuart SG, Udove J, Ullrich A, et al. Studies of the HER-2/neu proto-oncogene in human breast and ovarian cancer. Science. 1989;244(4905):707–12.

49. McGuire WP, Rowinsky EK, Rosenshein NB, Grumbine FC, Ettinger DS, Armstrong DK, Donehower RC. Taxol: a unique antineoplastic agent with significant activity in advanced ovarian epithelial neoplasms. Ann Intern Med. 1989;111(4):273–9.

50. Antoniou A, Pharoah PD, Narod S, Risch HA, Eyfjord JE, Hopper JL, Loman N, Olsson H, Johannsson O, Borg A, et al. Average risks of breast and ovar-ian cancer associated with BRCA1 or BRCA2 mutations detected in case Series unselected for family history: a combined analysis of 22 studies. Am J Hum Genet. 2003;72(5):1117–30.

51. Garfield E. The evolution of the science citation index. Int Microbiol. 2007;10(1):65–9.

52. Groneberg-Kloft B, Scutaru C, Kreiter C, Kolzow S, Fischer A, Quarcoo D. Institutional operating figures in basic and applied sciences: scientomet-ric analysis of quantitative output benchmarking. Health Res Policy Syst. 2008;6:6.

53. Parkin DM, Bray F, Ferlay J, Pisani P. Global cancer statistics, 2002. CA Cancer J Clin. 2005;55(2):74–108.

54. Wang B, Liu SZ, Zheng RS, Zhang F, Chen WQ, Sun XB. Time trends of ovarian cancer incidence in China. Asian Pac J Cancer Prev APJCP. 2014;15(1):191–3.

55. Adams J. Collaborations: the rise of research networks. Nature. 2012;490(7420):335–6.

56. Ferlay J SI, Ervik M, Dikshit R, Eser S, Mathers C, Rebelo M, Parkin DM, Forman D, Bray, F: GLOBOCAN 2012 v1.1, Cancer Incidence and Mortality Worldwide: IARC CancerBase No. 11 [Internet]. Lyon, France: International Agency for Research on Cancer, http://globocan.iarc.fr/Pages/bar_pop_sel.aspx. Accessed 01 Oct 2016.

57. Testa J. The Thomson Scientific journal selection process. Int Microbiol. 2006;9(2):135–8.

58. Durieux V, Gevenois PA. Bibliometric indicators: quality measurements of scientific publication. Radiology. 2010;255(2):342–51.

59. Merton RK. The Matthew Effect in Science: the reward and communication systems of science are considered. Science. 1968;159(3810):56–63.

7

Using Google Location History data to quantify fine-scale human mobility

Nick Warren Ruktanonchai[1,2]* ⓘ, Corrine Warren Ruktanonchai[1,2], Jessica Rhona Floyd[1,2] and Andrew J. Tatem[1,2]

Abstract

Background: Human mobility is fundamental to understanding global issues in the health and social sciences such as disease spread and displacements from disasters and conflicts. Detailed mobility data across spatial and temporal scales are difficult to collect, however, with movements varying from short, repeated movements to work or school, to rare migratory movements across national borders. While typical sources of mobility data such as travel history surveys and GPS tracker data can inform different typologies of movement, almost no source of readily obtainable data can address all types of movement at once.

Methods: Here, we collect Google Location History (GLH) data and examine it as a novel source of information that could link fine scale mobility with rare, long distance and international trips, as it uniquely spans large temporal scales with high spatial granularity. These data are passively collected by Android smartphones, which reach increasingly broad audiences, becoming the most common operating system for accessing the Internet worldwide in 2017. We validate GLH data against GPS tracker data collected from Android users in the United Kingdom to assess the feasibility of using GLH data to inform human movement.

Results: We find that GLH data span very long temporal periods (over a year on average in our sample), are spatially equivalent to GPS tracker data within 100 m, and capture more international movement than survey data. We also find GLH data avoid compliance concerns seen with GPS trackers and bias in self-reported travel, as GLH is passively collected. We discuss some settings where GLH data could provide novel insights, including infrastructure planning, infectious disease control, and response to catastrophic events, and discuss advantages and disadvantages of using GLH data to inform human mobility patterns.

Conclusions: GLH data are a greatly underutilized and novel dataset for understanding human movement. While biases exist in populations with GLH data, Android phones are becoming the first and only device purchased to access the Internet and various web services in many middle and lower income settings, making these data increasingly appropriate for a wide range of scientific questions.

Keywords: Human mobility, Mobile phone data, GPS tracker data

Background

Understanding human mobility and how it manifests across temporal and spatial scales is important across the health and social sciences [1], as mobility patterns drive important spatial processes from infrastructure and land use to infectious disease spread [2]. The health sciences have increasingly focused on human movement in recent decades, accounting for the importance of geographical context in driving health inequalities and exposure to environmental risks [3]. Geographical context is strongly linked to the critical concept of "neighbourhood" [3], or the spatial context of a given individual. Within the social sciences, this temporally dynamic concept of incorporating an individual's experiences is foundational to informing how social inequalities persist through mechanisms such as racial segregation, how individuals are exposed to environmental hazards, and how accessibility varies to social and health resources [4]. Traditionally, studies

*Correspondence: nrukt00@gmail.com
[1] WorldPop Project, Geography and Environment, University of Southampton, Southampton SO17 1BJ, UK
Full list of author information is available at the end of the article

examining geographical context have used the charac-teristics of the administrative unit that individuals reside within to quantify their exposure to risks or accessibil-ity to various rather than an emergent understanding of exposure [3]. This ignores individual-level spatial and temporal variation in where people spend time [5], how-ever, potentially smoothing over the unique mobility pat-terns of marginalized populations and subgroups.

More recently, these issues have been addressed using the concept of an individual's activity space (defined as encompassing all the locations a person interacts with over time) [6, 7], yielding a much more accurate picture of risk and social context than residence alone. Along these lines, recent studies have found that using place of residence rather than actual activity space underesti-mated exposure to spatial risks by 16 and 7% in Vancou-ver and Southern California respectively [8]. Further, using an individualized understanding of activity space can uncover sources of social patterns and inequalities that would not be observed using a static, administrative-boundary-based understanding of neighbourhood, such as accessibility to healthcare services [9, 10], personal exposure to spatial risks [11], and social networks [12]. In particular, populations that are highly segregated will have strongly disparate activity spaces [13], which will cause geographically close groups of people to experience dramatically different realities.

Utilizing such activity-based approaches in the health and social sciences, however, requires a precise and broad understanding of geographical context and envi-ronmental exposure across time [14]. Because locations for certain activities are often very close in space (for example, work and commercial activity), data used to inform activity space should be ideally be spatially refined enough to enable identification of different location types [14]. These data should also be temporally broad enough to capture regular behaviour patterns across long peri-ods with sufficient certainty [14]. Though various disci-plines have explored how activity spaces over weekly and monthly periods affect transit and exposure to frequently visited areas such as physical activity spaces, schools, workplaces, and otherwise [6], the extent of exposures experienced over a more broad timescale such as years and decades have been less explored. This owes partly to lacking data on long-term mobility patterns at suf-ficient spatial resolutions, and remains a critical gap in our understanding of exposure to risks that lead to spatial outcomes such as cancer, obesity, and various inequali-ties that arise from long-term differences in accessibility between populations.

With recent technological advancements, a number of data sources on human movement have been used to inform activity space across temporal scales [15, 16]

(Fig. 1). Traditionally, travel diaries have been an invalu-able source of mobility information to inform activity spaces [13], as respondents can identify the specific loca-tions used for various activities, which can then be iden-tified in the context of the respondent's residence. While data from personal GPS trackers provide information on short-distance, circulatory movement and can directly inform activity spaces [17], census-derived and popula-tion stock data inform longer-distance migratory move-ment, and exposure over longer periods [18]. Other data inform mobility at intermediate spatial and temporal scales, such as remotely sensed night-time light data that help infer where people are within cities over the course of a year [16, 19, 20], or social media data, which record the location where various social media services are used [21]. In some countries, data from mobile phones (call data records, or CDRs) provide national-scale coverage, recording the cell tower that calls and texts are routed through and the associated times over months or years [11, 22].

These sources of mobility data can also be significantly biased or have other drawbacks. Travel diaries are labo-rious to collect, for example, and subject to recall bias, especially when requesting the respondent to recall beyond several months [23]. Further, while CDRs have facilitated a national-level understanding of activity space and mobility, these data remain particularly difficult to obtain and use at present, however, requiring oner-ous data-sharing agreements with mobile operators, are treated as proprietary due to privacy concerns, and are spatially coarse as towers can be many kilometres apart in rural areas, and cannot typically track international movement. Social media and CDR data collection can also be highly biased, only recording location when calls and texts occur, or when social media services are used, causing CDRs to underestimate total travel distance and movement entropy [24].

Because of these drawbacks in current data, and a broader need to understand activity spaces across tempo-ral scales, novel data are needed that can be easily col-lected with social and demographic information, cover long time periods, and identify locations of travel with high spatial precision. We explore here Google Location History (GLH) data as an underused source of human mobility information that could fill this niche in numer-ous research contexts. These data consist of geographic coordinates routinely recorded by Android phones, and are associated with a consolidated user account, allow-ing for location data that are recorded across all mobile devices that an individual has owned. GLH data have been collected in an opt-out, passive fashion for Android users since location services have been fully integrated into Android in 2012 [25]. Each user can quickly and

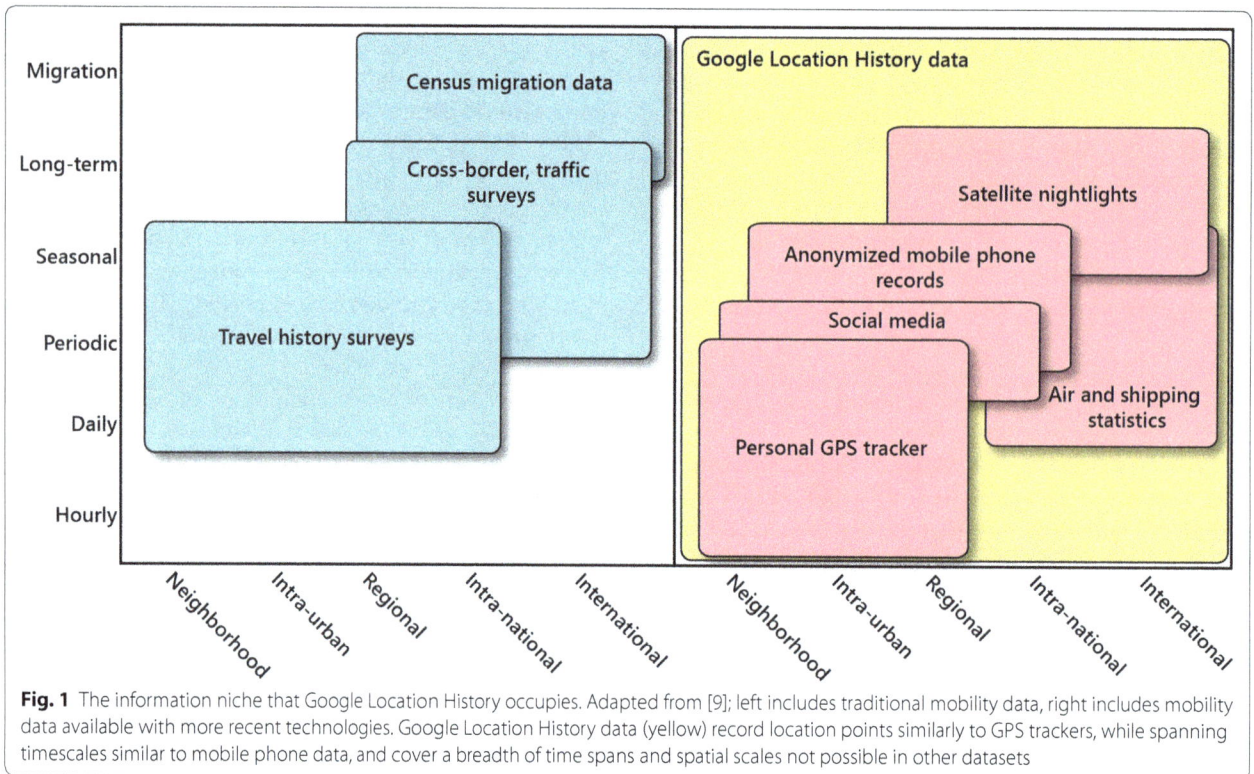

Fig. 1 The information niche that Google Location History occupies. Adapted from [9]; left includes traditional mobility data, right includes mobility data available with more recent technologies. Google Location History data (yellow) record location points similarly to GPS trackers, while spanning timescales similar to mobile phone data, and cover a breadth of time spans and spatial scales not possible in other datasets

freely access their own data through a web browser. In studies that use GLH data, users can download their associated data and provide it to researchers during surveys that include an appropriate informed consent process. Because location is identified using a combination of the phone's internal GPS and connected WiFi devices and cell towers, we show that these data are as spatially refined as GPS tracker data while spanning years (Fig. 1). Further, the passively-collected nature of GLH data avoids many known biases from compliance issues in studies that use GPS trackers, and avoids recall bias found in self-reported travel history data.

Though potentially biased towards wealthier populations, GLH data are available from an increasingly large proportion of the world, as the Android user base has increased dramatically since 2012 [26], reaching over 1.4 billion active devices in 2015 [27]. In particular, these devices are popular as an affordable way to access the Internet in low and middle income settings [27], and worldwide, Android market share for accessing the Internet has surpassed Microsoft Windows [26].

As they have only become recently available, GLH data have not previously been used to understand patterns of human mobility in social science research. Therefore, critical questions must be addressed before they can be used to examine important issues in the social sciences. Here, we conducted a pilot study among Android users in the United Kingdom to address: (1) what proportion

of Android users have GLH data enabled, and whether this correlates with use of various Google services; (2) how much data are typically available for a given Android user; (3) whether GLH recording rates depended on cell signal, and (4) whether GLH location points are spatially accurate compared to established GPS tracking units. To address these questions, we collected GLH data among Android users and administered a survey addressing recent international movement, use of Google services, and technology use among individuals recruited through the University of Southampton in the United Kingdom. Among a subsample of these participants, we further validated the feasibility and accuracy of the GLH data by comparing GLH data to GPS data, and by correlating points recorded by the GPS and Android phone. Finally, we independently administered Google Surveys to Android users in several countries to address the proportion of users that have GLH data across high and middle-income countries.

Methods

Data collection

For the GLH and survey data collection, we recruited 25 individuals throughout the University of Southampton (ethics approval ERGO ID 23647) from October to December 2016, targeting people who use an Android device as their primary mobile device. After administering informed consent, participants were randomly assigned to one of two possible study groups: "GLH only" or "+GPS". The "GLH only" group involved a single study visit where participants accessed and downloaded their GLH data and completed a self-administered survey. The survey included questions about phone model and Android version installed, past and present use of GLH and other Google services, opinions on data privacy, recent self-reported international travel, and health related questions. For those randomized to the "+GPS" group, the initial study visit consisted of the same process, in addition to carrying a GPS logger unit (i-gotU model GT-600) for the following 7 days. Technical details and validation of the i-gotU GPS unit are outlined elsewhere [28]. After one week, participants returned for a final study visit, where they returned the GPS logger unit and downloaded their GLH data again, providing GLH data for the 7 days corresponding to GPS tracker carriage. Study design is outlined in more detail in Additional file 1, including the GLH data download process and questionnaire.

We measured how much GPS and GLH data we obtained from each user, quantifying temporal and spatial extent of data and recording rates. We associated these measures with survey data to determine if data availability depended on technical details such as phone model and the version of Android installed. We also examined the correlation between data availability/breadth and a user's utilisation of various Google services and data privacy perceptions more generally.

Google surveys

To address the likelihood of Android users having GLH data across different countries, we administered online Google Surveys in Brazil, the USA, the UK, Japan, and Mexico to 250 Android users in each country (1250 total). These surveys are administered to users through the Google Opinion Rewards app. This service provides nationally population-representative results to researchers using weights based on self-reported age and gender, and location based on browsing history and IP address. Further details on the Google Survey weighting methodology can be found at https://www.google.com/analytics/resources/whitepaper-how-google-surveys-works.html. In each of these surveys, we asked users if their Google account has GLH reporting enabled ("Yes", "No", or "Don't Know"), instructing users that they are able to check under "Your Timeline" in the Google Maps app.

Comparison with common types of mobility data

To better contextualize the temporal breadth and resolution of GLH data, we performed a rapid literature review in PubMed using the following search terms in the title/abstract: 'human mobility', 'travel patterns', 'human movement', 'GPS tracker', 'Call Data Records', 'migration', 'population dynamics' or 'mobility networks'. This search resulted in 36,982 publications, which we further restricted to studies on humans published within the past 10 years, resulting in 2203 articles. Papers were selected for inclusion if they met the following criteria: (1) the study was published after 2008, (2) the study captured data on individual-level human mobility (i.e., social media check-ins, Call Data Records, GPS trackers, and travel history surveys), and (3) the study reported information on temporal resolution of analysis. We did not include review articles or studies modelling human movement using agent-based models or aggregate data, such as air traffic or commuter data. Some datasets had several associated articles (for example, CDRs provided for Senegal and the Ivory Coast through the D4D Challenge initiative); we therefore removed articles reporting on data previously included in the literature review. After reviewing article abstracts and methods, we identified a total of 43 suitable articles to include in our literature review [2, 6, 17, 22, 23, 28–65]. The table of studies used in this literature review is provided as Additional file 2.

Cell tower comparison

To determine whether GLH recording rates depended on cell coverage, we quantified the relationship between rate of GLH data recording and distance from the nearest cell tower using a generalized linear model, including a randomly varying individual-level intercept to control for individual-level differences in ping rate. We obtained cell tower locations from OpenCellID.org, which synthesizes cell tower locations inferred from various smartphone apps and donated by mobile operators to build a database on cell towers throughout the world. This database was used previously to map hospital catchment areas [66]. Because Android devices occasionally stopped recording location history points for long periods, we restricted these analyses to points where the time between the last point collected was 1 week or less and to points within the United Kingdom, yielding a total sample size of 1,821,728 data points. We restricted the analysis to 1 week or less to account for very long periods when users may have either disabled the internal GPS functionality on their phone, or switched to a phone without an internal GPS, removing 43 data points in total.

GPS validation

To validate whether the GLH data are as spatially accurate and frequently-collected as established GPS tracker data, we compared ping rates between users with both GLH and GPS tracker data, distance between recorded location points, and other metrics to address whether the GLH data were accurate and representative of overall movement. Specifically, we calculated the distance between GPS and GLH points for all minutes where both GPS and GLH data were recorded. If multiple coordinates were recorded in a given minute, we assigned the mean latitude and longitude for that minute.

We also aggregated both datasets to gridded surfaces of varying resolution (ranging from grid squares of 100 m by 100 m to 2500 m by 2500 m) and determined if GLH and GPS points were recorded within the same grid squares for each hour. We used gridded surfaces because researchers often combine location data with gridded spatial data that informs the risk of interest, such as malaria prevalence [67], healthcare accessibility [9], or air pollution [68]. We calculated percentage agreement for each hour by dividing the number of grid squares with points in both datasets by the total number of grid squares with points across both datasets. For each hour, if $C_{GLH} \cap C_{GPS}$ is the number of grid squares with points in both the GPS and GLH data and $C_{GLH} \cup C_{GPS}$ is the number of grid squares with points from either dataset, then the percent agreement a for that hour is $a = \frac{C_{GLH} \cap C_{GPS}}{C_{GLH} \cup C_{GPS}}$. Therefore, if all the grid squares with GLH points also had GPS points and vice versa for a given hour, we recorded 100% agreement for that hour at that gridded surface resolution.

We repeated this analysis after interpolating linearly between points for minutes where no data were recorded. Linear interpolation is commonly used to fill in location information [69, 70], as GPS tracker data often have large gaps with no data recorded, particularly when the device is not moving, which we also observed in the GLH data.

We also determined if one dataset captured more travel than the other during the week that the GPS trackers were carried, by comparing the numbers of trips away from the previous night's residence recorded in each dataset. We accomplished this by assigning a residence using the last location point from the GPS tracker data from the previous night. This assumes that the GPS trackers provided an accurate location for where that person spent the night, and we then calculated numbers of trips in the GPS and GLH data by counting the number of times people more than 100 m away from their daily assigned residence. Here, 100 m was chosen to define travel away from home due to the apparent accuracy of the GLH data compared to the GPS tracker data. We compared these using different definitions of trips away from home, ranging from at least 10 min away from home to two hours.

Results
GLH data
Among the 25 participants in our pilot study, two individuals reported that their GLH was disabled. A further two

participants had no GLH data, suggesting they thought GLH recording was enabled, but was disabled in reality. This resulted in GLH data from a total of 21 participants, or approximately 85% of our sample. Among all participants, 20% (n = 5) reported that they had ever disabled GLH services, while a further 28% (n = 7) reported not knowing if they had ever disabled it. Among those who had previously disabled the service, two reported doing so for privacy reasons, two reported not feeling the need to enable it, and one reported disabling it to save battery life. Two participants further reported turning GLH services back on specifically to utilise the Google Maps feature.

Our sample included a variety of Android phone models, with a plurality (n = 9) of respondents owning a Samsung Galaxy device. Other models included Huawei, Lenovo, Tecno, Infinix, Medion, Xiaomi, Asus, LG Nexus, Motorola, Blue Diamond, and OnePlus phones. The current Android operating system version on these phones varied between versions 4.4.2 through 7.0, and we found no significant difference in ping rate over the last three months of data collection with different Android versions or with different phone models (Additional file 3).

For the 21 participants with GLH data, we obtained a mean 205,000 location history points per user across an average of 367 days, yielding 4.32 million total geographic coordinates (Fig. 2). This often included days without any recorded data. On average, the beginning and end dates of location history points were 556 days apart, suggesting that phones did not record data during roughly 1/3 of days. This may be due to study participants not using an Android smartphone for the entire period, or due to study participants turning off location history collection or the GPS service on their smartphone. The actual proportion of days with no data ranged from 0% to 90% across the 21 users, which did not appear to correlate with Android version or phone model (Additional file 3) but did negatively correlate strongly with total number of points collected, suggesting no-data days were due to other factors.

We identified numerous occasions of international travel, with locations recorded in 41 different countries across the 21 individuals. In the questionnaire, we asked participants the last country they visited outside of the UK, and 17 users reported traveling internationally in the past year. After excluding very short periods recorded in other countries (less than one day), the GLH data accurately captured the last visited country for 14 out of these 17 users. We excluded travel to a country for less than one day, as that likely indicates stopovers and would not typically be counted as international travel. For the three cases where GLH data did not capture the last country

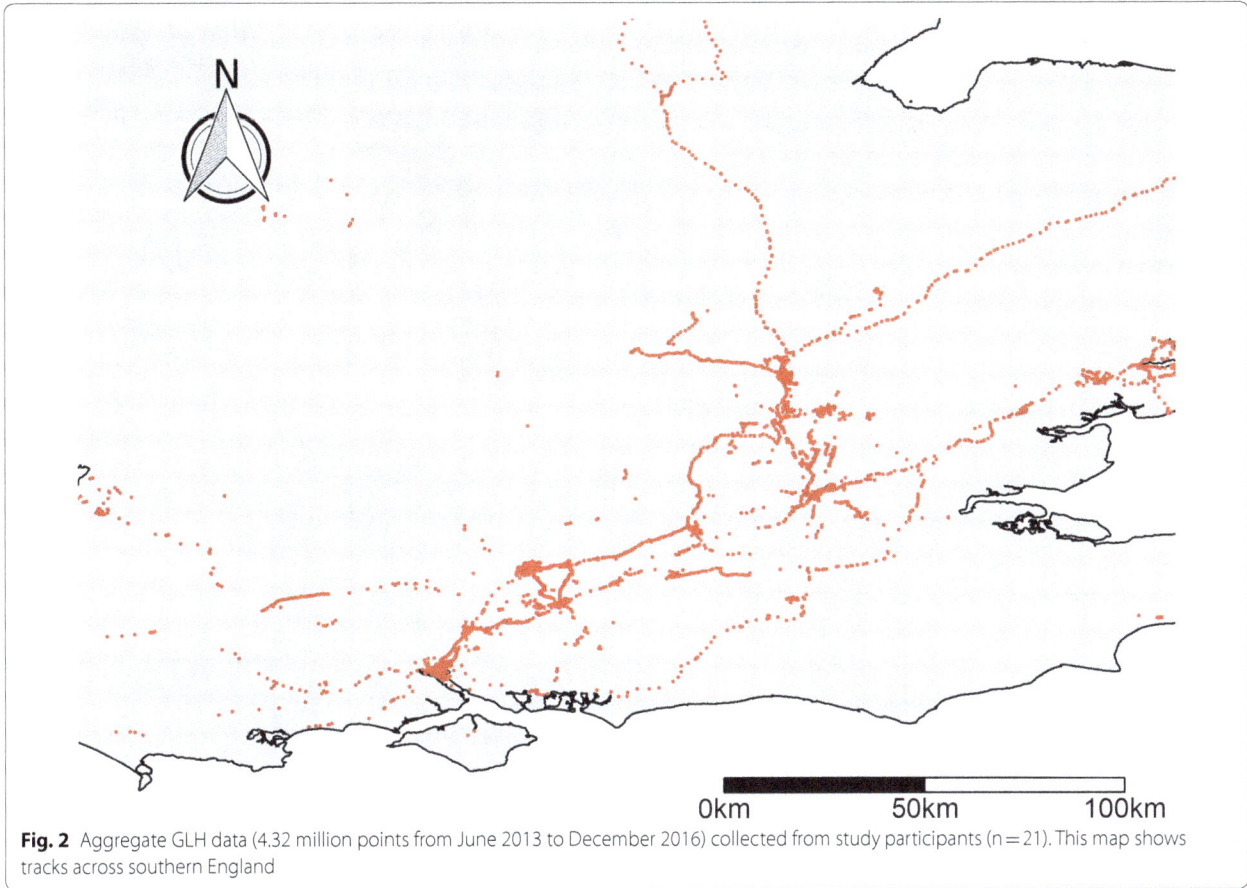

Fig. 2 Aggregate GLH data (4.32 million points from June 2013 to December 2016) collected from study participants (n = 21). This map shows tracks across southern England

visited, two participants reported disabling data/GPS regularly.

Figure 3 shows GLH and GPS tracker data for a randomly chosen subset of individuals from the +GPS group, and differences in data collected at various spatial scales between the GLH data and the GPS trackers. This figure also shows simulated mobile phone (CDR) data, assuming each GLH location point corresponded with a call or text event, and using the OpenCellID dataset to inform cell tower locations, yielding Voronoi polygons around cell towers roughly 242.8 m^2 in size on average after isolating the OpenCellID dataset to the mobile operator with the most towers. As location point recording occurred often every minute or more frequently during travel, this is likely a very large overestimation of call and text rates. Because CDR data generally only include calls and texts within networks that do not cross national borders, we excluded any international travel from the simulated CDR data. This figure also includes the countries reported as visited during the in-person questionnaire.

Notably, the GLH data recorded 41 international trips across 21 individuals (excluding countries where the

person spent less than one day, to account for stopovers during travel), while the GPS data captured zero international trips for six individuals in the +GPS group due to the short duration covered, and the travel history data captured 18 international trips due to the questionnaire recording the most recent country visited in the past year. When comparing numbers of trips recorded during the week when the +GPS group carried GPS trackers, we found similar trips in both datasets regardless of the minimum amount of time away required to count a trip. Specifically, for the six individuals where we compared this analysis, if the minimum duration to qualify as a trip was 10 min away from home, the mean number of trips identified was 10 (minimum 6, maximum 15) in the GPS data, and 10 (minimum 7, maximum 15) in the GLH data. If the duration was set to 120 min, the GPS data recorded 7.2 trips (minimum 5, maximum 10), while the GLH data recorded 7.4 trips (minimum 4, maximum 10).

Google surveys

Among 1250 Android users, most countries had the highest proportion of users reporting having GLH reporting enabled, ranging from 43% in Japan to 72% in Mexico.

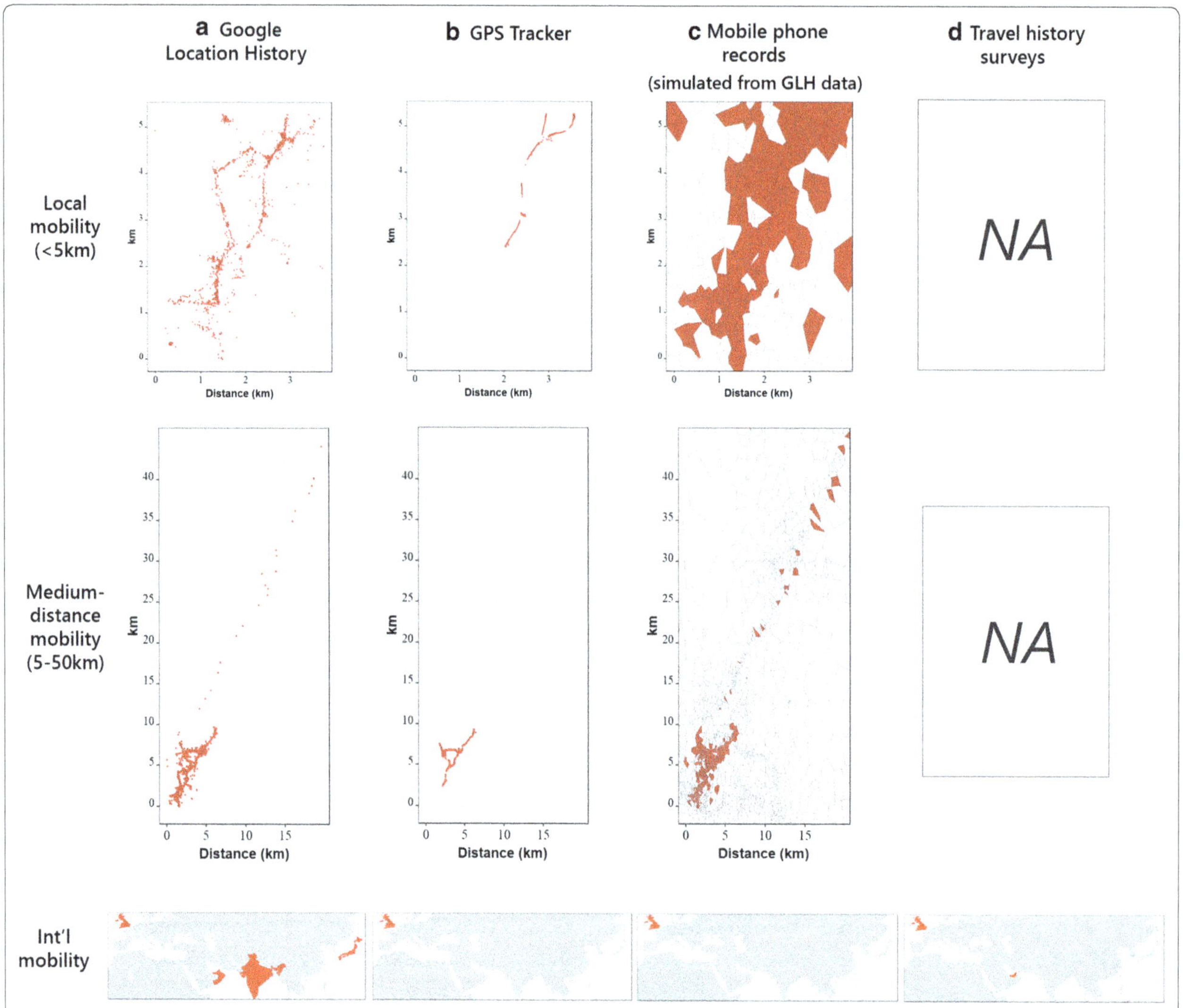

Fig. 3 Location information available at different spatial scales from the **a** GLH, **b** GPS, **c** simulated mobile phone data, and **d** survey data collected during this study. **c** Mobile phone data shown here were simulated using the GLH data, assuming each GLH location point was a call or text event routed through the nearest cell tower. In the simulated mobile phone data, polygons represent Voronoi polygons drawn around cell towers from the OpenCellID dataset, and are colored red if any simulated call/text events were routed through the associated tower

In comparison, the proportion of users reporting having GLH reporting disabled (as measured by a 'No' response to the question) ranged from 5.6% in Brazil to 17.5% in the UK. Other users reported not knowing whether this feature is enabled, ranging from 20% in Mexico to 51% in Japan. Additional file 3 includes more detail on these survey results.

Comparison with common types of mobility data

Figure 4 visualizes the temporal resolution and duration of travel period by data type, with the GLH data collected during this study included. We found that generally, GPS tracker data captured trips at the highest temporal resolution, while travel history surveys did not often capture shorter-term (less than 1 day) travel, and social media

and call detail records enabled by new technologies had the longest travel periods recorded, frequently spanning many months or years. We also found that the GLH data fill a unique niche spanning travel periods of many years similar to CDRs, while also having high temporal resolution similar to GPS tracker data.

Cell tower comparison

We found a statistically significant positive relationship between time since the last GLH data point and distance from the nearest cell tower ($p < .0001$) in a generalized mixed model that included user ID as a random effect to account for individual-level differences in recording behaviour. In this model, we only included points where the time since the previous recording point was less than

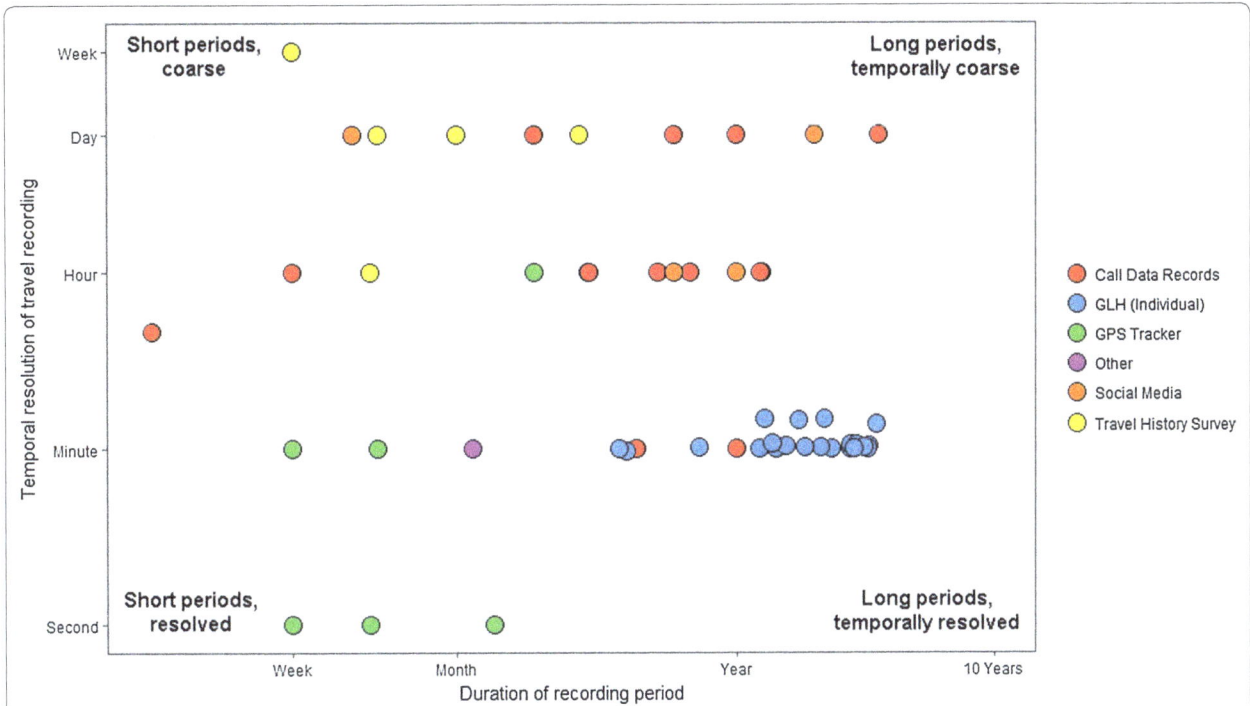

Fig. 4 Temporal breadth and resolution of various data types, from studies found through a rapid literature review. The temporal breadth is the period of time over which travel was reported for that study, and the resolution is the greatest accuracy in mobility (i.e. for CDR and GPS data, the average frequency that location points were recorded, while for travel history surveys, the minimum trip duration for a trip to be recorded). GLH points (in blue) represent individuals in our study, to illustrate the range of breadth and resolution of the collected data

1 week, to account for participants potentially using a phone without GPS functionality or disabling their Android phone's internal GPS. Overall, GLH recording rate increased by 1 s for every additional 7.5 m from the nearest cell tower (regression coefficient .1325). This relationship appeared to be partly driven by high recording rates (every 30 s or less) less than 1 km from the nearest cell tower. When repeated using only points separated by 30 s or more, this relationship became a non-significant positive trend between cell tower distance and ping rate ($p = .2721$). Additional file 3: Fig. S5 shows the relationship between time since last recorded point and distance from the nearest cell tower in more detail.

GPS validation

To validate GLH data as compared to established methods such as GPS trackers, we quantified the spatial percent agreement of GLH and GPS data points. In total, there were 1267 min where both GPS and GLH data were recorded. For these minutes, the GLH data were typically less than 100 m away from the GPS data in the corresponding minute, with a median distance of 64 m separating the GLH and GPS data.

We compared percentage agreement across varying grid cell sizes, which helps identify the spatial resolutions at which GLH data are functionally equivalent to GPS tracker data. We found that the two datasets had roughly 85% agreement when using a gridded surface of cells that were 100×100 m. As expected, this percentage increased with larger grid cells (Fig. 5). The linearly interpolated data generally agreed less, with only 60% agreement using a gridded surface of 100 m $\times$ 100 m cells. At 500 m $\times$ 500 m, the interpolated data began to agree similarly to the non-interpolated data, with roughly 85% agreement between the two datasets.

Two individuals in the GPS+group contained days both with and entirely without GLH data collection, critically allowing us to examine travel patterns on days without GLH data, thereby making inferences about whether these data are not collected as a function of movement. Importantly, the qualitative patterns as measured by the GPS tracker in days with and without GLH data did not appear to differ for these individuals. Specifically, the radius of gyration, a common aggregate measure of movement [2], was .586 decimal-degrees during days without GLH data versus .677 during days with GLH data, suggesting that gaps in the GLH data may not

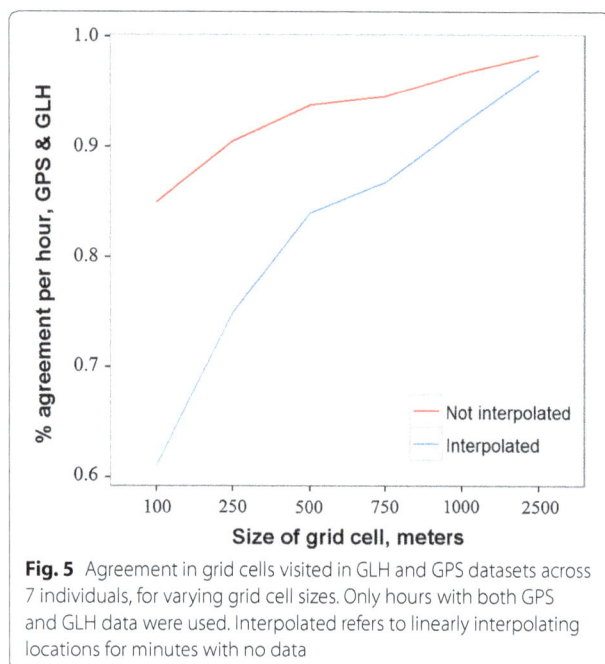

Fig. 5 Agreement in grid cells visited in GLH and GPS datasets across 7 individuals, for varying grid cell sizes. Only hours with both GPS and GLH data were used. Interpolated refers to linearly interpolating locations for minutes with no data

depend on mobility, and are due to user behaviour or other non-mobility related factors.

Discussion

Our results suggest that GLH data could provide unmatched individualized human movement information and address key gaps in currently-available data, including many trips over long periods of time while being spatially resolved (Fig. 3). These data are functionally similar to GPS tracker data (Figs. 3, 4), but are easier to collect in a survey-based study than GPS data and less prone to participant usage issues, as they are passively collected and are easily retrieved by users. We collected these data in conjunction with a questionnaire that addressed self-reported international movement patterns, use of Android phones and various Google services, and provide our study materials for further use in Additional file 3. Other surveys may similarly collect broad demographic information to link with GLH movement data, which currently represents an important gap in human mobility research.

We found that GLH data can provide mobility data over periods and at a resolution infeasible from other typical sources of movement information (Figs. 3, 4) [15, 71], and were more temporally resolved and broad than data used in most recent studies (Fig. 4). We collected roughly two years of data on average from study participants, while studies using GPS trackers generally are only able to collect 1–2 weeks of location data at a time due to battery life issues [28]. Because the GLH data covered

much longer periods, we were able to identify not only very short-distance, circulatory movements (top, Fig. 3a), but also numerous international trips (bottom, Fig. 3a). Furthermore, GLH data contain more fine-scale information than CDR data, since CDR data only identify the cell tower used (top, Fig. 3c), and in this case, cell towers covered an area of 242.8 m^2, suggesting lower accuracy than the GLH data. In reality, CDR data provide less location information than Fig. 3 implies, as calls and texts occur typically much less frequently than the GLH recording average of once per minute, and towers are typically less densely placed than in urban centers like Southampton. On larger spatial scales (bottom, Fig. 3), the GLH data recorded more information than could be reasonably expected to be collected through travel history surveys, collecting information on travel to up to countries, where travel history surveys are generally treated as unreliable after the first few recollected locations. Importantly, the GPS tracker data recorded no international mobility due to the short time span of data collection, and CDR data generally do not include international movement due roaming on cell networks in other countries.

The GLH data were as accurate and representative as GPS tracker data from the same period if aggregated to an appropriate temporal and spatial resolution, such as 500 m or greater (Fig. 5; Additional file 3: Fig. S3). Even still, we found recorded GLH points were generally within 100 m of the corresponding recorded GPS data point, which is significantly better than the best-case scenario of 250 m found with the CDR data in Southampton (Fig. 3). Across a weeklong timescale, these data also generally strongly agreed both when interpolated between minutes and when non-interpolated on grids of 500 m × 500 m or coarser. These are conservative estimates as they assume the GPS tracker data were perfectly accurate, where GPS tracker points are known to vary up to 20 m even when the GPS unit is stationary [28]. While we did observe gaps in GLH data collection, these gaps did not appear to correlate with movement in the two individuals where gaps occurred during GPS data collection and therefore allowed for location tracking when no GLH points were recorded. GLH data collection did appear to correlate with distance from the nearest cell tower, but found that this source of bias can be mitigated by aggregating location points to each minute or longer.

Broad applications

Understanding how people move throughout their daily activities within the context of spatial risks will be important for the health and social sciences, as this would enable a better understanding of the environmental drivers of chronic disease, socioeconomic inequalities, and other issues that involve long-term differences in exposure and mobility. GLH data could yield important insights into disparities in health, wealth, and wellbeing in settings where these analyses were previously impossible, such as in urban centres when considering risks associated with long-term exposure. Because these data are opt-out and are passively-collected as an Android user carries their smartphone, they will often include locational information over longer periods than it is possible to obtain from other sources that collect data at a similar spatial resolution (Fig. 3). While wealthier urban populations tend to have better access to resources such as green spaces [72] and high quality food [73, 74], nearby poorer populations often experience worse social outcomes due in part to the effective inaccessibility of such resources, and use of these resources is best measured across long periods. In these settings, small distances separate populations that spend time in very different places, but GPS trackers generally cannot cover the periods needed. The high resolution of GLH data mean they are one of few viable sources of information for better understanding and mapping these differences towards mapping activity spaces and travel routes across long periods (Fig. 2, 4). These inferences can assist infrastructure and intervention planning, as identifying routes used to access various social and health-oriented resources could identify the most important routes for ensuring equitable infrastructure access [75]. By providing urban planners with better context on not only which infrastructure is most used, but which populations are using various resources, could help promote socially sustainable transport [76], and could help inform urban planning in the context of historically socially-isolated communities [77].

The directly collected nature of obtaining a user's GLH data also means the data pair well with other useful information such as demographics and health related outcomes. As fine scale mobility can differ greatly between people based on income, gender, and other sociodemographic factors, survey data combined with GLH data could determine whether important travel patterns depend on socioeconomic factors, to help target and account for vulnerable populations. Due to their uniquely identifiable nature, however, linking sociodemographic and health information with high resolution mobility data such as GLH raises important privacy considerations, necessitating an ethical obligation to protect participant confidentiality. Confidentiality of sensitive geographic data has been similarly faced by household survey programmes such as the Demographic and Health Surveys (DHS) who release publicly available georeferenced data. Towards this, the DHS outlines common practices in ensuring participant confidentiality, using established techniques such as aggregate data disclosure and geographic masking techniques such as displacement

[78]. By employing these measures, researchers may ensure the benefits of their study do not outweigh individual risk of identification.

Limitations

Critically, GLH data can only be obtained by the user, necessitating a study design similar to typical survey-based research and similar sample sizes. Future work could facilitate faster data collection, by providing an automated process for participants to easily view, download and provide their GLH data to researchers. While this requirement increases the cost of studies that collect GLH data, actively engaging participants during data download also permits simultaneous collection of other demographic or health related information, such as recent infection status of various diseases.

Though the active nature of data retrieval makes large sample sizes difficult to obtain, this makes GLH data complementary with CDRs where both are available. Where GLH data provide fine-scale and international travel and can be collected with individual-level socioeconomic data, CDR data provide comprehensive travel patterns for all people across a country but do not include international movement or locations between call and text events. The two could be directly linked by recording phone numbers when collecting GLH data and linking individuals with their corresponding CDR data. In lieu of directly linked data, relationships between risk, socioeconomic status, location, and mobility in GLH data could help predict risk or socioeconomic characteristics for individuals in CDR data.

We enrolled study participants using non-representative recruitment methods, potentially biasing participants towards those more engaged with new smartphone technologies. This may therefore result in an overrepresentation of GLH data than would be expected in other settings. Further, our study population is comprised of residents within the United Kingdom, which may be more likely to own smartphones and frequently use app-based services such as Google Location History. We confirm that Android users are likely to have GLH data in a variety of countries using Google Surveys (Additional file 3: Fig. S1), but future work will need to better describe smartphone-owning populations and quantify how long various populations are likely to have owned smartphones in areas where GLH data may be collected.

Along these lines, GLH data are currently impossible to collect for many populations, as data collection requires that populations have Android smartphones, and have reliable mobile infrastructure and Internet connection for data retrieval. While these data will likely not be relevant for some of the most vulnerable populations in low income settings, Android phone use is increasing globally and becoming available to more people each year [21, 26]. In many middle income countries, Android has surpassed Windows and all other operating systems as the most common OS for accessing the Internet, and in many of these countries, people are opting to use mobile phone primarily as computing devices over desktop or laptop computers [26].

It is also possible that Android users do not have GLH data, most likely due to having GLH data reporting disabled. In our Southampton sample and in our Google Survey results, we found that this likely does not affect data collection, as a majority of Android users reported having GLH reporting enabled in all countries but Japan in our Google Survey results. Across these surveys, typically 10% or less reported having GLH reporting disabled (Additional file 3: Fig S1). While 20–51% of respondents did not know whether GLH reporting was enabled, because GLH reporting is opt-out, it is likely most of these users have it enabled.

Ultimately, GLH data are a greatly underutilized and novel dataset for understanding human movement, and for mapping activity spaces. While there is a strong bias in populations with GLH data to be wealthier than those without, Android phones are becoming the first and only device purchased to access the Internet and various web services in many middle and lower income settings, making these data increasingly appropriate for a wide range of scientific questions.

Additional files

> **Additional file 1.** Study materials.
>
> **Additional file 2.** Literature review data.
>
> **Additional file 3.** Google Surveys and other Google Location History data (GLH) analysis.

Authors' contributions
NWR CWR JRF: Conception or design of the work. NWR CWR: Data collection. NWR CWR JRF AJT: Data analysis and interpretation. NWR CWR JRF AJT: Drafting the article. NWR CWR JRF AJT: Final approval of the version to be published. All authors read and approved the final manuscript.

Author details
[1] WorldPop Project, Geography and Environment, University of Southampton, Southampton SO17 1BJ, UK. [2] Flowminder Foundation, Roslagsgatan 17, 11355 Stockholm, Sweden.

Acknowledgements
This work forms part of the output of WorldPop (www.worldpop.org) and the Flowminder Foundation (www.flowminder.org). The authors would like to thank the members of the WorldPop Project for helping confirm data collection was possible by viewing their own Google Location History data prior to the study. NWR would also like to thank OP for support and for lending an open ear throughout the data analysis process.

Competing interests
The authors declare that they have no competing interests.

Funding
A.J.T. is supported by funding from the Bill & Melinda Gates Foundation (OPP1182408, OPP1106427, 1032350, OPP1134076), the Clinton Health Access Initiative, National Institutes of Health, a Wellcome Trust Sustaining Health Grant (106866/Z/15/Z), and funds from DFID and the Wellcome Trust (204613/Z/16/Z). N.W.R. is supported by funding from the Bill & Melinda Gates Foundation (OPP1170969). This work was supported by the UK Economic and Social Research Council's Doctoral Training Programme which funds CWR.

References
1. Sturrock HJW, Roberts KW, Wegbreit J, Ohrt C, Gosling RD. Tackling imported malaria: an elimination endgame. Am J Trop Med Hyg. 2015;93:139–44.
2. González MC, Hidalgo CA, Barabási A-L. Understanding individual human mobility patterns. Nature. 2008;453:779–82.
3. Perchoux C, Chaix B, Cummins S, Kestens Y. Conceptualization and measurement of environmental exposure in epidemiology: accounting for activity space related to daily mobility. Health Place. 2013;21:86–93.
4. Kwan M-P. Beyond space (as we knew it): toward temporally integrated geographies of segregation, health, and accessibility. Ann Assoc Am Geogr. 2013;103:1078–86.
5. Järv O, Müürisepp K, Ahas R, Derudder B, Witlox F. Ethnic differences in activity spaces as a characteristic of segregation: a study based on mobile phone usage in Tallinn, Estonia. Urban Stud. 2015;52:2680–98.
6. Perkins TA, Garcia AJ, Paz-Soldán VA, Stoddard ST, Reiner RC, Vazquez-Prokopec G, et al. Theory and data for simulating fine-scale human movement in an urban environment. J R Soc Interface. 2014;11:20140642. https://doi.org/10.1098/rsif.2014.0642.
7. Horton FE, Reynolds DR. Effects of urban spatial structure on individual behavior. Econ Geogr. 1971;47:36–48.
8. Setton E, Marshall JD, Brauer M, Lundquist KR, Hystad P, Keller P, et al. The impact of daily mobility on exposure to traffic-related air pollution and health effect estimates. J Expo Sci Environ Epidemiol. 2011;21:42–8.
9. Ruktanonchai CW, Ruktanonchai NW, Nove A, Lopes S, Pezzulo C, Bosco C, et al. Equality in maternal and newborn health: modelling geographic disparities in utilisation of care in five east African countries. PLoS ONE. 2016;11:e0162006.
10. Gabrysch S, Campbell OM. Still too far to walk: literature review of the determinants of delivery service use. BMC Pregnancy Childbirth. 2009;9:34.
11. Wesolowski A, O'Meara WP, Tatem AJ, Ndege S, Eagle N, Buckee CO. Quantifying the impact of accessibility on preventive healthcare in Sub-Saharan Africa using mobile phone data. Epidemiol Camb Mass. 2015;26:223–8.
12. Phithakkitnukoon S, Smoreda Z. Influence of social relations on human mobility and sociality: a study of social ties in a cellular network. Soc Netw Anal Min. 2016;6:42.

13. Huang Q, Wong DWS. Activity patterns, socioeconomic status and urban spatial structure: what can social media data tell us? Int J Geogr Inf Sci. 2016;30:1873–98.

14. Matthews SA, Yang T-C. Spatial polygamy and contextual exposures (SPACEs): promoting activity space approaches in research on place and health. Am Behav Sci. 2013;57:1057–81.

15. Pindolia DK, Garcia AJ, Wesolowski A, Smith DL, Buckee CO, Noor AM, et al. Human movement data for malaria control and elimination strategic planning. Malar J. 2012;11:205.

16. Tatem AJ. Mapping population and pathogen movements. Int Health. 2014;6:5–11.

17. Vazquez-Prokopec GM, Bisanzio D, Stoddard ST, Paz-Soldan V, Morrison AC, Elder JP, et al. Using GPS technology to quantify human mobility, dynamic contacts and infectious disease dynamics in a resource-poor urban environment. PLoS ONE. 2013;8:e58802.

18. Abel GJ, Sander N. Quantifying global international migration flows. Science. 2014;343:1520–2.

19. Bharti N, Lu X, Bengtsson L, Wetter E, Tatem AJ. Remotely measuring populations during a crisis by overlaying two data sources. Int Health. 2015;7:90–8.

20. Stathakis D, Baltas P. Seasonal population estimates based on night-time lights. Comput Environ Urban Syst. 2018;68:133–41.

21. Burton SH, Tanner KW, Giraud-Carrier CG, West JH, Barnes MD. "Right time, right place" health communication on Twitter: value and accuracy of location information. J Med Internet Res. 2012;14:e156.

22. Lu X, Wetter E, Bharti N, Tatem AJ, Bengtsson L. Approaching the limit of predictability in human mobility. Sci Rep. 2013;3:2923.

23. Paz-Soldan VA, Reiner RC Jr, Morrison AC, Stoddard ST, Kitron U, Scott TW, et al. Strengths and weaknesses of Global Positioning System (GPS) data-loggers and semi-structured interviews for capturing fine-scale human mobility: findings from Iquitos, Peru. PLoS Negl Trop Dis. 2014;8:e2888.

24. Zhao Z, Shaw S-L, Xu Y, Lu F, Chen J, Yin L. Understanding the bias of call detail records in human mobility research. Int J Geogr Inf Sci. 2016;30:1738–62.

25. MacLean D, Komatineni S, Allen G. Exploring maps and location-based services. In: MacLean D, Komatineni S, Allen G, editors. Pro Android 5. Berkeley: Apress; 2015. p. 405–49. https://doi.org/10.1007/978-1-4302-4681-7_19.

26. StatCounter Global Stats. StatCounter Global Stats. StatCounter Global Stats. http://gs.statcounter.com/. Accessed 4 Apr 2018.

27. Poushter J. Smartphone ownership and internet usage continues to climb in emerging economies. Pew Research Center's Global Attitudes Project. 2016. http://www.pewglobal.org/2016/02/22/smartphone-ownership-and-internet-usage-continues-to-climb-in-emerging-economies/. Accessed 4 Apr 2018.

28. Vazquez-Prokopec GM, Stoddard ST, Paz-Soldan V, Morrison AC, Elder JP, Kochel TJ, et al. Usefulness of commercially available GPS data-loggers for tracking human movement and exposure to dengue virus. Int J Health Geogr. 2009;8:68.

29. Bengtsson L, Gaudart J, Lu X, Moore S, Wetter E, Sallah K, et al. Using mobile phone data to predict the spatial spread of cholera. Sci Rep. 2015;5:8923. https://doi.org/10.1038/srep08923.

30. Brucker DL, Rollins NG. Trips to medical care among persons with disabilities: evidence from the 2009 National Household Travel Survey. Disabil Health J. 2016;9:539–43.

31. Calabrese F, Lorenzo GD, Ratti C. Human mobility prediction based on individual and collective geographical preferences. In: 13th international IEEE conference on intelligent transportation systems. 2010. p. 312–7.

32. Cho E, Myers SA, Leskovec J. Friendship and mobility: user movement in location-based social networks. In: Proceedings of the 17th ACM SIGKDD international conference on knowledge discovery and data mining. New York: ACM; 2011. p. 1082–1090. https://doi.org/10.1145/2020408.2020579.

33. Deville P, Linard C, Martin S, Gilbert M, Stevens FR, Gaughan AE, et al. Dynamic population mapping using mobile phone data. Proc Natl Acad Sci. 2014;111:15888–93.

34. Dewulf B, Neutens T, Lefebvre W, Seynaeve G, Vanpoucke C, Beckx C, et al. Dynamic assessment of exposure to air pollution using mobile phone data. Int J Health Geogr. 2016;15:14.

35. Finger F, Genolet T, Mari L, de Magny GC, Manga NM, Rinaldo A, et al. Mobile phone data highlights the role of mass gatherings in the spreading of cholera outbreaks. Proc Natl Acad Sci. 2016;113:6421–6.

36. Garske T, Yu H, Peng Z, Ye M, Zhou H, Cheng X, et al. Travel Patterns in China. PLOS ONE. 2011;6:e16364.

37. Giannotti F, Nanni M, Pedreschi D, Pinelli F, Renso C, Rinzivillo S, et al. Unveiling the complexity of human mobility by querying and mining massive trajectory data. VLDB J. 2011;20:695–719.

38. Hine J, Kamruzzaman M. Journeys to health services in Great Britain: an analysis of changing travel patterns 1985–2006. Health Place. 2012;18:274–85.

39. Jaeger VK, Tschudi N, Rüegg R, Hatz C, Bühler S. The elderly, the young and the pregnant traveler: a retrospective data analysis from a large Swiss Travel Center with a special focus on malaria prophylaxis and yellow fever vaccination. Travel Med Infect Dis. 2015;13:475–84.

40. Jurdak R, Zhao K, Liu J, AbouJaoude M, Cameron M, Newth D. Understanding human mobility from Twitter. PLoS ONE. 2015;10:e0131469.

41. Li L, Yang L, Zhu H, Dai R. Explorative analysis of wuhan intra-urban human mobility using social media check-in data. PLoS ONE. 2015;10:e0135286.

42. Marshall JM, Wu SL, Kiware SS, Ndhlovu M, Ouédraogo AL, et al. Mathematical models of human mobility of relevance to malaria transmission in Africa. Sci Rep. 2018;8:7713.

43. Padgham M. Human movement is both diffusive and directed. PLoS ONE. 2012;7:e37754.

44. Palmer JRB, Espenshade TJ, Bartumeus F, Chung CY, Ozgencil NE, Li K. New approaches to human mobility: using mobile phones for demographic research. Demography. 2013;50:1105–28.

45. Peng C, Jin X, Wong K-C, Shi M, Liò P. Collective human mobility pattern from taxi trips in urban area. PLoS ONE. 2012;7:e34487.

46. Phithakkitnukoon S, Smoreda Z, Olivier P. Socio-geography of human mobility: a study using longitudinal mobile phone data. PLoS ONE. 2012;7:e39253.

47. Ruktanonchai NW, Bhavnani D, Sorichetta A, Bengtsson L, Carter KH, Córdoba RC, et al. Census-derived migration data as a tool for informing malaria elimination policy. Malar J. 2016;15:273.

48. Ruktanonchai NW, DeLeenheer P, Tatem AJ, Alegana VA, Caughlin TT, zu Erbach-Schoenberg E, et al. Identifying malaria transmission foci for elimination using human mobility data. PLoS Comput Biol. 2016;12:e1004846.

49. Song C, Qu Z, Blumm N, Barabási A-L. Limits of predictability in human mobility. Science. 2010;327:1018–21.

50. Stoddard ST, Forshey BM, Morrison AC, Paz-Soldan VA, Vazquez-Prokopec GM, Astete H, et al. House-to-house human movement drives dengue virus transmission. Proc Natl Acad Sci. 2013;110:994–9.

51. Tatem AJ, Qiu Y, Smith DL, Sabot O, Ali AS, Moonen B. The use of mobile phone data for the estimation of the travel patterns and imported *Plasmodium falciparum* rates among Zanzibar residents. Malar J. 2009;8:287.

52. Tizzoni M, Bajardi P, Decuyper A, King GKK, Schneider CM, Blondel V, et al. On the use of human mobility proxies for modeling epidemics. PLoS Comput Biol. 2014;10:e1003716.

53. Toole JL, Herrera-Yaqüe C, Schneider CM, González MC. Coupling human mobility and social ties. J R Soc Interface. 2015;12:20141128.

54. Wang D, Pedreschi D, Song C, Giannotti F, Barabasi A-L. Human mobility, social ties, and link prediction. In: Proceedings of the 17th ACM SIGKDD international conference on knowledge discovery and data mining. New York: ACM; 2011. p. 1100–8. https://doi.org/10.1145/2020408.2020581.

55. Wang Q, Taylor JE. Quantifying human mobility perturbation and resilience in hurricane sandy. PLoS ONE. 2014;9:e112608.

56. Wang Q, Taylor JE. Patterns and limitations of urban human mobility resilience under the influence of multiple types of natural disaster. PLoS ONE. 2016;11:e0147299.

57. Wesolowski A, Buckee CO, Pindolia DK, Eagle N, Smith DL, Garcia AJ, et al. The use of census migration data to approximate human movement patterns across temporal scales. PLoS ONE. 2013;8:e52971.

58. Wesolowski A, Qureshi T, Boni MF, Sundsøy PR, Johansson MA, Rasheed SB, et al. Impact of human mobility on the emergence of dengue epidemics in Pakistan. Proc Natl Acad Sci. 2015;112:11887–92.

59. Wesolowski A, Stresman G, Eagle N, Stevenson J, Owaga C, Marube E, et al. Quantifying travel behavior for infectious disease research: a comparison of data from surveys and mobile phones. Sci Rep. 2014;4:5678. https://doi.org/10.1038/srep05678.

60. Wiehe SE, Carroll AE, Liu GC, Haberkorn KL, Hoch SC, Wilson JS, et al. Using GPS-enabled cell phones to track the travel patterns of adolescents. Int J Health Geogr. 2008;7:22.

61. Wu J, Jiang C, Jaimes G, Bartell S, Dang A, Baker D, et al. Travel patterns during pregnancy: comparison between Global Positioning System (GPS) tracking and questionnaire data. Environ Health. 2013;12:86.

62. Wu L, Zhi Y, Sui Z, Liu Y. Intra-urban human mobility and activity transition: evidence from social media check-in data. PLoS ONE. 2014;9:e97010.

63. Yen IH, Leung CW, Lan M, Sarrafzadeh M, Kayekjian KC, Duru OK. A pilot study using Global Positioning Systems (GPS) devices and surveys to ascertain older adults' travel patterns. J Appl Gerontol. 2015;34:NP190–201.

64. Yukich JO, Taylor C, Eisele TP, Reithinger R, Nauhassenay H, Berhane Y, et al. Travel history and malaria infection risk in a low-transmission setting in Ethiopia: a case control study. Malar J. 2013;12:33.

65. zu Erbach-Schoenberg E, Alegana VA, Sorichetta A, Linard C, Lourenço C, Ruktanonchai NW, et al. Dynamic denominators: the impact of seasonally varying population numbers on disease incidence estimates. Popul Health Metr. 2016;14:35.

66. Resch B, Arif A, Krings G, Vankeerberghen G, Buekenhout M. Deriving hospital catchment areas from mobile phone data. In: International Conference on GIScience Short Paper Proceedings, vol. 1. 2016. https://doi.org/10.21433/b31154n7c1z2.

67. Hay SI, Guerra CA, Gething PW, Patil AP, Tatem AJ, Noor AM, et al. A world malaria map: *Plasmodium falciparum* endemicity in 2007. PLOS Med. 2009;6:e1000048.

68. Beelen R, Hoek G, Pebesma E, Vienneau D, de Hoogh K, Briggs DJ. Mapping of background air pollution at a fine spatial scale across the European Union. Sci Total Environ. 2009;407:1852–67.

69. Kuhn C, Johnson D, Ream R, Gelatt T. Advances in the tracking of marine species: using GPS locations to evaluate satellite track data and a continuous-time movement model. Mar Ecol Prog Ser. 2009;393:97–109.

70. Li J, Taylor G, Kidner DB. Accuracy and reliability of map-matched GPS coordinates: the dependence on terrain model resolution and interpolation algorithm. Comput Geosci. 2005;31:241–51.

71. Stoddard ST, Morrison AC, Vazquez-Prokopec GM, Soldan VP, Kochel TJ, Kitron U, et al. The role of human movement in the transmission of vector-borne pathogens. PLoS Negl Trop Dis. 2009;3:e481.

72. Matthew McConnachie M, Shackleton CM. Public green space inequality in small towns in South Africa. Habitat Int. 2010;34:244–8.

73. Larsen K, Gilliland J. Mapping the evolution of "food deserts" in a Canadian city: supermarket accessibility in London, Ontario, 1961–2005. Int J Health Geogr. 2008;7:16.

74. Battersby J. Urban food insecurity in Cape Town, South Africa: an alternative approach to food access. Dev South Afr. 2011;28:545–61.

75. Keeling DJ. Transportation geography: local challenges, global contexts. Prog Hum Geogr. 2009;33:516–26.

76. Boschmann EE, Kwan M-P. Toward socially sustainable urban transportation: progress and potentials. Int J Sustain Transp. 2008;2:138–57.

77. Donaldson R. Mass rapid rail development in South Africa's metropolitan core: towards a new urban form? Land Use Policy. 2006;23:344–52.

78. Burgert CR, Colston J, Roy T, Zachary B. Geographic displacement procedure and georeferenced data release policy for the Demographic and Health Surveys. Calverton: ICF International; 2013. http://dhsprogram.com/pubs/pdf/SAR7/SAR7.pdf.

8

Does the edge effect impact on the measure of spatial accessibility to healthcare providers?

Fei Gao[1,3,5*], Wahida Kihal[2], Nolwenn Le Meur[1,3,5], Marc Souris[4] and Séverine Deguen[1,6]

Abstract

Background: Spatial accessibility indices are increasingly applied when investigating inequalities in health. Although most studies are making mentions of potential errors caused by the edge effect, many acknowledge having neglected to consider this concern by establishing spatial analyses within a finite region, settling for hypothesizing that accessibility to facilities will be under-reported. Our study seeks to assess the effect of edge on the accuracy of defining healthcare provider access by comparing healthcare provider accessibility accounting or not for the edge effect, in a real-world application.

Methods: This study was carried out in the department of Nord, France. The statistical unit we use is the French census block known as 'IRIS' (Ilot Regroupé pour l'Information Statistique), defined by the National Institute of Statistics and Economic Studies. The geographical accessibility indicator used is the "Index of Spatial Accessibility" (ISA), based on the E2SFCA algorithm. We calculated ISA for the pregnant women population by selecting three types of healthcare providers: general practitioners, gynecologists and midwives. We compared ISA variation when accounting or not edge effect in urban and rural zones. The GIS method was then employed to determine global and local autocorrelation. Lastly, we compared the relationship between socioeconomic distress index and ISA, when accounting or not for the edge effect, to fully evaluate its impact.

Results: The results revealed that on average ISA when offer and demand beyond the boundary were included is slightly below ISA when not accounting for the edge effect, and we found that the IRIS value was more likely to deteriorate than improve. Moreover, edge effect impact can vary widely by health provider type. There is greater variability within the rural IRIS group than within the urban IRIS group. We found a positive correlation between socioeconomic distress variables and composite ISA. Spatial analysis results (such as Moran's spatial autocorrelation index and local indicators of spatial autocorrelation) are not really impacted.

Conclusion: Our research has revealed minor accessibility variation when edge effect has been considered in a French context. No general statement can be set up because intensity of impact varies according to healthcare provider type, territorial organization and methodology used to measure the accessibility to healthcare. Additional researches are required in order to distinguish what findings are specific to a territory and others common to different countries. It constitute a promising direction to determine more precisely healthcare shortage areas and then to fight against social health inequalities.

Keywords: Edge effect, Potential spatial accessibility of healthcare professionals, E2SFCA algorithm, Geographic information systems, Spatial analyses, Pregnant women

*Correspondence: fei.gao@ehesp.fr
[5] Department of Quantitative Methods for Public Health, EHESP School of Public Health, Avenue du Professeur Léon Bernard, 35043 Rennes, France
Full list of author information is available at the end of the article

Background

Equitable distribution of health resources is a key priority for health professionals and policy makers worldwide; reducing health inequalities has long been of concern to community and public health planners [1–4]. Access to healthcare, as one potential driver of health inequalities, is at the heart of public health policy and is internationally recognized as a key goal in meeting the essential health needs of individuals [5–8].

Access to healthcare varies across space due to the uneven distribution of both healthcare providers and consumers, and the impact of geographical location on health is increasingly being examined. Various studies in Europe (including France) have shown unequal distribution of health service resources [9]. With heightened interest in residential neighborhood the characteristics that could influence health behaviors and outcomes, spatial accessibility and availability indices are being used in epidemiological studies more and more [10–15]. As a measure for determining those areas having inadequate levels of health service provision, spatial accessibility of health services refers to relative access to health services in a given location, which is influenced primarily by travel distance (or travel time) and the spatial distribution of health service providers and consumers [16–18]. Most studies examining the geographical accessibility of healthcare and health-related services have suggested a growing range of indices, including Physician Population Ratio, nearest distance, shortest time, cumulative opportunity and the gravity model [5, 19–26]. Recent methodological developments in this field have emerged in international research, including Enhanced 2-Step Floating Catchment Area method (E2SFCA) [27], which provides a summary measure of two important and related components of access: volume of services provided relative to population size, and proximity of services provided relative to population location.

In addition, one methodological limitation often mentioned in research considering accessibility concerns the fact that studies failed to include behavior outside the study area [17, 28–39]. Known as the edge effect, it is central to this paper. Edge effect occurs "when the study area is defined by a border which does not actually prevent travel across the border" [40] and people are free to travel beyond that border to receive healthcare goods and services. Arbitrary administrative boundaries (such as census tracts or block groups) are often used without consideration that resources beyond a given boundary are likely to affect behaviors within a given spatial unit [35]. This means that any geographic distribution or spatial interaction occurring within the spatial unit may extend beyond its boundaries [30]. More precisely, edge effects manifest when the boundaries of the study area

affect a given spatial measurement and lead to the distortion of estimates [35, 41]. Interestingly, although most studies do mention potential errors caused by the edge effect, many acknowledge their mistake in neglecting to consider this in the spatial analyses they have undertaken within a finite region [42]. Because this can result in areas close to the boundary being classified as having poor geographic access even though they may in fact be proximate to resources across the boundary, many research projects have hypothesized that failure to accounting for edge effect will lead to considerable biases [34–37], even under-reporting [17, 28, 29, 31, 43] of accessibility to facilities.

Although edge effect is a well-documented phenomenon, researches choosing this issue as the main subject used for most of the time distance/travel time measure [34, 35], or availability measures such cumulative index [28, 34, 35, 38, 43]. Focusing on E2SFCA method, the edge effect is frequently observed in studies measuring the spatial accessibility to healthcare providers. More and more studies have corrected for edge effects [32, 33]. However, to the best of our knowledge, very few studies based on E2SFCA have focused on edge effect in a real-world application with a view to quantifying its effect on the accuracy of defining health service access.

In this context, our study compares health service accessibility when accounting or not for the edge effect, taking into account that patients may overcome geographical boundaries, choosing to consult health professionals in neighboring departments. The geographical accessibility indicator used to quantify spatial accessibility is the *Index of spatial accessibility* (*ISA*), based on the E2SFCA algorithm. ISA was previously developed by our team for the pregnant women population, focusing on the three types of healthcare professionals (GP, midwife and gynecologist) involved during the pregnancy [44]. Conducted in the department of Nord at French census block spatial scale, our study aimed to quantify edge effect bias using the ISA index, and investigate the impact on spatial analysis results.

Besides, it is well documented that levels of accessibility and utilization of healthcare are related with socio-economic distress level and geographical factors [45–48]. Consequently, in our study, we investigated the urban–rural disparity of ISA as well as the relationship of ISA with socioeconomic distress variables, both when offer and demand beyond the area of study are excluded or included. The underlying questions are: Would the association between socioeconomic factor and accessibility be biased by ignoring spatial interaction occurring between the spatial unit and its neighborhood? Would the difference of accessibly between urban/rural areas be accentuated?

Methods
Data and measures
Study setting and statistical unit

This study was carried out in the department of Nord, located in the north of France, close to the Belgian border. Analysis was conducted at French census block level (known as IRIS: "Ilots Regroupés pour l'Information Statistique") defined by the National Institute of Statistics and Economic Studies (INSEE) [49], which is the smallest infra-urban level for which census data is available. There are 1346 IRIS in the department of Nord.

Neighborhood characteristics

Two types of neighborhood characteristic were used at census-block level:

(i) *Degree of urbanization (rural/urban)* Each IRIS was classified as urban or rural according to the classification established by the national census bureau. These data are openly available from (https://www.insee.fr/fr/information/2017499) [49].
(ii) *Level of socioeconomic distress* According to previous work on social health inequality [50], we selected five variables from the 2006 French census (https://www.insee.fr/fr/information/2017499) [49] to characterize the neighborhood socioeconomic level: low level of educational attainment, women's unemployment rate, single parent families, non-homeowner, and insecure employment situation (see variables definition in "Appendix I").

Health professionals

The postal addresses of GPs, midwives and gynecologists were obtained from the French state health insurance website (http://www.ameli-sante.fr) in 2014 [51]. To assess the edge effect, we considered the health professional offer both within and outside of the department of Nord. Service providers were represented by their geocoded professional addresses (latitude, longitude), obtained through Batch Geocoder (http://dehaese.free.fr/Gmaps/testGeocoder.htm). Eight general practitioners and one obstetrical gynecologist were excluded from the analysis due to low quality of professional postal addresses. No georeferencing quality difference was detected between adjacent department and Nord Department. Further methodological details are available elsewhere [44].

Index of spatial accessibility (ISA)

ISA is an indicator which measures healthcare service accessibility.

The ISA is based on the E2SFCA method, a method which maintains the advantages of a gravity model while

being easier to interpret, since it represents a derived form of a Physician Population Ratio. As the name suggests, two steps must be performed:

Step 1 For each provider in location k, look up all population locations of IRIS i within a catchment, and within a predefined distance d_{ik} from location k. A distance decay function is applied within a catchment. $w(d_{ik})$ is the weight quantifying travel time between IRIS i and healthcare provider k. Sum up all population sizes (Pi) within that catchment area to compute the provider-to-population ratio (R_k):

$$R_k = \frac{1}{\sum_{d_{jk}<d_{max}} P_i * w(d_{ik})} \quad (1)$$

Step 2 For each population location i, look up all provider locations k that are within the catchment from location i. Sum up all R_k for the catchment area to calculate the Index of spatial accessibility (ISA_i) at location i:

$$ISA_i = \sum_{d_{ij}\leq d_{max}} w(d_{ij})R_k \quad (2)$$

ISA takes into account:

(i) The latitude and longitude of each healthcare professional.
(ii) The centroids of residential buildings for each IRIS (Residential buildings came from BD TOPO® and was provided by the *Institut National de l'Information Géographique et Forestière (French National Geographic Institute)* [52]). And
(iii) Car travel time, calculated by Google Maps. We used the FILENAME statement and the URL access method within SAS to access Google Maps, and extracted both the driving time and distance each time the site was accessed [44, 53].

We estimated an ISA for GPs, gynecologists and midwives, separately. A composite ISA relying on principal component analysis was also calculated, describing overall accessibility of the three types of healthcare professionals. Further details of the method developed for ISA estimation are given in [44].

Decay function and travel time threshold

We defined the time threshold according to figures already published by *the French Institute for research and information in health economics* for general practitioners [54]:

- less than 5 min' travel: fully access to healthcare providers ($w = 1$)
- more than 15 min' travel: no access to healthcare providers ($w = 0$).
- between 5 and 15 min: partial access to healthcare providers (w is defined by a continuous decay function [Eq. (3)] with the weighting factor equal to 1.5 [55])

$$w = \frac{(15 - d)}{(15 - 5)} e^{1.5} \tag{3}$$

We based the threshold of the two other healthcare professionals on general practitioners' results: the nearest travel time to general practitioner is lower than 5 min and between 5 and 15 min for 88 and 12% of the population, respectively; we used these proportions to define the threshold for two other health professionals: 15 and 34 min for gynecologists and 17 and 34 min for midwives.

Figure 1 provides an illustration of the impact of including offers and demands outside the study area defining what we call the "patient area" or catchment. This illustration deals with gynecologists only for the IRIS named "Fournes-en-Weppes" (IRIS no. 592 500 000), with keys for reading.

Keys for reading Fig. 1 and fully understanding the principle of edge effect:

- Figure 1a—study area without consideration of offer and demand beyond the boundary
- All 218 gynecologists are represented by dark purple dots. The IRIS "Fournes-en-Weppes" is highlighted in fuchsia and circled in orange. We count 146 gynecologists accessible by car within 34 min of Fournes-en-Weppes, within the study area. The 1201 IRIS are highlighted in purple forms the "patient area" of the 146 gynecologists (circled in orange). Figure 1b—study area with consideration of offer and demand beyond the boundary

With edge effect, the residents of Fournes-en-Weppes could reach 181 gynecologists (an additional 35 from outside) within 34 min by car. However, they must share these with 2203 IRIS (1001 IRIS from outside). "Patient area" IRIS are colored purple.

GIS methods
We began by quantifying a global ISA spatial autocorrelation, separately with, and without, consideration of offer and demand beyond the department of Nord, based on Moran's I statistic (calculated by means of the distance matrix) [56–58]. Spatial autocorrelation can be defined as

the coincidence of value similarity and locational similarity [59]. Positive spatial autocorrelation therefore exists where the high or low values of a random variable tend to be spatially clustered, with negative spatial autocorrelation existing where geographical areas tend to be surrounded by neighbors having highly dissimilar values. The values of the Moran's I statistic range from -1 to $+1$.

Next, a Local Indicator of Spatial Autocorrelation (LISA) was applied. More precisely, Moran's diagram was produced in order to reveal the types of spatial relationship between a geographic unit and its neighboring area.

Four types of LISA can be detected: High–High (HH): high level of ISA in both a given IRIS and in its neighbors and Low–Low (LL): low level of ISA in both a given IRIS and in its neighbors, characterizing a positive association; High–Low (HL): high level of ISA in a given IRIS, whereas its neighbors have a low level of ISA and Low–High (LH): low level of ISA in a given IRIS, whereas its neighbors have high level of ISA, characterizing a negative association.

Statistical analysis
Classification
In order to analyze ISA variations when offer and demand outside are included, the 1346 IRIS making up the Nord department are divided into three classes, named *improved, unchanged* and *deteriorated*. These classes were constructed according to the results obtained using the simple linear regression model, where Y and X correspond to the ISA estimated with and without taking into account offer and demand across the boundary, respectively (see "Appendix II").

Statistical associations
ISA's composite values when offer and demand beyond the boundary were then cross-referenced with the individual variables of socioeconomic distress mentioned in the data section. The statistical significance of the relation was tested using a simple linear regression where Y and X were the ISA index and one of the socioeconomic variables, respectively. The α-risk was set at 5%.

Strategy and the statistical analysis plan
Preliminary work was carried out to study ISA variation when offer and demand outside are excluded or included, and the spatial distribution of this variation. To quantify overall and local autocorrelation of ISA in the two cases, the GIS method was then applied. Following this, we analyzed the ISA variation for urban and rural zones, separately. Finally, we compared the relationship between the socioeconomic distress variable and ISA, to find out whether there is an impact when studying the association,

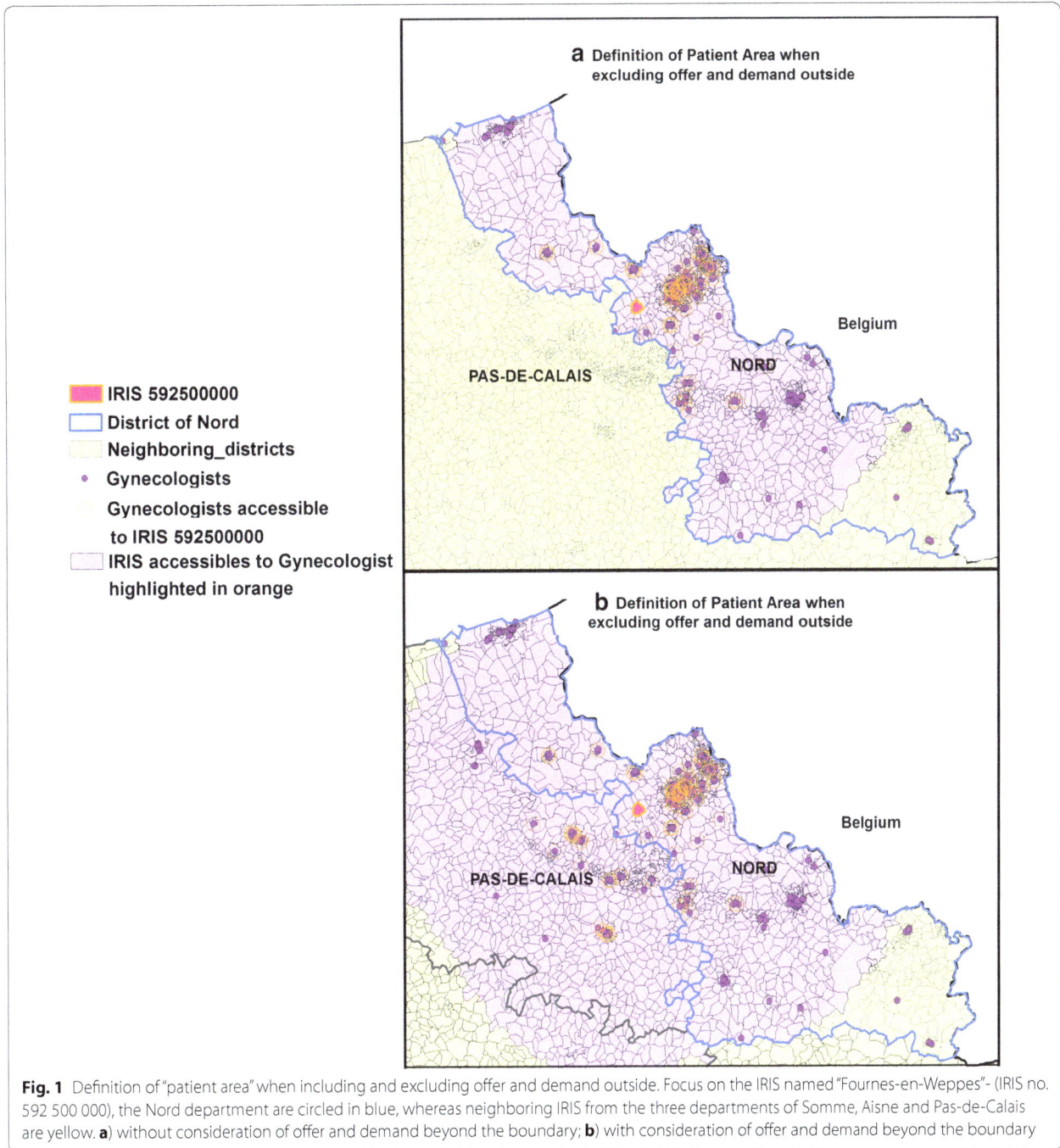

Fig. 1 Definition of "patient area" when including and excluding offer and demand outside. Focus on the IRIS named "Fournes-en-Weppes"- (IRIS no. 592 500 000), the Nord department are circled in blue, whereas neighboring IRIS from the three departments of Somme, Aisne and Pas-de-Calais are yellow. **a**) without consideration of offer and demand beyond the boundary; **b**) with consideration of offer and demand beyond the boundary

both when excluding and including healthcare offer and demand outside the area of study, to account for a deficiency in analysis termed the "edge effect".

Results
Descriptive results
When excluding healthcare providers outside the department boundary, we geolocalized 2590 GPs, 143 midwives and 218 gynecologists. In order to include offer and demand beyond outside, we added 493 GPs, 60 midwives and 78 gynecologists from the neighboring area who were capable of providing services to those residing in the department of Nord. Ignoring the offer beyond the department led to an 18% decrease in the total number of health professionals potentially available; this decrease reaches 30% when focusing on midwives (Table 1).

Table 1 Number of health professionals by medical specialty

Medical special-ity of health professional	Number of healthcare providers			Number of IRIS of "patient area"			
	Department of Nord	Neighboring IRIS	% increase	Department of Nord	Average popula-tion	Neighboring IRIS	Average popu-lation
GPs	2590	493	16	1346	1905	1362	1076
Midwives	143	60	30	1346	386	2425	187
Gynecologists	218	78	26	1346	986	2583	484
Total	2951	631	18	–	–	–	–

After calculation of travel time via Google Maps, when including offer and demand beyond the boundary, "patient area" is not restricted to the 1346 IRIS of the department of Nord. In all, 1362, 2425 and 2583 IRIS in the departments of Pas-de-Calais, Oise, Somme, Aisne and Ardennes are added to the ISA calculation for GPs, midwives and gynecologists respectively (Table 1). The "average population" columns show that les IRIS neighboring have lower population density than IRIS Nord.

The descriptive statistics of the ISA when offer and demand beyond the study area are included or excluded are presented in Table 2. Mean and standard deviation are slightly below when offer and demand outside are taken into account, whichever health professionals are included. The two-means comparison is only statistically different for ISA gynecologist ($p < 0.00$).

Spatial distribution of ISA at IRIS level

Spatial distributions of ISA for GPs (a), midwives (b) and gynecologists (c) considered separately, and combined in the composite index (d) when offer and demand beyond the department of Nord are included or not (Fig. 2). The maps show minor changes: ISA distributions in the two cases are fairly similar. Changes appear mainly in those IRIS located close to boundaries.

Accounting for edge effect

In order to focus on ISA variation when offer and demand beyond the study area were included, we distributed the 1346 IRIS into three classes: improved, unchanged and deteriorated according to simple linear regression results (presented with more detail in "Appendix II").

Figure 3 shows that when accounting for healthcare provider source and patient needs outside the area of Nord the percentage of IRIS having decreased ISA is larger than those with increased ISA (13.15 vs. 5.50% for GPs; 29.79 vs. 15.68% for midwives and 30.46 vs. 9.88% for gynecologists). Many past researches have hypothe-sized that failure to accounting for edge effect will lead to considerable under-reporting of accessibility to facilities. We obtain the exact opposite findings. The composite ISA which give an overall view of accessibility to various types of health professionals is subject to a slight edge effect (25.33% deteriorated and 21.55% improved). Those IRIS too far from boundaries to be affected are colored in grey ("outside service area" in the key).

It can be observed in Fig. 4 that IRIS where GPs ISA changed are mainly located close to the boundaries. Conversely, only 36 IRIS where midwives ISA are not impacted as a result of distance, and 2 IRIS for gynecol-ogists ISA. The white zone does not mean that they are not subject to edge effect, but rather reveal the existence

Table 2 Descriptive statistics of ISA when accounting or not for the edge effect—North department

	When not accounting for the edge effects			When accounting edge effects		
	Min[¥]	Mean (SD*)	Max[φ]	Min[¥]	Mean (SD*)	Max[φ]
GPs	1.67	93.42 (35.74)	245.88	1.67	92.98 (35.17)	245.88
Midwives	0	22.64 (11.57)	50.29	0	21.16 (11.06)	49.90
Gynecologists	0	22.47 (9.51)	43.76	0	20.20 (8.62)	41.46
Composite index**	0.40	39.38 (14.19)	91.43	0.41	39.40 (13.92)	91.98

ISA GPs is expressed per 100,000 inhabitants, ISA Midwives per 100,000 women inhabitants aged between 15 and 44 and ISA gynecologists per 100,000 women inhabitants

*Standard deviation

**Composite ISA resulting from the principal component analysis

[¥] Minimum

[φ] Maximum

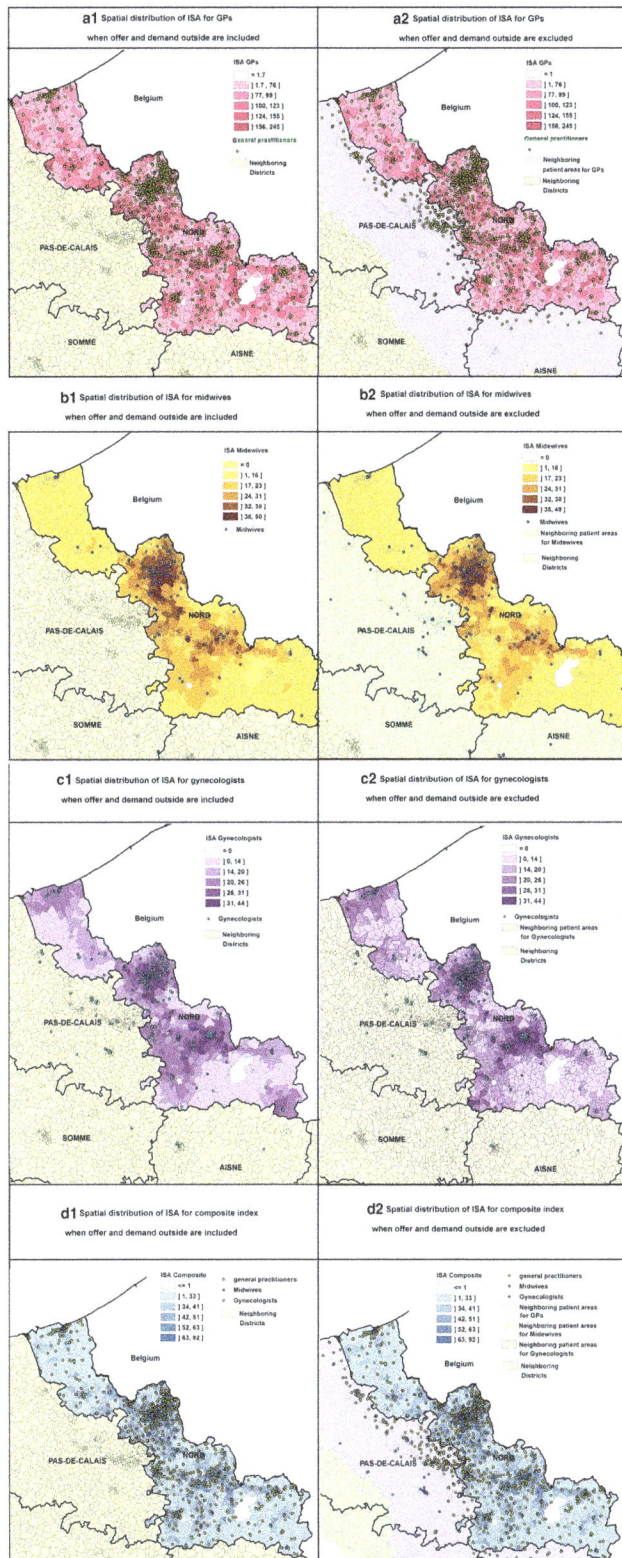

Fig. 2 Spatial distribution of ISA when offer and demand outside are included or excluded. ISA distribution is showed for GPs (**a**), midwives (**b**) and gynecologists (**c**) and combined in the composite index (**d**). For each map, neighboring departments are colored in yellow and the department of Nord is colored using a graduated approach (according to Jenks' Natural Breaks), showing different ISA scales at IRIS level, expressed per 100,000 inhabitants. The 1362, 2425 and 2583 Neighboring IRIS added to the ISA calculation for GPs, midwives and gynecologists when edge effect included are colored purple, green and khaki respectively

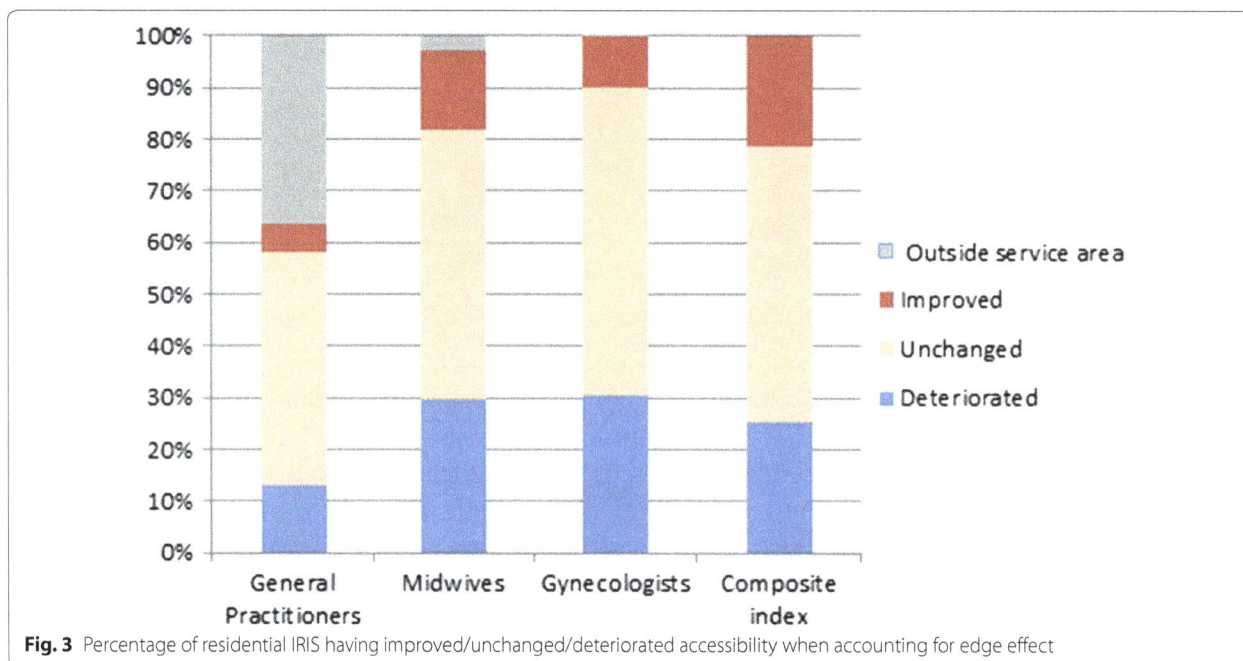

Fig. 3 Percentage of residential IRIS having improved/unchanged/deteriorated accessibility when accounting for edge effect

of a kind of "balance": people from this zone could reach more healthcare professionals beyond the department of Nord but at the same time they must share health resources with residents from neighboring departments. Their accessibility score therefore remains relatively stable.

When focusing on composite ISA, results reveal that all IRIS are subject to edge effect. Most of the IRIS located close to the border and in the agglomeration area (such as Roubaix, Anzin, Maubeuge and Saint-Pol-sur-Mer) saw their ISA improved. However, more IRIS have a deteriorated ISA (25.3%) than an improved ISA (21.5%).

Spatial analysis of ISA

The result of Moran's test for the composite ISA reveal significant spatial autocorrelation (I = 0.73 when offer and demand beyond the study area are included, and I = 0.74 when excluded—p = 0.0001, pseudo-significance values based on a permutation approach [56]). This means that the IRIS which have a high level of healthcare accessibility are more often located close to other IRIS having a high ISA score in the two cases than they were if this distribution were random.

Figure 5 shows the mapped results of the LISA statistics calculations. According to the results obtained from the LISA statistics, when excluding the offer and demand beyond the boundary, the 1346 IRIS are distributed as follows (Table 3): 287 HH-type (high level surrounded

by high levels), 273 LL-type (low level surrounded by low levels). Despite some minor differences, we found similar distribution of LISA statistics: 277 HH-type, 264 LL-type.

Comparative analysis of urban and rural ISA variation with edge effect

Figure 6 shows the ISA variation when accounting for the edge effect and the distribution of urban IRIS and rural (hatched) IRIS. Most IRIS in the department of Nord are urban (1030 urban vs. 336 rural), concentrated around several densely-populated areas close to major cities such as Lille, Roubaix, Tourcoing and Villeneuve d'Ascq (Fig. 6). Using a 10 km buffer zone around the boundaries, we estimated that 180 rural IRIS (54% of total rural IRIS) and 304 urban IRIS (just 29% of total urban IRIS) were near the Nord Pas-de-Calais and the Nord Aisne border.

Figure 7 shows the percentage of urban/rural IRIS variation separately, when offer and demand beyond the boundary were included. Overall, for ISA midwives and gynecologists, there is more variation in rural IRIS: only 16.14 and 26.25% of rural IRIS remain unchanged for ISA midwives and gynecologists respectively, compared with 48.35 and 62.82% of urban IRIS. Moreover, a sharp downward trend was observed in the rural zone; about 53.80% of rural IRIS have a deteriorated ISA midwife and gynecologist value.

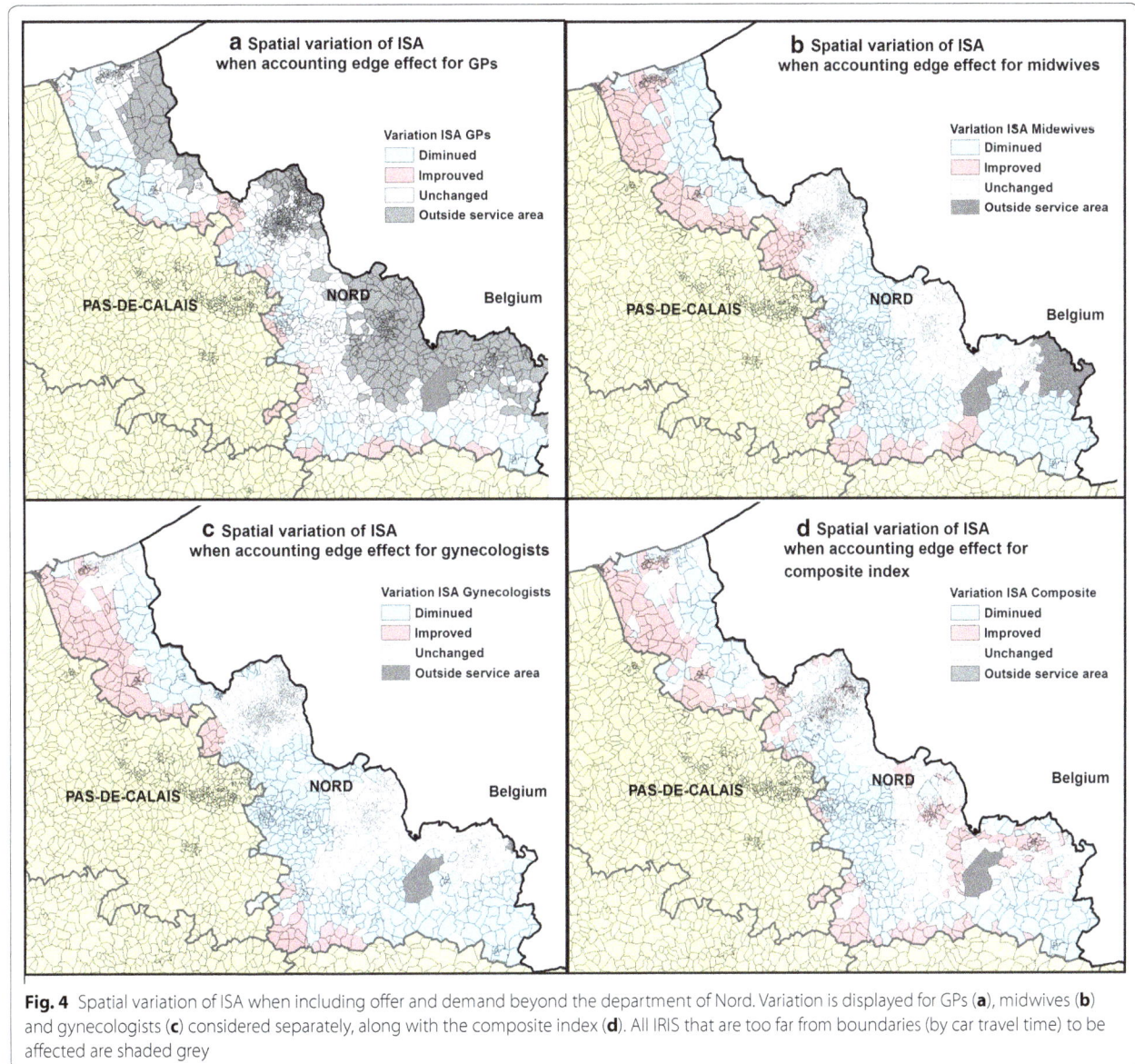

Fig. 4 Spatial variation of ISA when including offer and demand beyond the department of Nord. Variation is displayed for GPs (**a**), midwives (**b**) and gynecologists (**c**) considered separately, along with the composite index (**d**). All IRIS that are too far from boundaries (by car travel time) to be affected are shaded grey

Spatial variation of ISA according to socioeconomic distress level

The strength of the associations between the socioeconomic distress variable and composite ISA when offer and demand beyond the boundary were included or exclude are quite similar (Table 4): the association between socioeconomic factor and accessibility is therefore not impacted when offer and demand beyond the boundary Included. All the associations are positive and statistically significant ($p < 0.0001$) with the exception of the level of education; the association with women's unemployment is close to reaching statistical significance. Population residing in the more deprived neighborhoods have the highest level of accessibility

to healthcare providers, suggesting that there is no systematic absence of healthcare providers in impoverished areas.

Discussion

This work highlights the impacts of edge effect on spatial modelling of accessibility to healthcare professionals; this has been a matter of some concern to spatial analysts. Edge effect is one of the most commonly mentioned problems in studies dealing with spatial accessibility. We were interested in exploring the role of edge effect, to determine whether or not it has a relevant impact on healthcare provider accessibility in the department of Nord, using the "Index of Spatial Accessibility" previously

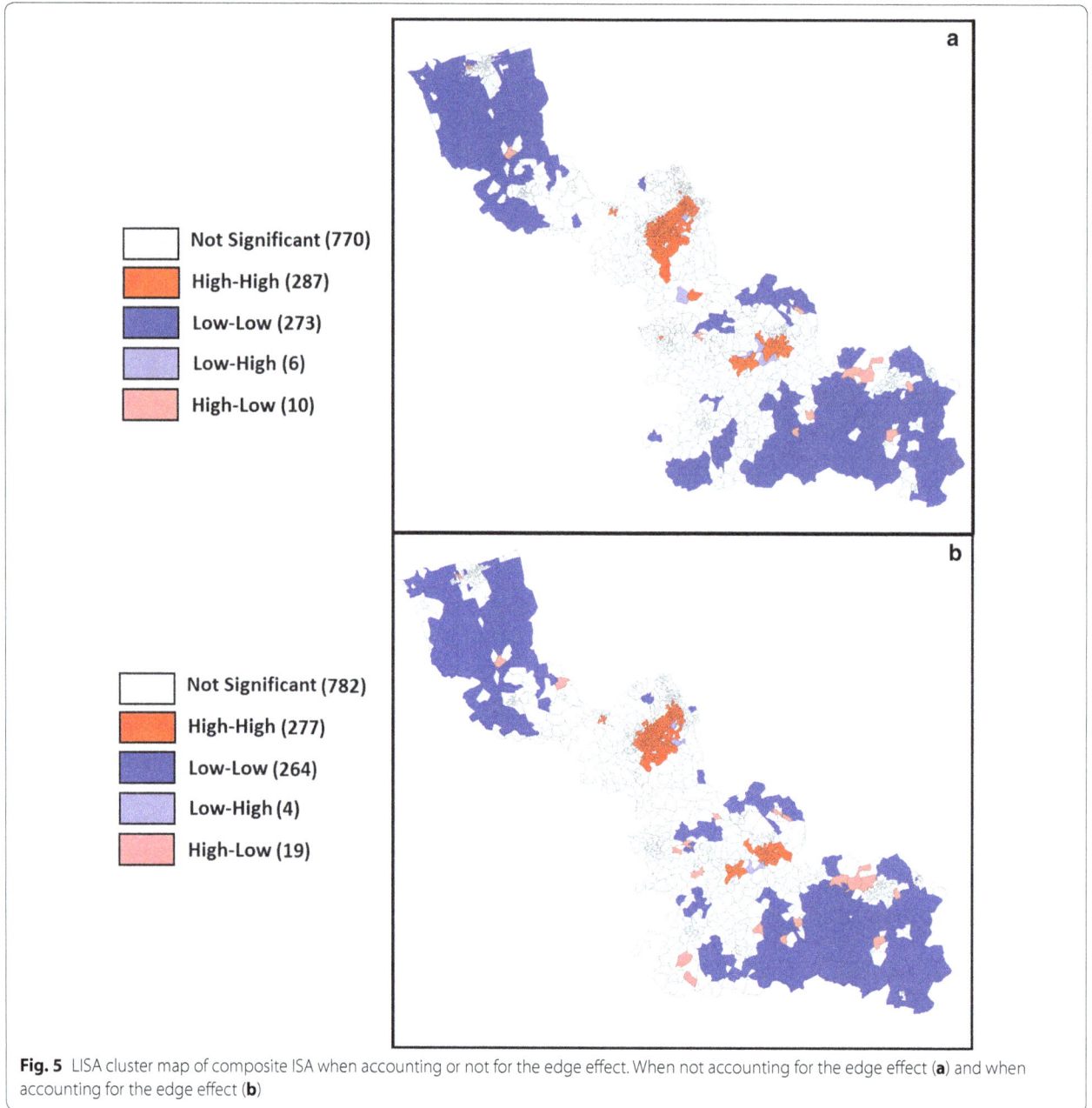

Not Significant (770)
High-High (287)
Low-Low (273)
Low-High (6)
High-Low (10)

Not Significant (782)
High-High (277)
Low-Low (264)
Low-High (4)
High-Low (19)

Fig. 5 LISA cluster map of composite ISA when accounting or not for the edge effect. When not accounting for the edge effect (**a**) and when accounting for the edge effect (**b**)

developed by our team [44]. Our study has shown that it is difficult to reach a general conclusion. Firstly, in many published studies, authors have argued that accessibility to facilities (including healthcare providers) will lead to considerable biases [34–37], even under-reporting [17, 28, 29, 31, 43] when not accounting for the edge effect. Our work has revealed that on average, the Index of Spatial Accessibility is only slightly lower with edge effect accounted, than without. In addition, when accounting for the edge effect, our study suggests that more IRIS see their value reduced than see it improved. Indeed, when

spatial analyses are not limited within a finite region, not only are facilities beyond the border disregarded, but the fact that patients from the neighboring area are also able to overcome geographical boundaries and consult a healthcare professional within the department of Nord is also ignored.

More specifically, the role of edge effect is largely linked to the method used to estimate accessibility. A range of methods exists for measurement of spatial accessibility to healthcare professionals—including Physician Population Ratio, distance/time (Euclidean, Manhattan, or network)

Table 3 Descriptive statistics of composite ISA in the IRIS types obtained by LISA statistics

LISA statistic level types	HH	LL	LH	HL	NS	Total
Number of IRIS when accounting for the edge effect	*287*	*273*	*6*	*10*	*770*	*1346*
%	*21.3%*	*20.3%*	*0.4%*	*0.7%*	*57.2%*	
ISA composite						
Minimum	40.1	0.4	33.8	36.3	7.0	
Mean	57.0	24.3	36.3	45.1	38.1	
Standard deviation	8.7	7.9	2.0	5.2	10.1	
Maximum	91.4	39.8	38.8	58.8	77.8	
Number of IRIS when not accounting for the edge effect	*277*	*264*	*4*	*19*	*782*	*1346*
%	*20.6%*	*19.6%*	*0.3%*	*1.4%*	*58.1%*	
ISA composite						
Minimum	41.3	0.4	6	39.7	7.2	
Mean	57.2	24.6	33.5	45.2	38.2	
Standard deviation	8.7	7.7	36.3	4.2	9.7	
Maximum	92.0	39.2	2.6	54.4	76.7	

Results when accounting or not for the edge effects are shown separately

to the nearest healthcare professional, average distance/time to a certain number of healthcare professionals, cumulative opportunity (which counts the number of opportunities that can be reached within a travel time) [22, 54] and the gravity model [23, 24]. When the accessibility indicator is based on availability or proximity (such as distance/time or cumulative opportunity) taking facilities beyond the border into account can improve the accessibility score. However, when the availability measure is weighted by population size (as our ISA indicator is), so that the volume of services available (relative to the population's size and the proximity of services available relative to the location of the population) is taken into account, it is also important to consider demand from the population on the other side of the border. The population living either side of the study border must share the healthcare supply. As a result, the impact of edge effect on this type of accessibility indicator is more subtle; variation occurs in a balanced way, and should not be subject to arbitrary conclusions.

Secondly, our study shows that depending on health professional type, edge effect impact may vary considerably. We found that changes to GPs ISA are mainly in those IRIS located close to the boundaries. One explanation is that the "patient area" of GPs is limited ($\leq$ 15 min) [44, 54]. Moreover, GP numbers are much higher than specialist doctor numbers, leading to more homogenous distribution. Consequently, supply and demand beyond the border will not have a very significant impact. Conversely, midwife and gynecologist numbers are very limited. People may be willing to travel further/longer to access a specialist doctor. This is why almost all IRIS are impacted by distance. Yet

variations in ISA values are minor, because of the 'balance' of edge effects.

Healthcare accessibility is especially vital for rural populations; a matter that has long been of concern to community and health planners [17, 31–33]. Typically, these populations experience restricted access to healthcare and other resources due to the spatial inequality of living in rural or impoverished areas. ISA comparisons between urban and rural zones reveal a greater variability within the group of rural IRIS than within the group of urban IRIS. This finding may be partially explained by the spatial distribution of the rural IRIS located close to the border of the study area: 54% of rural IRIS are located within ten kilometers (as the crow flies) from the frontier (as against only 29% of urban IRIS). However, the fact that a steep downward trend was observed in the rural zone when offer and demand beyond the boundary were included is both unexpected and related specifically to the distribution of healthcare providers and consumers in the department of Nord and its neighboring areas. This result should therefore be analyzed and interpreted with caution, since it is study-area dependent. One of the explanations is that the physicians' density of district Nord (436.2 per 100,000 inhabitants) is greater than its neighboring districts: 307.2 for Pas-de-Calais, 271.1 for Oise, 401.1 for Somme, 280.2 for Aisne and 288.5 for Ardennes [60]. On the other hand, in most cities in the Nord department, when edge effect is corrected, the ISA score is mainly classified as 'unchanged'—thanks to well-balanced offer and demand.

We found a positive correlation between socioeconomic distress levels and composite ISA. This finding suggests that areas of high socioeconomic distress tended

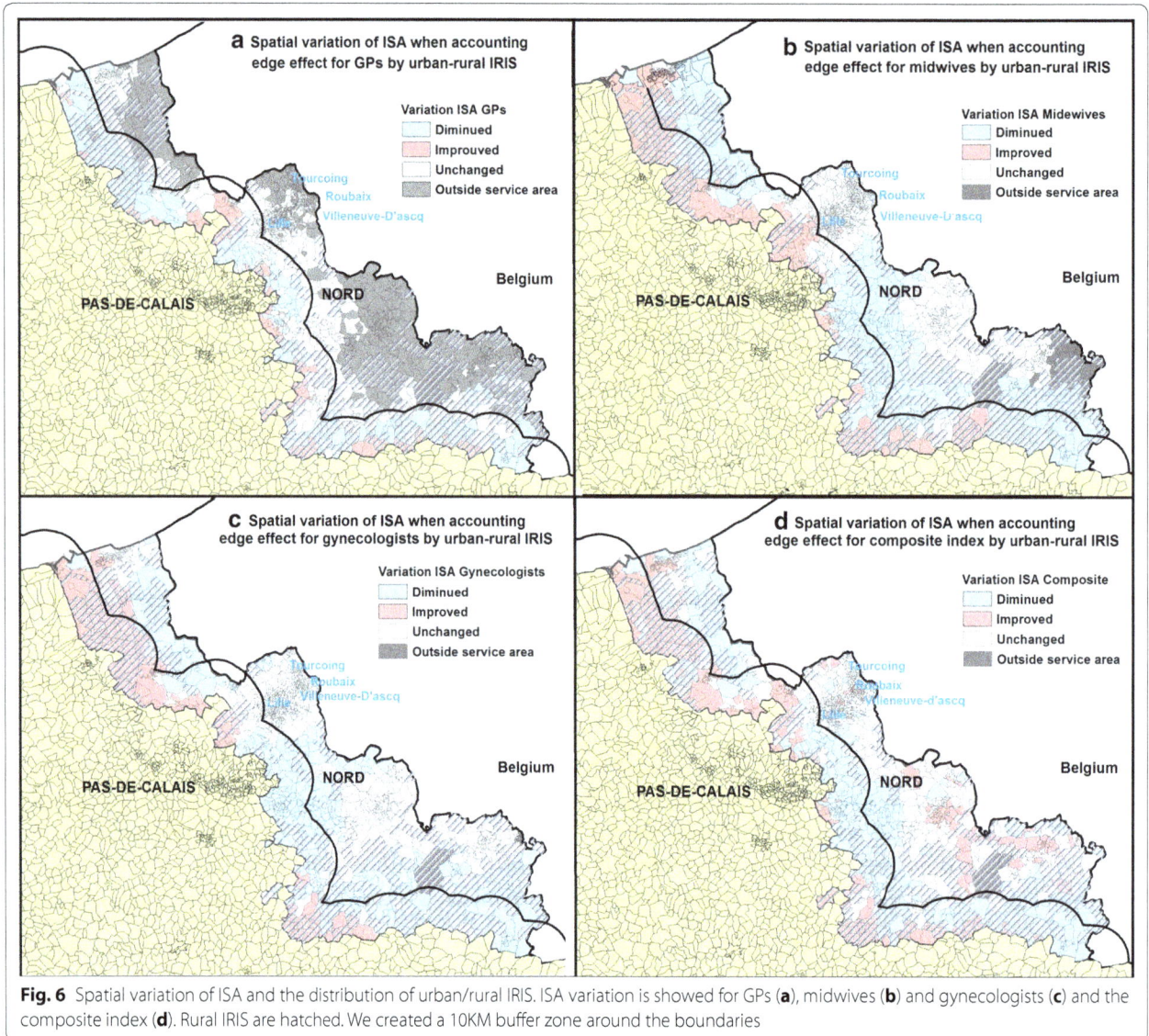

Fig. 6 Spatial variation of ISA and the distribution of urban/rural IRIS. ISA variation is showed for GPs (**a**), midwives (**b**) and gynecologists (**c**) and the composite index (**d**). Rural IRIS are hatched. We created a 10KM buffer zone around the boundaries

to have better access than low socioeconomic distress areas. This result is not surprising, given the spatial planning of the Nord department: lower-income residents are more likely to live in urban areas in which social housing and services are concentrated. This significant association is quite similar to the result when offer and demand beyond the boundary were excluded: inclusion of offer and demand beyond the boundary did not impact the relationship between distress levels and composite ISA within our study area. These findings tend to demonstrate that the impact of edge effect is dependent on both the spatial distribution of healthcare providers and territorial organization.

Our study aims to provide additional evidence to the existing scientific literature in the field of spatial accessibility to healthcare by carrying out a detailed examination

of the impact of edge effect. To our knowledge, this is the first work assessing edge effect based on algorithm E2SFCA. No research has explicitly demonstrated access differences when outside healthcare sources and patient demand are excluded or included. This study highlights the fact that there is a inaccuracy in hypothesizing that accessibility will be considerably and systematically under-reported where external healthcare providers are excluded. Indeed, our study found IRIS in which the ISA was reduced when offer and demand beyond the boundary were included. The result of this study will be useful to both health resource planners and other researchers in the public health field.

Several limitations of this study should be addressed here. Despite its relative popularity of algorithm, the E2SFCA method remained highly debated. The choice

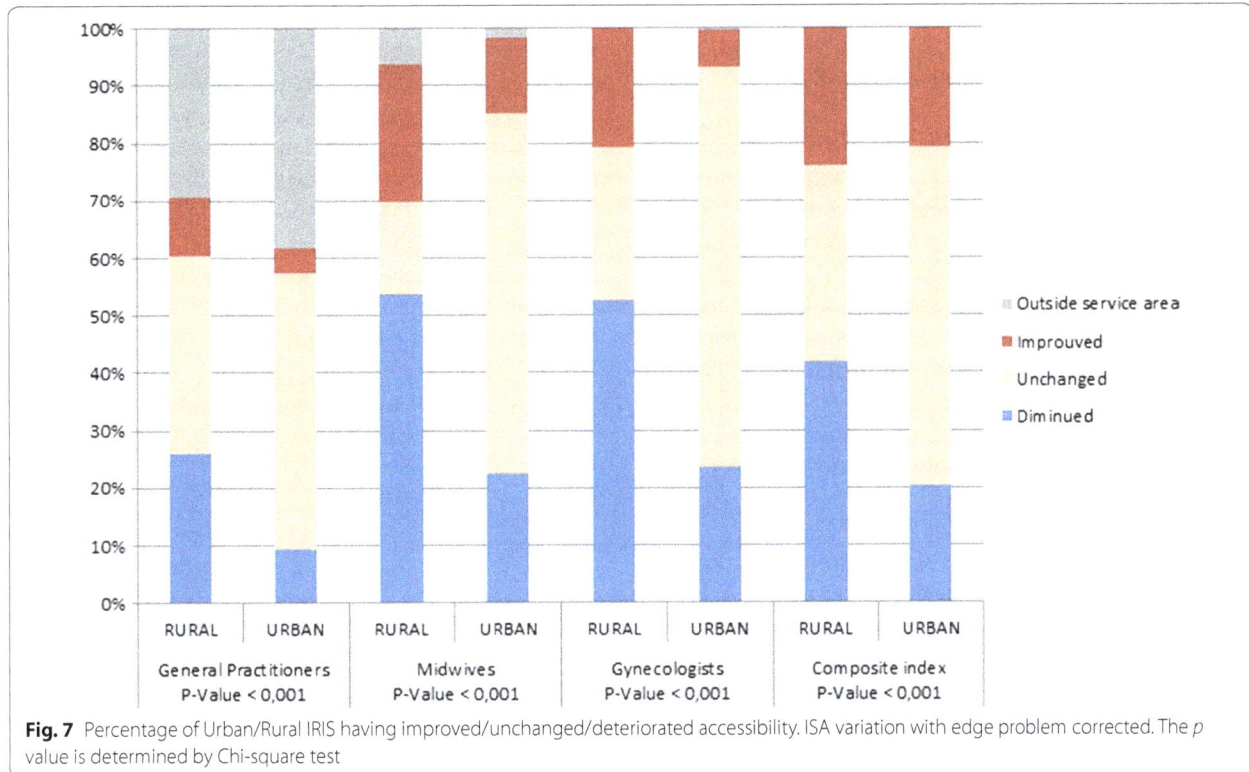

Fig. 7 Percentage of Urban/Rural IRIS having improved/unchanged/deteriorated accessibility. ISA variation with edge problem corrected. The *p* value is determined by Chi-square test

Table 4 Simple linear regression between Socioeconomic variables and composite ISA when accounting or not edge effect

	ISA composite when not accounting edge effects			ISA composite when accounting edge effects		
	β	CI 95%*	*p* value	β	CI 95%*	*p* value
Single parent families	81.3	[72.8, 89.9]	< 0.0001	79.7	[71.3, 88.1]	< 0.0001
Non-homeowner	26.5	[23.6, 29.4]	< 0.0001	26.2	[23.4, 29.0]	< 0.0001
Insecure employment	24.9	[13.1, 36.6]	< 0.0001	27.0	[15.5, 38.5]	< 0.0001
Women's unemployment rate	8.7	[−.3, 17.8]	0.058	9.3	[.5, 18.2]	0.04
Low level of educational attainment among women	5.0	[−3.3, 13.4]	NS 0.24	5.9	[− 2.3, 14.0]	NS 0.16

*Confidence interval at 95%

of the best decay function or the right size for catchment areas needs rigorous modeling to derive the best fitting parameters [61]. In the absence of appropriate empirical evidence, it was necessary to make a number of estimations during the definition of distance-decay function and the threshold for healthcare professionals other than general practitioners.

Another limitation is aggregation error, which arises when measuring distance from aggregated areal units to facilities, and results from the use of a single point as a proxy for the locations of individuals within the area units [5]. We have attempted to reduce aggregation error by considering the spatial distribution of the living building, since it better reflects the spatial distribution of individuals [5, 62].

In this study, we were not interested in the interaction across the border between France and Belgium. Even though the European Health Insurance Card (EHIC) gives the right to access state-provided healthcare during a temporary stay in another European Economic Area, a pregnant woman have make a specific request. This request must then be accepted to be able to benefit from health care during the pregnancy and to avoid advancing their own funds to cover expenses, which do add an extra layer of administrative complexity. We assumed therefore that the offer and demand of pregnancy-related healthcare across this border is limited.

In addition, it is also worth noting that (as in many other studies dealing with spatial accessibility) our method concerns only potential spatial accessibility, rather than revealed access (actual utilization of health-care). Only complex and expensive investigations would be capable of providing the complementary information that would allow us to distinguish the difference between spatial and real access and use of healthcare services. Finally, our study addresses difficulties arising from the use of a large amount of data and distance calculation prior to application of the algorithm, which is time consuming and calls for technical know-how. However, this is the price to be paid for a more accurate indicator.

Conclusion

Access to healthcare services will continue to be one of the most important public health preoccupations, especially in the context of the increase of social health inequalities worldwide. Our study gave a real illustration of what could be the impact of edge effect in healthcare access in a French context. Our results did not support the "under-report" hypothesis discussed in many published studies. On the whole, our research has revealed only minor average value variations of ISA as a result of including interactions across the border. One explanation is that a kind of balance patient and healthcare professionals when considering neighboring department. However, it is not possible to set up general statement because intensity of impact varies according to healthcare provider type, urbanization level and territorial organization; in addition, we also know that the methodology implemented to measure the healthcare access combined with the size of the spatial unit may influence how the edge effect could impact the measure of healthcare accessibility. For these reason, we plan to carry out this study for another study area with a different territorial organization, to compare ISA variation in two cases in order to get a conclusion more general, at the France scale. Additional researches are required in different countries in order to improve our level of understanding about the influence of the edge effect on the accessibility to healthcare. Following the same methodology to measure the accessibility to healthcare, these different studies will help to distinguish what findings are specific to the characteristics and organization of the country and what findings are common to the different counties. It constitute a promising direction to determine more precisely healthcare shortage areas and then to fight against social health inequalities.

In conclusion, edge effect must be considered on a case-by-case basis, because it relies on choice of indicator, spatial distribution of facilities and urban organization of the territory studied.

This study represents an important step. It will serve not only to assist current researchers by identifying the common methodological hypothesis bias of edge effect in spatial accessibility studies, but will also be helpful to planners and other researchers in the public health field. This paper has presented high-quality geographic data and advanced GIS techniques. In order to examine whether the results are generalizable to different spatial scales and distribution, we hope to contribute to other areas of study in the near future.

Abbreviations

E2FCA: enhanced two-step floating catchment area; INSEE: National Institute of Statistics and Economic Studies; ISA: spatial accessibility index; IRIS: L'Îlot Regroupé pour des Indicateurs Statistiques.

Authors' contributions

Work presented here was conceived, carried out and analyzed by FG, SD and WK. MS and NL gave important suggestions and supervised the study. All authors read and approved the final manuscript.

Author details

[1] EHESP Rennes, Sorbonne Paris Cité, Paris, France. [2] LIVE UMR 7362 CNRS (Laboratoire Image Ville Environnement), University of Strasbourg, 6700 Strasbourg, France. [3] L'équipe REPERES, Recherche en Pharmaco-épidémiologie et recours aux soins, UPRES EA-7449, Rennes, France. [4] IRD, UMR_D 190 "Emergence des Pathologies Virales" (IRD French Institute of Research for Development, Aix-Marseille University, EHESP French School of Public Health), Marseille, France. [5] Department of Quantitative Methods for Public Health, EHESP School of Public Health, Avenue du Professeur Léon Bernard, 35043 Rennes, France. [6] Department of Social Epidemiology, Sorbonne Universités, UPMC Univ Paris 06, INSERM, Institut Pierre Louis d'Epidémiologie et de Santé Publique (UMRS 1136), Paris, France.

Acknowledgements

This research is supported by EHESP Rennes, Sorbonne Paris Cité and Institut de recherche sur la santé l'environnement et le travail. Points of view or opinions in this article are those of the authors and do not necessarily represent the official position or policies of the EHESP Rennes, Sorbonne Paris Cité and IRSET.

Competing interests

The authors declare that they have no competing interests.

Funding

Not applicable.

Appendix I

Socioeconomic variables	Definition
Low level of educational attainment	Proportion of women aged 25 and over not having graduated from high school
Women's unemployment rate	Proportion of unemployed women eligible to work
Single parent families	Proportion of all households with children headed by lone parents
Non-homeowner	Proportion of all households not owning their main residence
Insecure employment situation	Proportion of those on short-term or temporary contracts, in state-funded posts, or apprenticeship/internship

Appendix II
See Fig. 8.

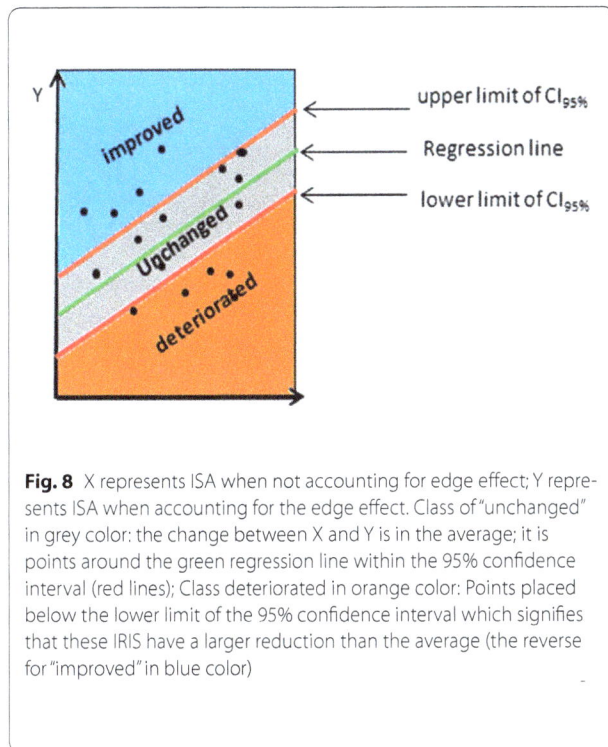

Fig. 8 X represents ISA when not accounting for edge effect; Y represents ISA when accounting for the edge effect. Class of "unchanged" in grey color: the change between X and Y is in the average; it is points around the green regression line within the 95% confidence interval (red lines); Class deteriorated in orange color: Points placed below the lower limit of the 95% confidence interval which signifies that these IRIS have a larger reduction than the average (the reverse for "improved" in blue color)

References

1. Sasaki S, Comber AJ, Suzuki H, Brunsdon C. Using genetic algorithms to optimise current and future health planning-the example of ambulance locations. Int J Health Geogr. 2010;9:4. https://doi.org/10.1186/1476-072X-9-4.

2. Walsh SJ, Page PH, Gesler WM. Normative models and healthcare planning: network-based simulations within a geographic information system environment. Health Serv Res. 1997;32:243–60.

3. Patel AB, Waters NM, Ghali WA. Determining geographic areas and populations with timely access to cardiac catheterization facilities for acute myocardial infarction care in Alberta, Canada. Int J Health Geogr. 2007;6:47. https://doi.org/10.1186/1476-072X-6-47.

4. Parker EB, Campbell JL. Measuring access to primary medical care: some examples of the use of geographical information systems. Health Place. 1998;4:83–193.

5. Hewko J, Smoyer-Tomic KE, Hodgson MJ. Measuring neighbourhood spatial accessibility to urban amenities: does aggregation error matter? Environ Plan A. 2002;34(7):1185–206.

6. Talen E. Visualizing fairness: equity maps for planners. J Am Plan Assoc. 1998;64(1):22–38.

7. Talen E, Anselin L. Assessing spatial equity: an evaluation of measures of accessibility to public playgrounds. Environ Plan A. 1998;30(4):595–613.

8. Lawrence D, Kisely S. Inequalities in healthcare provision for people with severe mental illness. J Psychopharmacol. 2010;24(Suppl 4):61–8. https://doi.org/10.1177/1359786810382058.

9. Charreire H, Combier E. Poor prenatal care in an urban area: a geographic analysis. Health Place. 2009;15(2):412–9.

10. Smoyer-Tomic KE, Spence JC, Raine KD, Amrhein C, Cameron N, Yasenovskiy V, Cutumisu N, Hemphill E, Healy J. The association between neighborhood socioeconomic status and exposure to supermarkets and fast food outlets. Health Place. 2008;14:740–54. https://doi.org/10.1016/j.healthplace.2007.12.001.

11. Ball K, Timperio A, Crawford D. Neighbourhood socioeconomic inequalities in food access and affordability. Health Place. 2009;15:578–85. https://doi.org/10.1016/j.healthplace.2008.09.010.

12. Galvez MP, Hong L, Choi E, Liao L, Godbold J, Brenner B. Childhood obesity and neighborhood food-store availability in an inner-city community. Acad Pediatr. 2009;9:339–43. https://doi.org/10.1016/j.acap.2009.05.003.

13. Spence JC, Cutumisu N, Edwards J, Raine KD, Smoyer-Tomic K. Relation between local food environments and obesity among adults. BMC Public Health. 2009;9:192. https://doi.org/10.1186/1471-2458-9-192.

14. Macdonald L, Ellaway A, Macintyre S. The food retail environment and area deprivation in Glasgow City, UK. Int J Behav Nutr Phys Act. 2009;6:52. https://doi.org/10.1186/1479-5868-6-52.

15. Feng J, Glass TA, Curriero FC, Stewart WF, Schwartz BS. The built environment and obesity: a systematic review of the epidemiologic evidence. Health Place. 2010;16:175–90. https://doi.org/10.1016/j.healthplace.2009.09.008.

16. Hu R, Dong S, Zhao Y, Hu H, Li Z. Assessing potential spatial accessibility of health services in rural China: a case study of Donghai County. Int J Equity Health. 2013;12:35. https://doi.org/10.1186/1475-9276-12-35.

17. Wang F, Luo W. Assessing spatial and nonspatial factors for healthcare access: towards an integrated approach to defining health professional shortage areas. Health Place. 2005;11(2):131–46. https://doi.org/10.1016/j.healthplace.2004.02.003.

18. Wang F. Quantitative methods and applications in GIS. Boca Raton: Taylor & Francis Group; 2005.

19. Matsumoto M, Inoue K, Noguchi S, Toyokawa S, Eiji K. Community characteristics that attract physicians in Japan: a cross-sectional analysis of community demographic and economic factors. Human Resour Health. 2009;7:12.

20. Ranga V, Panda P. Geospat Spatial access to inpatient health care in northern rural India. Health. 2014;8(2):545–56.

21. Talen E. Neighborhoods as service providers: a methodology for evaluating pedestrian access. Environ Plan B. 2003;30:181–200. https://doi.org/10.1068/b12977.

22. Apparicio P, Abdelmajid M, Riva M, Shearmur R. Comparing alternative approaches to measuring the geographical accessibility of urban health services: distance types and aggregation-error issues. Int J Health Geogr. 2008;7:7. https://doi.org/10.1186/1476-072X-7-7.

23. Guagliardo MF. Spatial accessibility of primary care: concepts, methods and challenges. Int J Health Geogr. 2004;3:3.

24. Martin D, Williams HCWL. Market-area analysis and accessibility to primary health-care centres. Environ Plan. 1992;24:1009–19.

25. Bamford EJ, Dunne L, Taylor DS, Symon BG, Hugo GJ, Wilkinson D. Accessibility to general practitioners in rural South Australia. Med J Aust. 1999;171(11–12):614–6.

26. Apparicio P, Cloutier M-S, Shearmur R. The case of Montréal's missing food deserts: evaluation of accessibility to food supermarkets. Int J Health Geogr. 2007;6(1):4.

27. Luo W, Qi Y. An enhanced two-step floating catchment area (E2SFCA) method for measuring spatial accessibility to primary care physicians. Health Place. 2011;17(1):394.

28. Sadler RC, Gilliland JA, Arku G. An application of the edge effect in measuring accessibility to multiple food retailer types in Southwestern Ontario, Canada. Int J Health Geogr. 2010;10:34.

29. Salze P, Banos A, Oppert J-M, Charreire H, Casey R, Simon C, Chaix B, Badariotti D, Weber C. Estimating spatial accessibility to facilities on the regional scale: an extended commuting-based interaction potential model. Int J Health Geogr. 2011. https://doi.org/10.1186/1476-072X-10-2.

30. Vidal Rodeiro CL, Lawson AB. An evaluation of the edge effects in disease map modelling. J Comput Stat Data Anal. 2005;49:45–62.

31. Sharkey JR, Horel S. Neighborhood socioeconomic deprivation and minority composition are associated with better potential spatial access to the ground-truthed food environment in a large rural area. J Nutr. 2008;138(3):620–7.

32. Wan N, Zhan FB, Zou B, Chow E. A relative spatial access assessment approach for analyzing potential spatial access to colorectal cancer services in Texas. Appl Geogr. 2012;32:291–9. https://doi.org/10.1016/j.apgeog.2011.05.001.

33. Ngui AN, Apparicio P. Optimizing the two-step floating catchment area method for measuring spatial accessibility to medical clinics in Montreal. BMC Health Serv Res. 2011;11:166. https://doi.org/10.1186/1472-6963-11-166.

34. Fortney PD, Rost J, Warren J. Comparing alternative methods of measuring geographic access to health services. Health Serv Outcomes Res Methodol. 2000;1(2):173–84.

35. Van Meter EM, Lawson AB, Colabianchi N, Nichols M, Hibbert J, Porter DE, Liese AD. An evaluation of edge effects in nutritional accessibility and availability measures: a simulation study. Int J Health Geogr. 2010;9:40. https://doi.org/10.1186/1476-072X-9-40.

36. Bissonnette L, Wilson K, Bell S, Shah TI. Neighbourhoods and potential access to health care: the role of spatial and aspatial factors. Health Place. 2012;18(4):841–53. https://doi.org/10.1016/j.healthplace.2012.03.007.

37. Donohoe J, Marshall V, Tan X, Camacho FT, Anderson R, Balkrishnan R. Evaluating and comparing methods for measuring spatial access to mammography centers in Appalachia (Re-Revised). Health Serv Outcomes Res Methodol. 2016;16(1):22–40.

38. Jordan H, Roderick P, Martin D, Barnett S. Distance, rurality and the need for care: access to health services in South West England. Int J Health Geogr. 2004;3:21. https://doi.org/10.1186/1476-072X-3-21.

39. Luo J, Tian LL, Luo L, Yi H, Wang FH. Two-step optimization for spatial accessibility improvement: a case study of health care planning in rural China. BioMed Res Int. 2017. https://doi.org/10.1155/2017/2094654.

40. Fortney J, Rost K, Warren J. Health services & outcomes research. Methodology. 2000;1:173. https://doi.org/10.1023/A:1012545106828.

41. Pipley BD. Spatial statistics. New York: Wiley; 1981.

42. Iredale R, Jones L, Gray J, Deaville J. 'The edge effect': an exploratory study of some factors affecting referrals to cancer genetic services in rural Wales. Health Place. 2005;11(3):197–204. https://doi.org/10.1016/j.healthplace.2004.06.005.

43. Zhang XY, Lu H, Holt JB. Modeling spatial accessibility to parks: a national study. Int J Health Geogr. 2011;10:31. https://doi.org/10.1186/1476-072X-10-31.

44. Gao F, Kihal W, Le Meur N, Souris M, Deguen S. Assessment of the spatial accessibility to health professionals at French census block level. Int J Equity Health. 2016;15(1):125. https://doi.org/10.1186/s12939-016-0411-z.

45. Jin C, Cheng JQ, Lu YQ, Huang ZF, Cao FD. Spatial inequity in access to healthcare facilities at a county level in a developing country: a case study of Deqing County, Zhejiang, China. Int J Equity Health. 2015;14:67. https://doi.org/10.1186/s12939-015-0195-6.

46. Zhou Z, Su Y, Gao J, Campbell B, Zhu Z, Xu L, Zhang Y. Assessing equity of healthcare utilization in rural China: results from nationally representative. Int J Equity Health. 2013;12:34. https://doi.org/10.1186/1475-9276-12-34.

47. McGrail MR, Humphreys JS. Measuring spatial accessibility to primary care in rural areas: improving the effectiveness of the two-step floating catchment area method. Appl Geogr. 2009;29(4):533–41.

48. Strasser R. Rural health around the world: challenges and solutions. Fam Pract. 2003;20(4):457–63. https://doi.org/10.1093/fampra/cmg422.

49. Institut national de la statistique et des études économiques. http://www.insee.fr/fr/. Accessed 2 May 2014.

50. Lalloué B, Monnez JM, Padilla C, Kihal W, Le Meur N, Zmirou-Navier D, Deguen S. A statistical procedure to create a neighborhood socio-economic index for health inequalities analysis. Int J Equity Health. 2013;12:21. https://doi.org/10.1186/1475-9276-12-21.

51. French health insurance. http://annuairesante.ameli.fr/. Accessed 12 Mar 2014.

52. Institut national de l'information géographique et forestière: http://www.ign.fr/.

53. Zdeb M. Driving distances and times using SAS® and Google Maps. SAS Global Forum 2010.

54. Barlet M, Coldefy M, Collin C, Lucas-Gabrielli V. L'Accessibilité potentielle localisée (APL): une nouvelle mesure de l'accessibilité aux médecins généralistes libéraux. Institut de recherche et documentation en économie de la santé. Question d'économie de la santé n° 174; 2012.

55. McGrail MR. Spatial accessibility of primary health care utilising the two step floating catchment area method: an assessment of recent improvements. Int. J. Popul Geogr. 2012. https://doi.org/10.1186/1476-072X-11-50.

56. Griffith DA. What is spatial autocorrelation? L'Espace Géographique. 1992;21:265–80.

57. Anselin L. Local indicator of spatial association—LISA. Geogr Anal. 1995;27:93–115. https://doi.org/10.1111/j.1538-4632.1995.tb00338.x.

58. Jacquez GM, Greiling DA. Local clustering in breast, lung and colorectal cancer in Long Island, New York. Int J Health Geogr. 2003;2:3. https://doi.org/10.1186/1476-072X-2-3.

59. Talen E. Neighborhoods as service providers: a methodology for evaluating pedestrian access. Environ Plann B. 2003;30:181–200. https://doi.org/10.1068/b12977.

60. https://demographie.medecin.fr/#l=fr;v=map2. Accessed June 2017.

61. Wang F. Measurement, optimization, and impact of health care accessibility: a methodological review. Ann Assoc Am Geogr Assoc Am Geogr. 2012;102(5):1104–12. https://doi.org/10.1080/00045608.2012.657146.

62. Zhao P, Batta R. Analysis of centroid aggregation for the Euclidean distance p-median problem. Eur J Oper Res. 1999;113(1):147–68. https://doi.org/10.1016/S0377-2217(98)00010-1.

9

Analysis of big patient mobility data for identifying medical regions, spatio-temporal characteristics and care demands of patients on the move

Caglar Koylu[1]*[iD], Selman Delil[2], Diansheng Guo[3] and Rahmi Nurhan Celik[2]

Abstract

Background: Patient mobility can be defined as a patient's movement or utilization of a health care service located in a place or region other than the patient's place of residence. Mobility provides freedom to patients to obtain health care from providers across regions and even countries. It is essential to monitor patient choices in order to maintain the quality standards and responsiveness of the health system, otherwise, the health system may suffer from geographic disparities in the accessibility to quality and responsive health care. In this article, we study patient mobility in a national health care system to identify medical regions, spatio-temporal and service characteristics of health care utilization, and demands for patient mobility.

Methods: We conducted a systematic analysis of province-to-province patient mobility in Turkey from December 2009 to December 2013, which was derived from 1.2 billion health service records. We first used a flow-based region-alization method to discover functional medical regions from the patient mobility network. We compare the results of data-driven regions to designated regions of the government in order to identify the areas of mismatch between planned regional service delivery and the observed utilization in the form of patient flows. Second, we used feature selection, and multivariate flow clustering to identify spatio-temporal characteristics and health care needs of patients on the move.

Results: Medical regions we derived by analyzing the patient mobility data showed strong overlap with the designated regions of the Ministry of Health. We also identified a number of regions that the regional service utilization did not match the planned service delivery. Overall, our spatio-temporal and multivariate analysis of regional and long-distance patient flows revealed strong relationship with socio-demographic and cultural structure of the society and migration patterns. Also, patient flows exhibited seasonal patterns, and yearly trends which correlate with implemented policies throughout the period. We found that policies resulted in different outcomes across the country. We also identified characteristics of long-distance flows which could help inform policy-making by assessing the needs of patients in terms of medical specialization, service level and type.

Conclusions: Our approach helped identify (1) the mismatch between regional policy and practice in health care utilization (2) spatial, temporal, health service level characteristics and medical specialties that patients seek out by traveling longer distances. Our findings can help identify the imbalance between supply and demand, changes in mobility behaviors, and inform policy-making with insights.

Keywords: Patient mobility, Health care, Spatial data mining, Regionalization, Flow mapping

*Correspondence: caglar-koylu@uiowa.edu
[1] Department of Geographical and Sustainability Sciences, University of Iowa, Iowa City, USA
Full list of author information is available at the end of the article

Background

Designing a well-functioning health care system that is accessible, high quality and affordable is challenging as it requires balancing supply and demand for quantity, quality and variety of specialized medical care. Patient mobility can be defined as a patient's movement or utilization of a health care service located in a place or region other than the patient's place of residence. Mobility provides patients a wider choice of providers and increases the competition in health care market [1] and the efficiency of the health system [2]. Patients who are in search for immediate, affordable, and unusual treatments travel long distances, and often go beyond the conventional territorial boundaries [3, 4]. Patient mobility has been used as a policy to provide accessible and equitable care across the world. For example, the European Union have implemented policies to support free movement of patients across the countries in the EU [5].

Patient mobility research has typically focused on transnational patient movements across countries and continents within the context of medical tourism [6, 7]. A growing body of research is increasingly recognizing the importance of patient mobility to address the issues such as high cost of long waiting list at home, new technology, and skills in destination areas and countries [8, 9]. Furthermore, reduced transport costs resulted in increased medical tourism that go beyond the borders of countries and even continents. Health care providers and planners have implemented policies and various techniques to create and implement medical regions in order to efficiently allocate resources and services [10–12]. Each medical region includes a hub which provides both quantity and variety of care for patients for the surrounding areas. The health system can function more efficiently if it is organized into functional regions where the size and characteristics of the population, the quantity of providers and type of health care needs are known. In this article, we study interregional patient mobility in Turkish Health System.

Glinos et al. [3] identify availability, affordability, familiarity, and perceived quality as the four major motivations for patients that seek health care elsewhere. Availability refers to both timely access to services (i.e., short waiting list) and types of specialized care services within the residents' area. Affordability allows patients to choose the most economical care. Familiarity represents the cultural closeness or the availability of family and social ties in destination location. Lastly, perceived quality refers to the patient's perception of the quality and safety of services, technology and methods used at the destination location. Additionally, indicators of geographic accessibility to health care [13, 14], and financial accessibility

and acceptability [15] have been considered to impact the choice of patients [4].

Although mobility increases competition in the market, it is essential to monitor the patterns and shifts in patient choices in order to identify the gap between what patients need and what the health system offers in terms of quality care and services [6, 16, 17]. Otherwise, the health system may suffer from geographic disparities in the access to quality and responsive health care. Furthermore, monitoring changes in mobility behaviors can help identify the imbalance between supply and demand and inform policy-making with insights.

Analysis of mobility data is challenging due to the large volume and number of flow variables (e.g., hundreds of variables including service levels, types and medical specialization); and the complexity of patterns in multiple spaces (e.g., geographic space, network space, multivariate space) and time, and at multiple scales (e.g., national patterns, regional patterns, local patterns). Analysis of mobility networks can be grouped into four major themes: (1) using network measures [18] to identify locational characteristics such as prominent nodes and popular destinations; (2) using community detection methods to identify functional regions such as medical regions [11], habitat territories [19], or migration regions [20, 21] where there are more flows within a spatial community (a set of locations) than the rest of the network; (3) using flow clustering, edge bundling and visualization [22, 23] to identify common characteristics of flows (4) using global statistical and network models such as power-law, and gravity to describe the governing laws behind the network construction, evolution, and distributional characteristics [24, 25].

In this article, we present a systematic approach to analyzing large and high dimensional (i.e., large number of variables) patient mobility data in order to evaluate the effectiveness of regional health care utilization and identify the characteristics and demands for long-distance patient mobility. To demonstrate, we analyze patient mobility in the Turkish National Health System across a 4-year period from December 2009 to December 2013. Mobility data is derived from 1.2 billion monthly aggregated health service records, which include locations of patients and health service facility as well as multivariate information on service provider, type of institution, and level and specialization of medical service received. We construct a province-to-province patient mobility network, one for each month, where nodes represent locations of patient residences and health service facilities, and edges represent monthly-aggregated movement of patients from the province of their residences (origin) to the province of health facilities (destination). We first derive functional regions of health service delivery by applying a flow-based regionalization approach [26] to the province-to-province mobility network. We compare the data-driven regions to the designated regions from the Turkish Ministry of Health in order to capture the mismatch between the implemented regional policy and observed choices of patients. Functional regions derived from patient mobility data can help evaluate the effectiveness of the regional health system. Second, we identify the spatio-temporal characteristics and health care demands of moving patients by performing feature selection and multivariate clustering on a large set of patient flow variables which include time (e.g., month, season, and year), type, level and specialization of medical services received by patients. Such information can help identify the imbalance between supply and demand, changes in mobility behaviors, and inform policy-making with insights.

Methods
Context and data
In this section, we introduce the details of the Turkish Healthcare system and the patient mobility data. Health providers in Turkey are organized into three levels (Table 1): (1) primary health centers staffed by family physicians (2) public and private health facilities and hospitals, and (3) training and research hospitals and independent university hospitals.

Turkish health system
Turkey's health system has radically changed with the Turkish Health Transformation Program (THTP) in 2003, which aimed to improve governance, efficiency and quality in the health care sector, with significant investments and the establishment of a family-physician system [27]. Employees in both public and private sectors were combined under the newly created Social Security Institution (SSI) and almost the entire population was covered by social insurance with universal health coverage. After many legislative changes, the SSI has become the sole buyer of health care services and the Ministry of Health (MoH) has become the main health care service provider in the country. With the implementation of THTP, citizens were given the freedom to choose where they are treated, whether in a private or a public institution without referral requirement or out-of-network coverage. In 2011, MoH released a new region-centered planning policy and family physician system, which combined eighty one provinces into twenty nine health regions. Figure 1 shows the regions and the health care hub designated for each region. According to the new policy, each patient was assigned to a family physician, and patients in each region were advised to seek specialized medical care from their regional hub before considering hubs in other regions. However, since there are no referral requirements, and citizens are free to choose health services with their universal health insurance, it is not clear whether the MoH regions and hub structure function effectively in practice. One of the objectives of this paper is therefore to identify the functional regions directly from the patient mobility data, and compare them to the designated regions by MoH to assess the effectiveness of the implemented policy.

Patient mobility data
After the health care reform, health care utilization has increased dramatically and patient mobility has continued to rise in Turkey. Main drivers of patient mobility are the search for better treatment or treatment affordability, and the availability of specialized health care services [28]. After the Social Security Institution (SSI) became the single buyer for health care services, different databases of providers and related insurance coverage were merged into a single database. The SSI health insurance covers 90% of the entire population in Turkey, a total of about 70 million. On average 400 million admissions are provisioned annually by health service providers. These records include the number of patients admitted to health care units on a monthly basis, and are verified and monitored by SSI using a single-center database. Both patients' residence location and health care unit or facility location are verified by the Turkish address-based population registration system (TABPRS). Because the data include all health service records, it potentially involve multiple trips from the same individual across 4 years. Because the data is aggregated by month and province and district to protect the privacy of patients, it is impossible to identify the individual trajectory of patients.

We acquired a 4-year dataset of patient mobility between December 2009 and December 2013, which includes more than 1.2 billion health service records. Each record has specific mobility information, including the visit time (year and month), the residence location

Table 1 Health care service levels in Turkey

	Primary	Secondary	Tertiary
Facility	Community health centers, family health centers	Public and private health facility and hospitals	Training and research, and university hospitals
Staff	Family physicians	Specialist physicians	Specialist physicians and medical residents

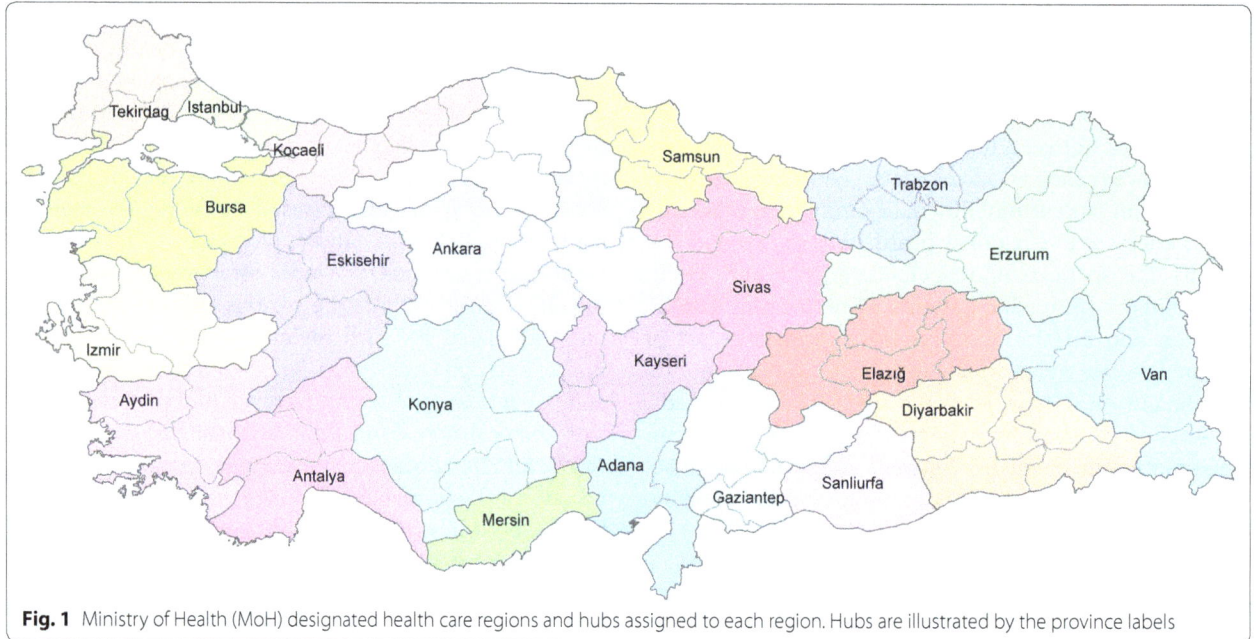

Fig. 1 Ministry of Health (MoH) designated health care regions and hubs assigned to each region. Hubs are illustrated by the province labels

Table 2 Patient admission records and attributes

Time period	December 2009 to December 2013 (48 months)
Origin	Patient's residence location at the district level
Destination	Health care unit location at the province level
Flow attributes	Institution: 12 types indicate the service provider and institution (e.g., public, private, university)
	Service level: (primary, secondary, and tertiary care)
	Service category: 120 medical specialties

of the patient at the district level, location of the health service facility at the province level, and service provider, type of institution, and category of medical service received (Table 2). Location information was not available for 11% of patients, who are either non-citizens from cross-border medical tourism or those that do not have a citizenship ID in the system. We excluded these records which do not have home residence information.

The patient mobility data naturally form a bipartite spatial network where there are two types of nodes: patient residences and health facilities. An edge (flow) in this network represents a patient's mobility from her/his residence (origin) to a health facility (destination). Provinces are divided into counties and counties are divided into districts in Turkey's hierarchy of administrative units. While the residence of a patient is provided at district level, the health facility that the patient was admitted is provided at province level. In order to match the spatial resolutions of origins and destinations, we generated a weighted and directed network of province-to-province

patient flows in which a node represents a province, whereas an edge represents monthly aggregated mobility of patients from the province of their residence to the province of the health facility. In addition to the total volume of each flow, we also aggregated the multivariate characteristics of each flow such as the type of service provider and the medical specialty by province-to-province pairs, with counts for each category.

Methods
Definitions
A longitudinal set of origin–destination (O–D) mobility network (graph) can be formulated by a sequence of non-overlapping time windows, each of which represents a snapshot of flows within that time window. Starting at time t_{min} and ending at t_{max}, we use the notation $M_t^w(t_{min}, t_{max})$ to describe a time-ordered sequence of mobility graphs, $M_{tmin}^w, M_{tmin+w}^w, \ldots, M_t^w t_{max}$, where w denotes the size of each time window in some time unit (i.e., hours, days, weeks, months). Each O–D graph M_t^w within the sequence is defined by a set of locations $P = \{p_1, \ldots, p_n\}$ and a set of flows (edges) $F = \left\{ f_{ij}^s \right\}$,

where $i \in P$, $j \in P$, $i \neq j$, $t \leq s \leq t + w$, and f_{ij}^s represents the flow from i to j within the time window s. In an O–D graph M_t^w, each location has fixed geographic coordinates, however, their existence depend on the existence of flows to and from that location within the given time window. By changing the size of the time window, one can obtain different levels of granularity in temporal scales. Selecting an appropriate size for time window is an application specific problem, as windows with different sizes may help capture different meaningful behavior, however, the maximum temporal resolution is preferred to be able to capture the finest differences between each graph [29]. On one end, the maximum temporal resolution results in each interval corresponding to the smallest time unit, or to the time between any two consecutive modification of the graph [30]. On the other hand, the minimum temporal resolution would correspond to a single graph which aggregates all interactions over time. In this paper, we first use the minimum temporal resolution, and consider the full dataset to identify consistent functional regions and multivariate flow patterns. Secondly, we use the maximum temporal resolution of monthly O–D graphs to identify spatiotemporal flow patterns that characterize the patient demands.

Locational measures of mobility

In order to identify the places of attraction and depletion, we compute locational measures of net-flow ratio and gross flow for the whole 4-year period, and the years 2010–2011 and 2012–2013.

$$Netflow_i = Inflow_i - Outflow_i$$

$$Gross\,flow_i = Inflow_i + Outflow_i$$

$$Netflow\,Ratio_i = \frac{Netflow_i}{Grossflow_i}$$

Net-flow ratio for a location i is calculated by dividing the net-flow (i.e., total patients in minus total patients out) by the total flow of patients in and out of a province.

Hierarchical regionalization of flows

We first derive functional regions of patient flows using a flow-based hierarchical regionalization, or in other words, spatially-constrained graph partitioning approach. A hierarchy of regions allows capturing mobility patterns at different scales such as the national scale, regional and provincial scale. For example, when looking at 4-region partition one can better understand patterns at national scale, while patient mobility at 23 regions helps understand patterns at regional scale and allow comparison with the designated regions of Ministry of Health. We compare the results of data-driven regions to designated regions of the government in order to identify the areas of mismatch between planned regional hub structure and the observed structure of the patient flows. Different from community detection in non-spatial networks, the objective of a spatially or contiguity constrained graph partitioning is to identify functional regions by grouping strongly connected and spatially adjacent nodes into clusters.

We adopt the flow-based hierarchical regionalization approach [26] which consists of the following steps. First, we convert raw flow matrix into a modularity matrix in order to remove the effect of size differences among the locations (nodes) in the O–D network. Each edge in the modularity matrix represents the modularity between a pair of provinces in two directions, which is derived by the difference between the actual flow and the expected volume of flow for each pair of locations. A variety of statistical measures can be used to calculate the expected volume of flows, we employ the following formula which is based on an adjusted flow volume:

$$EF\,(O,D) = F_O\,F_D\,f(O,D)\bigg/\left(F_S^2 - \sum_{i=0}^{n} F_i^2\right)$$

where F_O is the number of flows between area O and its connections, F_D is the number of flows between area D and its connections, $f(O, D)$ is the number of flows between area O and area D, F_S is the number of flows between all areas (provinces), and $\sum_{i=0}^{n} F_i^2$ is used to remove within-area expectations. Finally, modularity of a link O–D is calculated as:

$$MOD(O, D) = AF - EF$$

where AF is actual number of flows, and EF is expected number of flows on the link O–D. Using this formula, we transform the O–D network of raw counts of patient flows into an O–D modularity graph, in which the weight of a link represents the modularity between two locations. If modularity value is positive the link is considered to be above expectation, if the value is negative the link is below expectation.

Second, we perform a full-order average linkage clustering (ALK) in order to construct a set of spatially contiguous regions. ALK is a clustering method that builds a hierarchy of spatially contiguous clusters by iteratively merging the most connected clusters. The method first produces a spatially contiguous tree, where each edge connects two geographic neighbors and the entire tree is consistent with the cluster hierarchy. Then each region in the spatially contiguous tree is partitioned into two regions based on an objective function which maximizes within-region modularity for each region (community). The modularity is calculated by the sum of flow-expectation difference for each pair of units inside a region and for all regions. We used the software tools developed in Java for regionalization and flow mapping whose further details can be found in [26].

Feature selection

Visual analytics allows users to explore hidden patterns in the data by integrating computational methods with multiple perspectives provided by dynamically-linked visualization of patterns in geographic space, attribute space and time. We used visual analytics to capture the complex patterns of patient flows, where they are from, where they are going to, what characteristics they have, and what regions they form. The visual analytics tools used in this study can also be used in any flow analysis such as migration, commuting, traffic flows or waste flows.

We first identify the spatio-temporal characteristics and health care needs of moving patients by performing feature selection using a visual analytics environment. There are four main groups of patient flow variables: the visit time (i.e., month, season, year), service provider (i.e., public, private, university); service level (i.e., primary, secondary, tertiary), and service category which includes 120 medical specializations such as Cardiology, Urology, and Gynecology. Large number of variables pose a significant challenge for flow pattern analysis, and we initially do not know which variables are relevant and can be useful to characterize or predict the mobility behaviors. In order to provide a comprehensive analysis framework that take into account the interaction between various flow variables, we use a feature selection [31] and clustering methodology [26].

For selecting interesting group of variables, we use degree of correlation and clustering between every pair of attributes to determine bivariate attribute pairs that contain interesting patterns. While correlation quantifies the linear relationship between a pair of variables, maximum conditional entropy (MCE) provides a measure of "goodness of clustering" between two variables. We first construct a feature similarity matrix that illustrate bi-variate similarity between every pair of variables both in terms of correlation and clustering, we then reorder this matrix in a way that higher values of entropy are next to each other and closer to the diagonal section of the matrix (Fig. 2). In the feature matrix, each cell with a color illustrates a measure value between two attribute pairs. The pairwise conditional entropy values of all dimensions are shown in the bottom left part of the matrix in which lower entropy values (darker colors) represent more interesting subspaces. On the other hand, the pairwise correlation values of all dimensions are shown in the top right of the feature selection matrix, and higher correlation values (darker colors) represent strong relationship between variables. In both sides the darker colors illustrate more interesting relationships between each pair of variables. The ordering of the variables in the matrix is derived from the entropy matrix using a minimum spanning tree (MST) in order to group the cells with higher interestingness to reveal potentially interesting variable subspaces [31].

We selected five interesting subspaces from the feature matrix which are highlighted in red, green, purple, cyan, orange, and yellow in Fig. 2 in order to guide our analysis

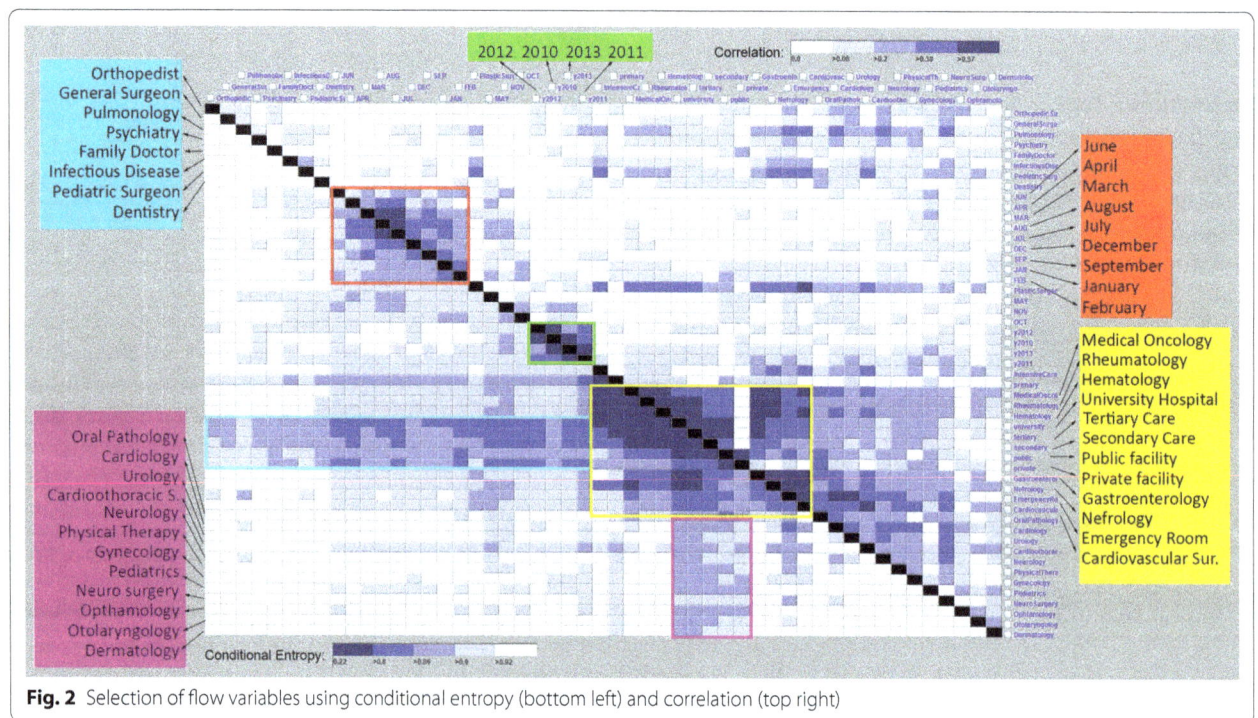

Fig. 2 Selection of flow variables using conditional entropy (bottom left) and correlation (top right)

of flow patterns. Red subspace consists of monthly variation of flows (i.e., January to December); green subspace consists of yearly aggregation of flows from 2010 to 2013; yellow subspace consists of a combination of flow variables that include type of institution and medical service; cyan subspace consists of variables of mostly monthly aggregations, some types of institution, and a few types of medical service; and purple subspace consists of types of institution, and certain types of medical service. In this paper, we provide a further analysis of flow patterns using the top four subspaces: red, green, and yellow in Fig. 2 which were identified as interesting by both conditional entropy and correlation measures. These subspaces illustrate the demands of patients that move long distances between regions.

Multivariate clustering
We use an integrated visual analytics framework [26] that combines flow mapping with multivariate clustering and visualization (Fig. 3). The integrated framework uses the pre-selected subspaces of variables in the first task (i.e., collection of variables included within red, green, cyan, yellow and purple rectangles), and help identify the multivariate relationships between the variables of each

subspace, and their spatial flow patterns. A self-organizing map (Fig. 3a) is used to order the multivariate clusters of flows in a two-dimensional layout in which nearby clusters are similar in terms of their flow attributes. Each SOM node (circle) illustrates a cluster of flows, and the size of each circle represents the number of flows the cluster contains. The hexagons that are drawn under each circle represent the multivariate dissimilarity between neighboring nodes, where darker tones illustrate greater dissimilarity. A 2D color scheme is used to assign each SOM cluster a unique color and similar clusters have similar colors. The colors created by the SOM are then passed onto a flow map that illustrates spatial patterns of flows (Fig. 3a) and a parallel coordinate plot (Fig. 3c) that reveals the meaning of each multivariate cluster. Figure 3 illustrates the multivariate clusters defined by the red subspace in Fig. 2 which corresponds to the monthly patterns of patient mobility. The flows are symbolized based on the proportion of the total volume of movement for a specific month to the total volume of flows for the whole time period. In Fig. 3, green clusters of patients who are residents of eastern regions and seek health services in large cities of Istanbul, Ankara, Izmir and Adana during the months from November to April. The purple clusters

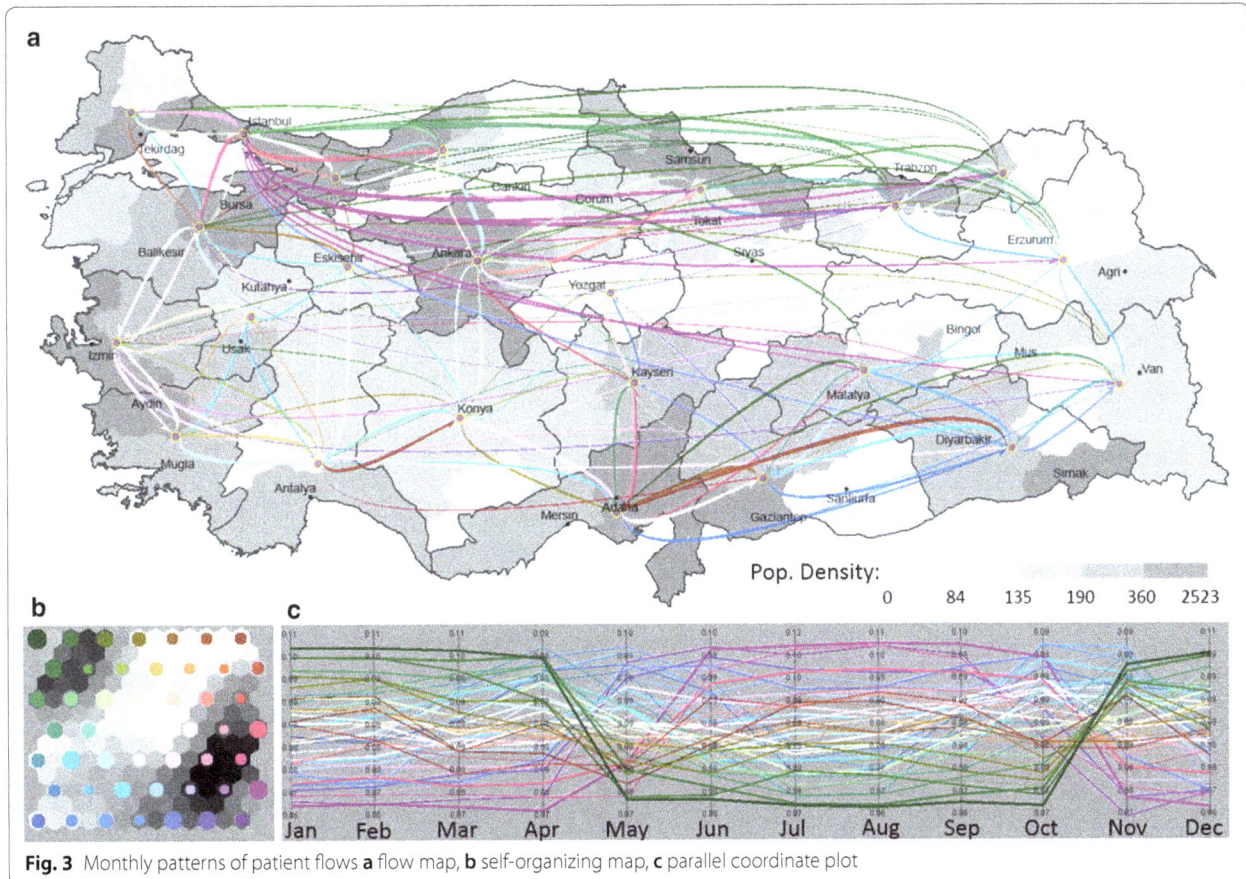

Fig. 3 Monthly patterns of patient flows **a** flow map, **b** self-organizing map, **c** parallel coordinate plot

of patients are residents of large cities that seek care in the north, north-eastern and south-eastern regions. In addition, blue clusters of patient flows in Fig. 3 characterizes the short-distance mobility of patients mostly in the South-East which peaks during spring and autumn months.

Results

We introduce the results of our analysis in three sections. The first section reports on the temporal and service level patterns. The second section introduces the functional regions derived from the patient mobility data, and compares the regionalization result to that of designated regions by Ministry of Health (MoH). The third section introduces the spatio-temporal and multivariate flow patterns that help characterize the demands of patients.

Temporal and service level patterns

In order to answer the question how has mobility changed over time?, we provide a summary of the total

Table 3 Health service records and mobility ratio by year

Time interval	# admissions	# mobility	Mobility ratio (%)
December 2009–November 2010	251,630,100	32,843,706	13.05
December 2010–November 2011	292,626,833	36,407,051	12.44
December 2011–November 2012	355,843,020	41,755,845	11.73
December 2012–November 2013	372,586,211	43,772,750	11.75

hospital admission records and mobility by year in Table 3, and we illustrate change in mobility by year and month in Fig. 4. Although health service use and mobility increased over time, yearly mobility ratio declined from December 2009 to December 2013. The volume of patient mobility between provinces follows an increasing trend with seasonal fluctuations and high volumes in summer months for the study period (Fig. 4a). Figure 4b illustrates monthly total mobility volumes across the 4-year period. The x-axis represents months, and the vertical lines on each month represents the yearly variation in monthly volume of mobility across the 4-year period. For example, for January and March, total volume of mobility increased steadily, however, it declined in year 2013 (see the declining lines in Fig. 4b). Horizontal lines are used to represent the average of the 4-year period for each month. Spring and summer months exhibit higher volume of mobility than autumn and winter. March and July are the peak months, whereas October and December exhibit the lowest patient mobility across the 4-year period. The range of values during each month of the 4-year period was between 100 thousand and 200 thousand. Although summer months resulted in more patient mobility, patient mobility in winter months increased greater than the summer months over the 4-year period.

Figure 5 illustrates the mobility by health care service levels such as primary, secondary and tertiary care, and by years. Secondary care includes most of patient mobility between provinces with an average of 232 million patient flows per year, and patient mobility demanding secondary care increased over years with a decline in 2013. Patients seeking tertiary care in other provinces

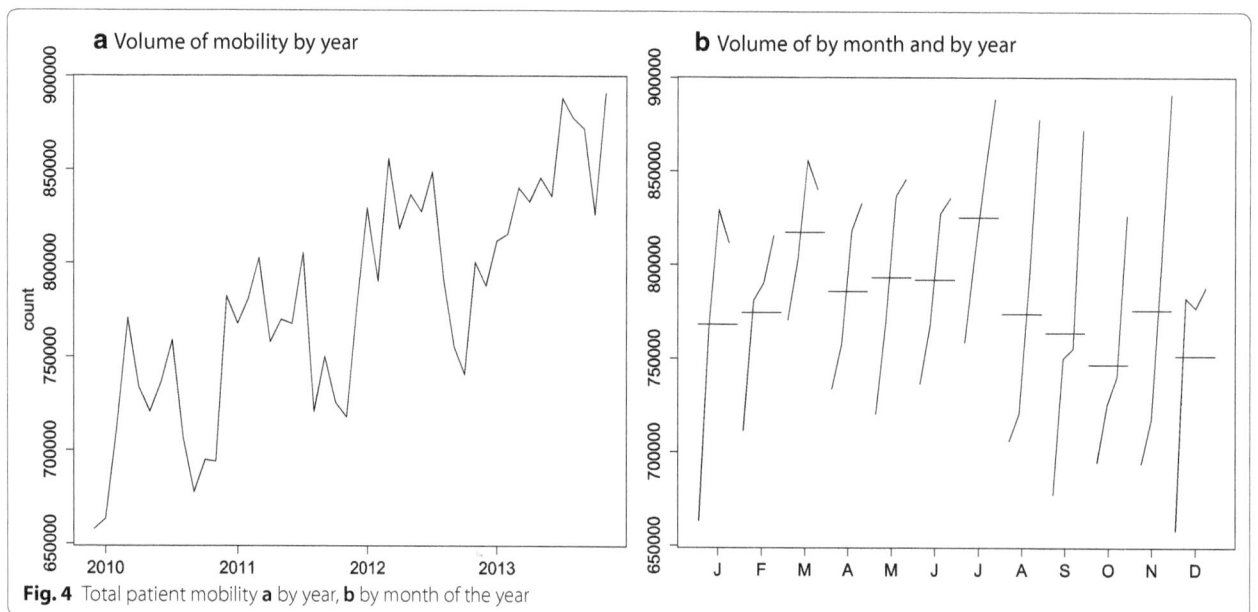

Fig. 4 Total patient mobility **a** by year, **b** by month of the year

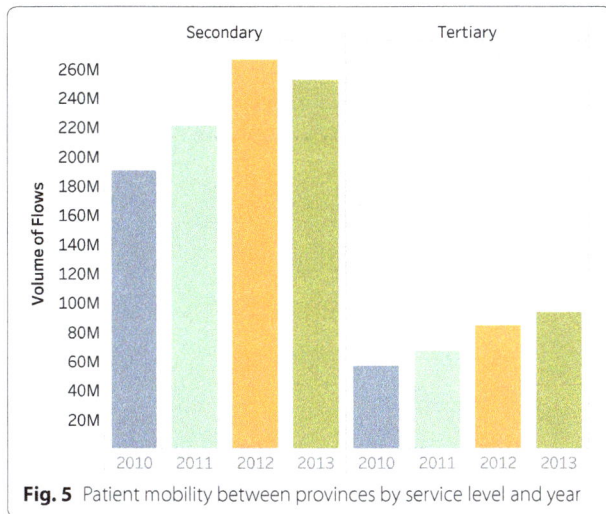

Fig. 5 Patient mobility between provinces by service level and year

steadily increased over time, however, the total number of patients for the 4 year average was around 75 million. Figure 5 does not display primary care patient flows between provinces since the numbers were very marginal as compared to secondary and tertiary care. In the years of 2010 and 2011, there was an average number of 713 thousand patients that received primary health care in a province other than the province of their residence. Strikingly, this number went down to only 86 and 128 for years 2012 and 2013 respectively. We can attribute this change to the policy change in 2011 that assigned each patient to a family physician.

Spatial patterns
Patterns of attraction and depletion
In order to reveal provinces that attract and push patients for health care service, we compute a series of patient flow ratio measures. Flow ratio is calculated by dividing the net flow (inflow–outflow) by the gross flow (the summation of total inflow and outflow) of patients per province. Figure 6 illustrates the net flow ratio for each province including all 4-year period (Fig. 6a), and net flow ratio and gross volume of flows per province for the time periods 2010–2011 (Fig. 6b) and 2012–2013 (Fig. 6c). These time periods correspond to the before and aftermath period of the policy change on the establishment of family physicians implemented in 2011 and put in place in 2012. Overall, orange colors highlight the provinces of Ankara and Eskisehir in central Anatolia, Isparta in south west; and Elazig in the east and Edirne in north west as major places of attraction for patients. It is remarkable to see that even though it has the largest number and variety of medical services, Istanbul has a negative net flow ratio, which highlight the excessive number of patients who reside in Istanbul but receive

health care elsewhere. On the other hand, Fig. 6 also highlights many small provinces such as Sinop, Kars and Erzincan where patients travel to other provinces to receive health care. These provinces cluster in the south east, north and north east. In addition to general patterns of health care utilization by province, Fig. 6b, c provide a comparison of the net flow ratio as well as gross flows in the first and second half of the dataset in order to reveal changes after the family physician policy implemented in 2011. A remarkable difference between the two time periods is that the values were stretched towards positive and negative outliers, and as a result we observe darker blue and darker red provinces that indicate increased attraction and depletion. It is clear from the two figures that patient mobility out of the eastern provinces increased in the period after the policy change, which is highlighted by large negative net flow ratio (dark blue colors). We attribute this change to the establishment of the family physician service which increased the number of referrals to specialist that are located elsewhere. On the other hand, central Anatolia including Ankara, Eskisehir and Bolu became central places of attraction for patients across the nation. We also observe an increase in net flow ratio in provinces such as Kayseri, Edirne, Bursa and Kocaeli.

Functional regions
We employed the Average Linkage Clustering (ALK) to derive a hierarchy of regions using the minimum temporal resolution, i.e., the mobility graph for the whole period $M_t^w(t_{min}, t_{max})$. We computed the total within-region modularity of the hierarchical partitions to evaluate the partitioning result at different levels up to twenty three regions which we used as a baseline to compare with the designated regions by MoH. While each partition level highlights patterns at different scales, the partition with four regions maximizes the total within-region modularity (Fig. 7a), therefore, suggests a stable partitioning of the patient mobility network for the discovery of community structures. As the number of regions increases, the percentage of flows between regions naturally increases. While 50% of flows were between regions for the four-region partition, 89% of flows were between regions for the twenty three-region partition (Fig. 7b). Among the four regions of Anatolia (i.e., the main land of Turkey), the northern region is formed by the provinces that are tightly connected to Istanbul (Fig. 7c). The inland and western regions are very consistent with the hinterlands of the two big cities Ankara and Izmir. The south-eastern region is formed by merging of the hinterland of Antalya and Diyarbakir. These two provinces were designated as major health care hubs by Ministry of Health (MoH) for the surrounding provinces in their allocated regions.

a Net patient mobility rate 2010 - 2013

b Net patient mobility rate 2010 - 2011

c Net patient mobility rate 2012 - 2013

Net Flow Ratio

Net Flow / Gross Flow

	-0.40 - -0.30
	-0.29 - -0.20
	-0.19 - -0.09
	-0.08 - 0.00
	0.01 - 0.11
	0.12 - 0.23
	0.24 - 0.34

Gross Flow

- 100,000
- 1,000,000
- 10,000,000

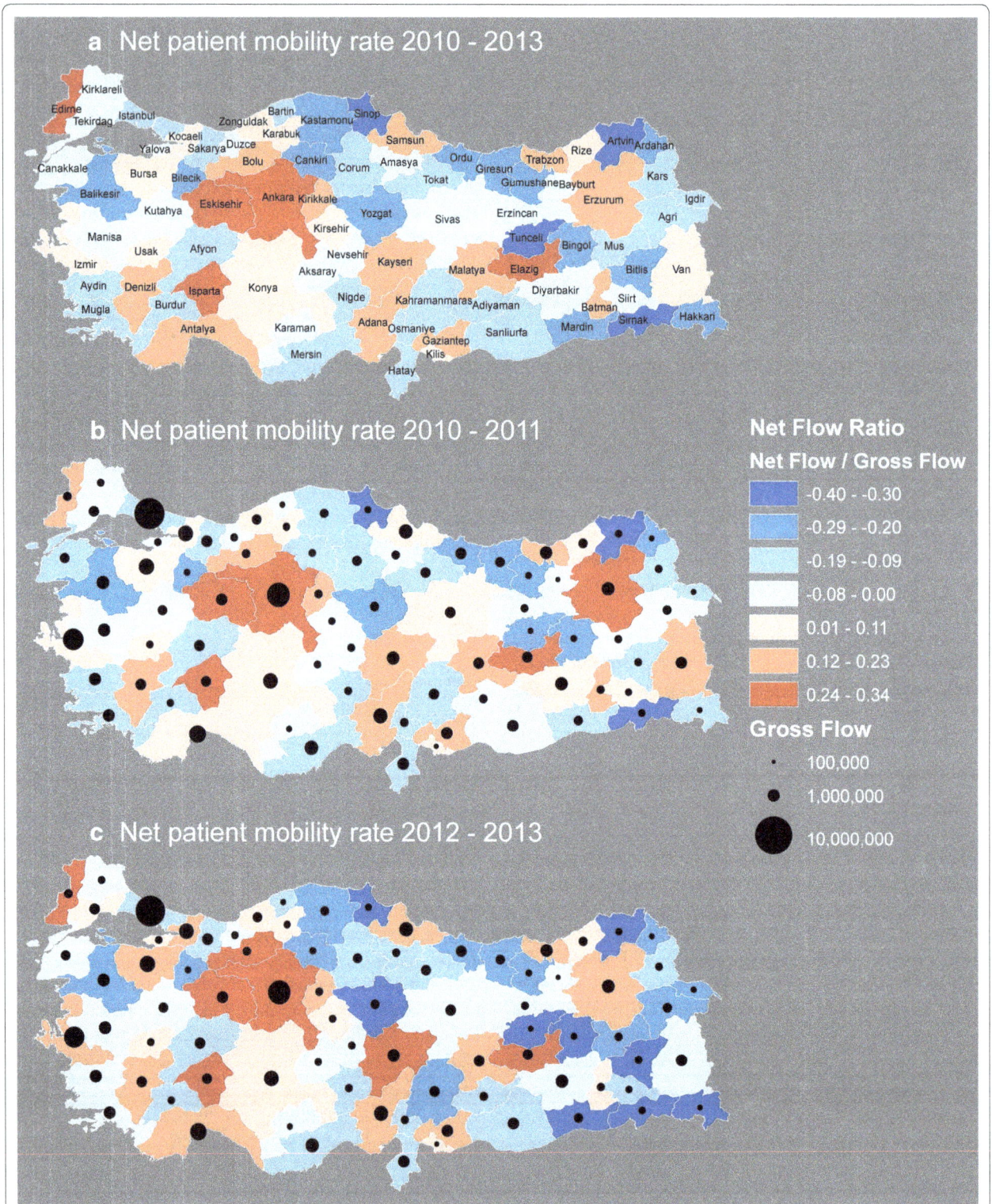

Fig. 6 a Net patient flow ratio for the 4-year period, **b** net flow ratio and gross flow in 2010–2011, **c** net flow ratio and gross flow in 2012–2013

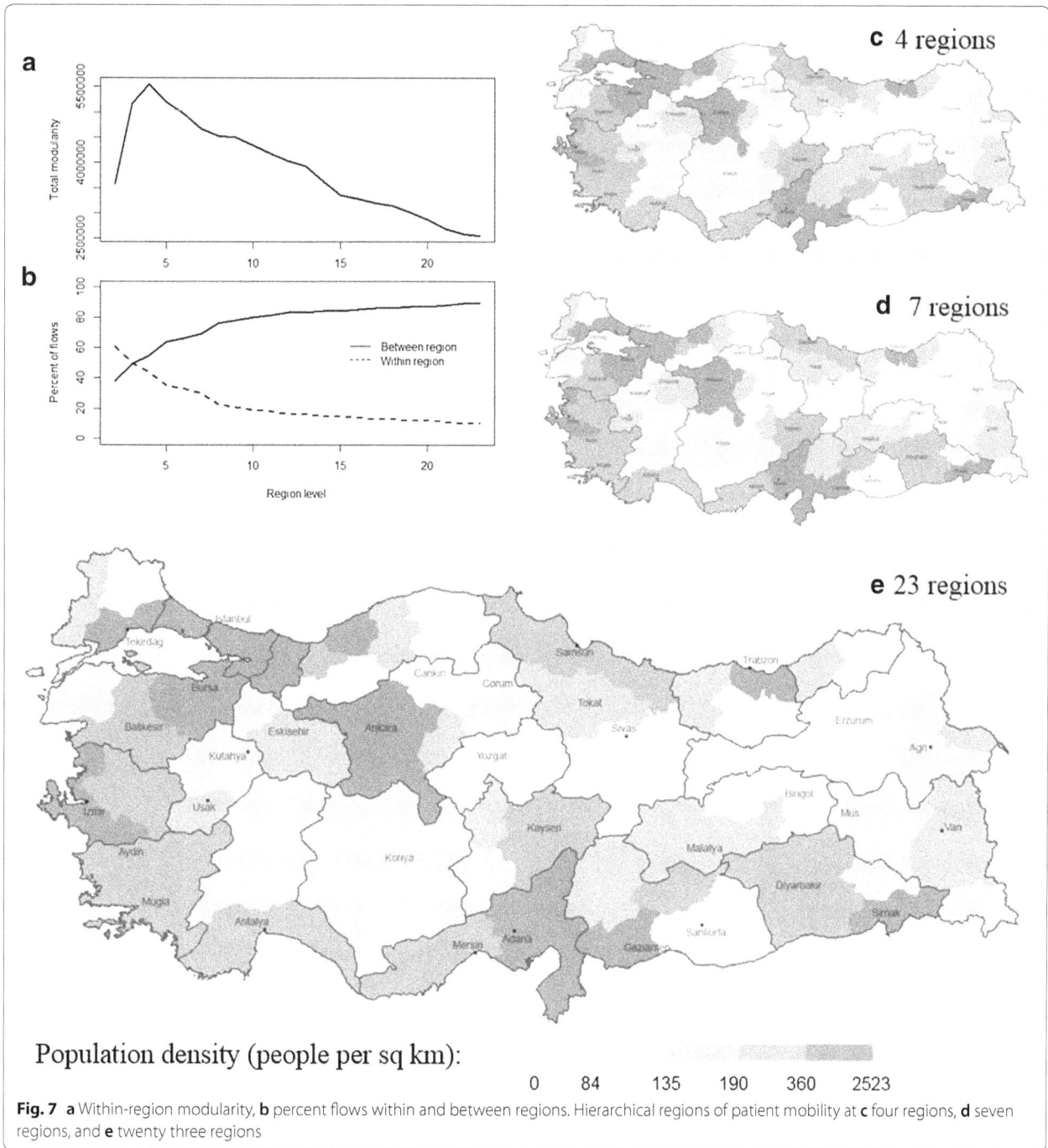

Fig. 7 **a** Within-region modularity, **b** percent flows within and between regions. Hierarchical regions of patient mobility at **c** four regions, **d** seven regions, and **e** twenty three regions

Seven-region partition results from further partitioning of the north, west, and south-east regions observed in the four-region partition (Fig. 7d). MoH designated health care regions, and assigned a hub for each region. These hubs were either already functioning as hubs or MoH planned these hubs as future hubs by investing in the health infrastructure to serve the surrounding provinces that lack capacities and certain specialized services.

The original designation by MoH consists of twenty nine regions which separates the metropolitan areas of Istanbul to six sub regions, Ankara to two regions. In order to compare the designated regions of MoH with the regions derived from flows of patients between provinces, we used Istanbul and Ankara in their own regions without splitting these provinces into sub-regions. As a result, the number of designated regions went from twenty nine down to twenty three. Figure 7e illustrates the twenty three-region partition in order to compare with the designated regions defined by MoH.

Figure 8 illustrates the comparison of Ministry of Health (MoH) designated regions and twenty three regions derived from patient mobility. Boundaries of designated regions by MoH are shown by thick black lines, whereas the boundaries of data-driven regions are illustrated by thinner red lines. The thick black lines that are overlayed by thin red lines illustrate the matching boundaries of designated and data-driven regions. On the other hand, thin black lines illustrate the province boundaries, and each hub city is labelled by its name within the provincial boundary. We compared the overlap between the two regionalizations by comparing the percentage of shared and mismatched boundaries. We excluded the bordering boundaries to the surrounding seas and other countries. Overall, 22% of the MoH region boundaries did not match the boundaries of the data-driven regions of patient mobility. Eastern and south eastern regions of Diyarbakir, Elazig, and Van; Marmara regions of Tekirdag and Bursa; and inner Anatolian regions such as Kayseri and Konya perfectly matched with the designated regions of MoH. Some of the MoH designated regions consists of only one province, which is a policy of MoH to establish those provinces as hubs that could serve the surrounding regions. However, these provinces were

merged with existing hubs and regions that are nearby in the data-driven regionalization. For example, Sanliurfa and Mersin, the two planned hubs, are merged with the existing hubs, Gaziantep and Adana, respectively. Also, Eskisehir province was considered as a major hub for the surrounding provinces by MoH. However, neighboring provinces of Eskisehir have stronger connections with other hubs such as Antalya and Izmir. The mismatch between the data-driven regionalization and designated regions by MoH can be used to implement policies that could strengthen the connection of provinces to their designated or planned regional hubs.

Flow patterns

In this section we report the results and discuss the patterns we captured using the integrated visual analytics framework presented in "Multivariate clustering" section. We first selected the variables defined by the red subspace in Fig. 2 and incorporated these variables into the flow mapping and multivariate clustering framework to capture the monthly variation of patient flows across the 4-year period (Fig. 3). Green clusters of patients who are residents of eastern regions and seek health services in large cities of Istanbul, Ankara, Izmir and Adana from November to April. Patients from the north and north east regions represent the largest portion of these patterns and they primarily target Istanbul and north

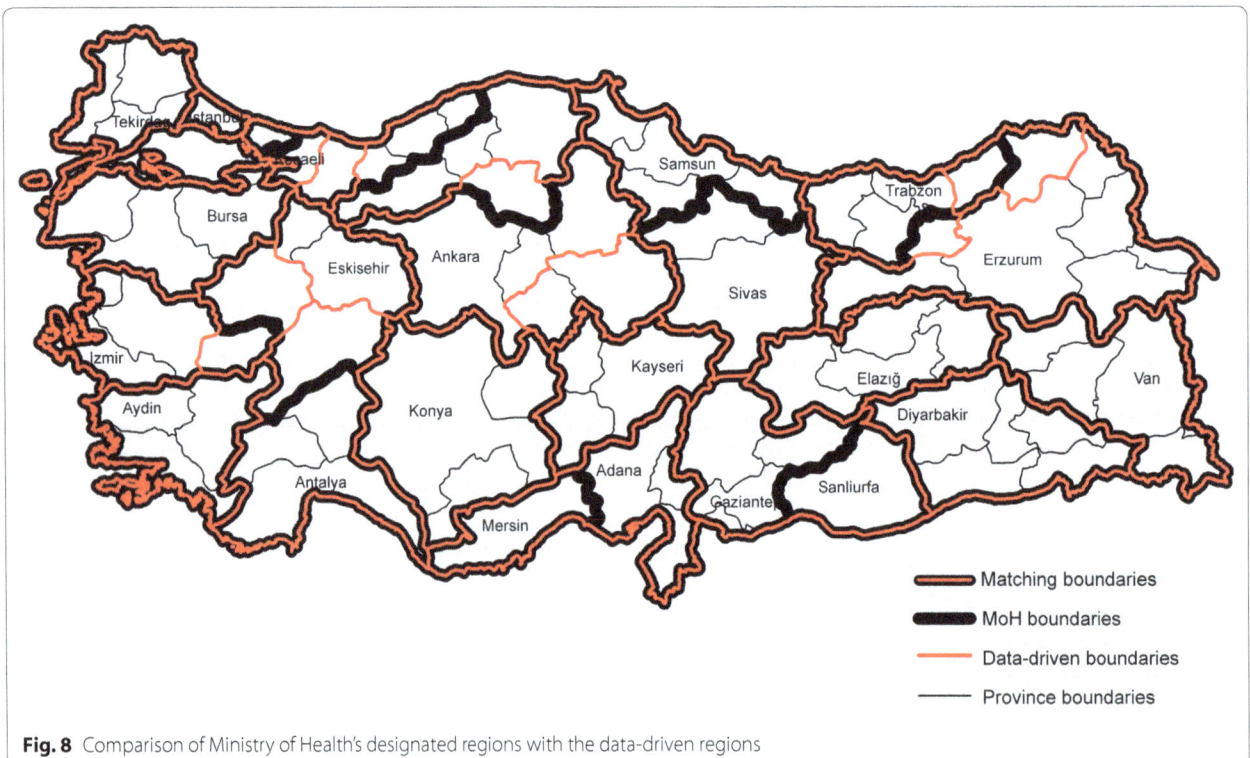

Fig. 8 Comparison of Ministry of Health's designated regions with the data-driven regions

western regions, whereas patients from the south east target Adana. Patient movements are tightly related to the general mobility patterns in Turkey, which is driven by sociodemographic structure of the society and its history of urbanization. Istanbul has the ability to pull patients from greater distances as a function of its large population, health care infrastructure, as well as other motivations such as familiarity in the form of cultural and family ties with the rest of the country, and perceived quality of care [3]. Residents of Istanbul who originally migrated from distant areas tend to keep their ties to where they migrated from, often own second homes, and have relatives in those provinces. Patients that seek health care in these large cities often stay with relatives or connections through home town organizations [32, 33] when they receive their specialized medical care [32, 34–36]. Ankara and Izmir, the second and the third largest city in Turkey, also attract migrants however, not from far locations, rather from the nearby provinces. In contrast to the green clusters of flows that seek health services in big cities during winter months, purple clusters of patients in Fig. 3 travel to acquire health services during months between May and October. The purple clusters of patients are residents of large cities that seek care in the north, north-eastern and south-eastern regions. During summer months when the school is over, these migrants visit their relatives and use health care facilities in their hometowns in the east and northeast provinces. In addition, blue clusters of patient flows in Fig. 3 characterizes the short-distance mobility of patients mostly in the South-East. Patients in the South-East continue to use the services in the regional hub of Diyarbakir throughout the year, while the demand peaks during spring and autumn months.

Second, we visualize and explore the green subspace defined in Fig. 2 into the flow mapping and clustering framework in order to discover annual changes in mobility patterns. Using the visual analytics interface explained in Fig. 3, we select the flows that were high in all years to identify whether these flows had distinct changes in time and geographic space (Fig. 9). While the selection leaves the high volume of flows on the maps with red and blue clusters, the rest of the flows are hidden in the map view in order to highlight the details-on-demand (i.e., high values in all years) as part of the visual information seeking mantra [37]. Correspondingly, the values of flows that were filtered out are still displayed on the parallel coordinate plot with grey color to show the overall distribution while highlighting the blue and red clusters with dynamic brushing and linking. When Fig. 9a illustrates the blue clusters of patients that are residents of large cities who seek for health services in the eastern as well as less populated regions. These flows significantly declined

after 2011. On the other hand, Fig. 9b illustrates the red clusters of patients are residents of south-eastern, eastern and southern regions that seek care in either the nearby hubs in the south and south-east or the north-west. These flows increased after 2011. We attribute the change in these mobility patterns after 2011 to the health care policy change implemented by the Turkish Health Transformation Program in 2011. The program was aimed to improve preventative care through family physicians, and thus, decrease the number of unnecessary admissions to secondary and tertiary care institutions. As a result, citizens were assigned to a family physician, and a considerable number of physicians in different specialties were assigned to the disadvantaged provinces in this period [28]. Our findings indicate that the program resulted in different outcomes across the country. The mobility of patients in the underdeveloped regions of the east and south east increased (Fig. 9b), while patient flows from the large cities to the eastern, south-eastern and other less populated areas across the country significantly decreased (Fig. 9a). The increasing mobility in the east and south east can be associated with the establishment of family doctors after 2011, which helped guide patients to seek for specialized care services in health care hubs.

Third, we explore the yellow subspace in Fig. 2 which consists of flow variables by institution and medical service (Fig. 10). Within this subspace of variables, the most distinct pattern is characterized by the blue clusters of patients who seek specialized services in Medical Oncology, Hematology and Rheumatology at university hospitals and at the tertiary level of care. Primary care demand for these patients were low, whereas secondary care and public institutions were utilized at medium level as compared to high level tertiary care and utilization of university hospitals. Unsurprisingly, these flows were targeted at urbanized and developed regions of Ankara, Istanbul, Izmir, and Adana where there are university hospitals and tertiary care institutions that provide sufficient services for those specialized care demands.

Discussion

We first discuss the implications of this study for the assessment of the health systems. Second, we discuss the limitations, challenges and future directions in the analysis of patient mobility. Our results agree with the findings of the previous work that analyze patient mobility data from European countries [5, 7, 38] in terms of the typology of patterns we discovered in our analysis. First, patient mobility correlates with provincial migration in the country. The provinces in western and eastern Marmara, Aegean, western and southern Anatolian regions have a relatively higher per capita income which attract migrants from the north-eastern Anatolian and

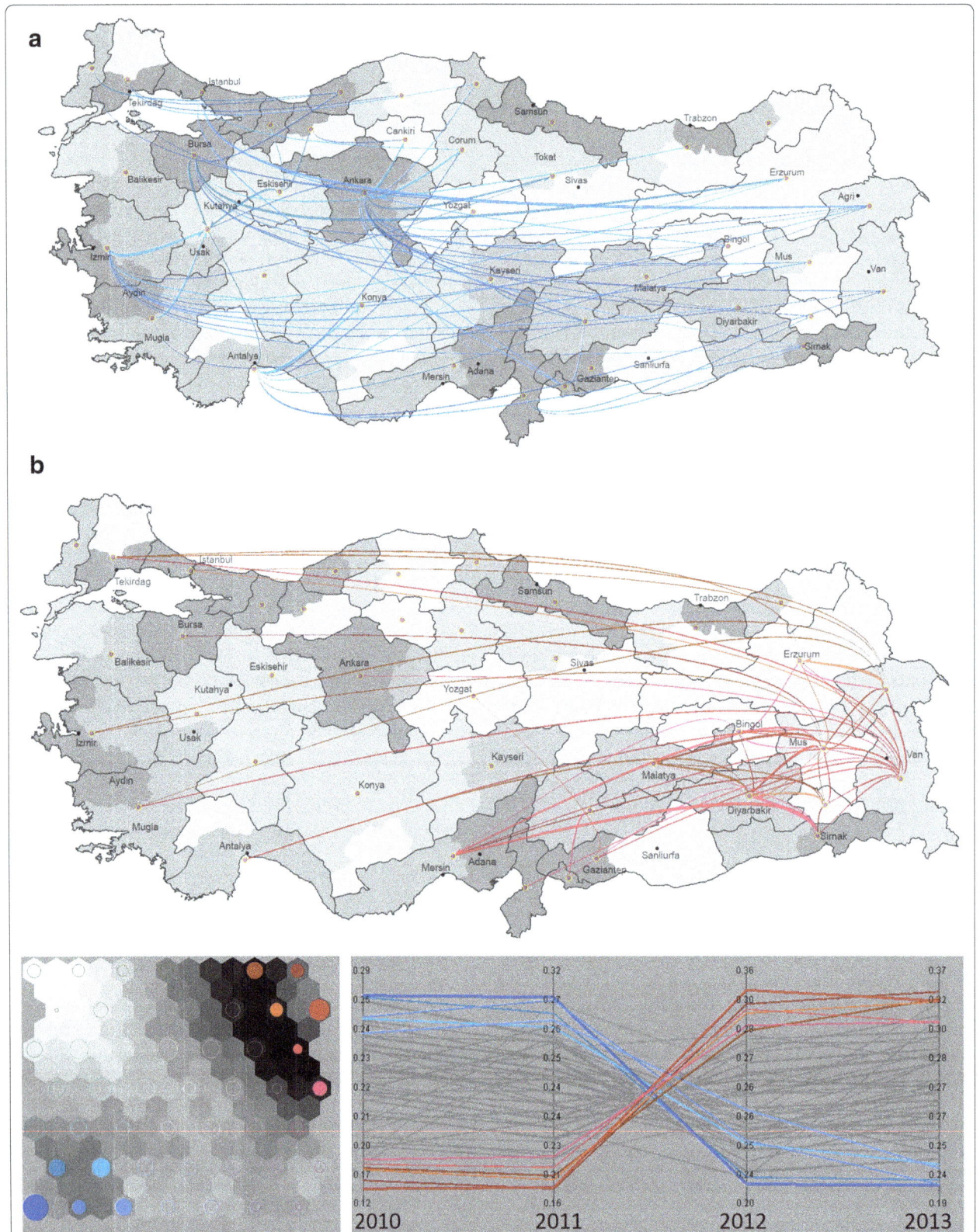

Fig. 9 Patients seeking care from **a** central and western regions, **b** the south-east

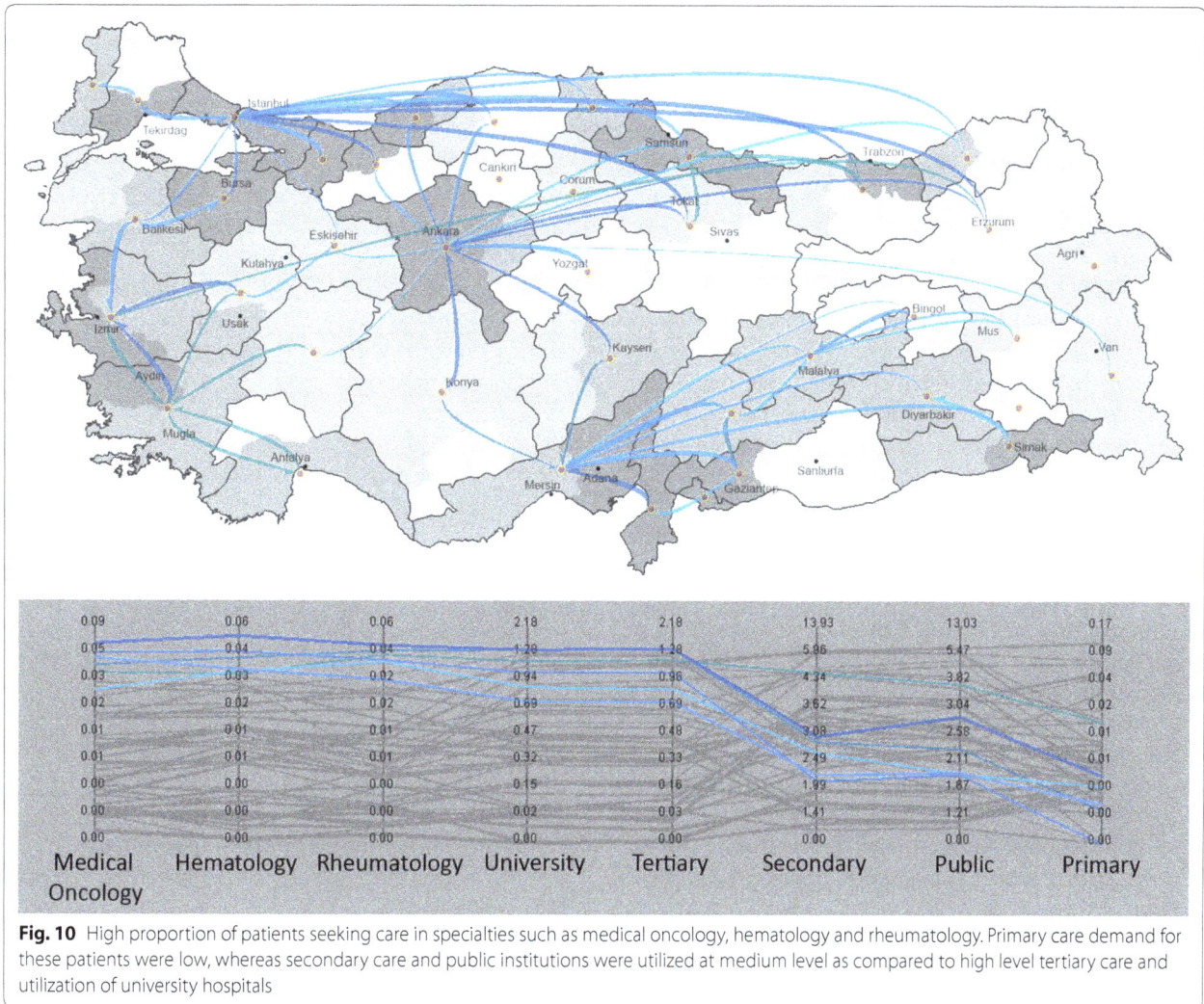

Fig. 10 High proportion of patients seeking care in specialties such as medical oncology, hematology and rheumatology. Primary care demand for these patients were low, whereas secondary care and public institutions were utilized at medium level as compared to high level tertiary care and utilization of university hospitals

mid-eastern Anatolian regions that are characterized by lower per capita income [20, 39]. The effect of social and geographical ties among various parts of the country is reflected in the use of health system. Patient movements to the large cities of Istanbul, Ankara and Izmir for receiving specialized medical care correlate with the migration patterns from the inner, north eastern and eastern parts of Anatolia, where the health infrastructure is inadequate in providing a comprehensive range of health services for the regional population. As a result of the lack of public policies and institutional support, patients from eastern Anatolia rely on family and kinship relationships to address their health care needs [40]. Second, different from the distant migratory ties, we identified a cluster of movements within the west, and south and south eastern regions, which may reflect strong cultural links. Patients living within these regions are more likely to look for treatment in areas that are culturally similar [3], and

geographically close by for keeping the travel and health care related costs as minimum as possible.

In addition to socio-demographic characteristics that impact patient mobility, our results correlate with the policies implemented by MoH. After the centralized health care system patients were given the ability to go to private or government (public) health care institutions, and as a result, private institutions in the regions that lack health care infrastructure received large number of patients from surrounding regions. We also found a distinct shift in the mobility patterns after 2011 which we attribute to the health care policy change implemented by the Turkish Health Transformation Program in 2011 [41]. This policy assigned each citizen to a family physician. Our findings indicate that the program resulted in different outcomes across the country. As a result of guidance from family physicians, seeking for specialized medical care expanded in the underdeveloped regions of the east after the implementation of the family physician system. On the contrary, patient flows from the large cities to the eastern and south-eastern regions significantly decreased.

A major limitation of this study is that we were able to identify when, and where patient travel to receive what type of care, but we do not know the actual motivation whether it is affordability, perceived quality, or familiarity. Further studies, in the form of interviews could be beneficial to identify the motives behind patients' choices. While our approach help identify flow patterns and trends, identifying main drivers of mobility requires comparing flow patterns to locational (node or regional) attributes such as socio-demographic and population characteristics and their spatiotemporal patterns. Patient mobility could result from a diverse set of reasons such as the number of hospitals/specialists, the number of beds, advanced health technology, lack of specialized centers, mistrust, comfort and cleaning of health care centers price, accessibility, seasonal migration and distances between origin and destination provinces [42–45]. Another factor is the presence of contact people through kinship and family ties at the destination as a result of past migration [36].

Because of high dimensionality (large number of attributes), and temporally varying characteristics, it is challenging to identify interesting relationships among the large number of flow and node attributes. There is a critical need for integrating feature selection methods to identify interesting relationships among a large number of both temporally varying variables such as health service capacity, population and patient characteristics. Also, in order to increase the quality of regionalization, and flow patterns, there is a need to increase the resolution of the dataset from province-to-province to district-to-district patient flows. While we hypothesize that the regional and national patterns would not change significantly, increasing the resolution of the dataset will allow capturing local patterns and fine details of regionalization.

Conclusion

Our data-driven approach has two major contributions. First, we can identify medical regions from the patient mobility network, and compare them to the designated or planned regional structure of the health care system. The mismatch between medical regions of patient mobility and the designated regions highlight the fact that the patient use of health care services do not overlap with the planned structure of health service delivery by Ministry of Health (MoH). By pointing out malfunctioning medical regions and underutilized regional hubs, our study can directly be

used in policy-making to improve the regional policy for health service delivery. Second, our study allows the identification of the demands, characteristics, and temporally varying patterns and shifts in patient mobility and health care utilization. Using such information, policies could be designed to satisfy varying needs of different regions such as the size, characteristics and health care demands of the population, and availability, quantity, quality and variety of health care providers. Implementing specific policies for different regions will allow addressing issues related to certain areas, and help close the gap between supply and demand for health service delivery.

Authors' contribution

The conceptual framework, computational, statistical and visual analysis of the patient mobility data was done by CK. Background research was mainly conducted by CK. SD contributed to the conceptual framework, background research, and interpretation of the results. DG contributed to the parameter selections for the adopted methodologies, and interpretation of the results. All authors read and approved the final manuscript.

Author details

[1] Department of Geographical and Sustainability Sciences, University of Iowa, Iowa City, USA. [2] Informatics Institute, Istanbul Technical University, Istanbul, Turkey. [3] Department of Geography, University of South Carolina, Columbia, USA.

Acknowledgements

The authors thank the anonymous reviewers for their constructive comments and suggestions.

Competing interests

The authors declare that they have no competing interests.

Availability of data and materials

The data used in this paper includes aggregated health service records, which were obtained from the Turkish Social Security Institution (TSSI) upon approval by the Data Sharing Committee following required legal procedures that protect patient and institutional privacy. The approval was granted on 01/15/2014 with the reference number 2014/146. The datasets generated and/or analyzed during the current study are not publicly available due to the policies of the Data Sharing Committee in the Turkish Social Security Institution (TSSI). The data can be acquired upon specific application to the Turkish Social Security Institution (TSSI).

Funding

The research reported here was not funded.

References

1. Andritsos DA, Tang CS. Introducing competition in healthcare services: the role of private care and increased patient mobility. Eur J Oper Res. 2014;234:898–909.
2. Mafrolla E, D'amico E. Patients' mobility as an indicator for (in) efficiency: a panel data analysis on Italian health care authorities. Health Econ Rev. 2013;3:3.
3. Glinos IA, Baeten R, Helble M, Maarse H. A typology of cross-border patient mobility. Health Place. 2010;16:1145–55.
4. Tang CF, Lau E. Modelling the demand for inbound medical tourism: the case of Malaysia. Int J Tour Res. 2017;19:584–93.
5. Rosenmöller, M, McKee, M, Baeten, R. Patient mobility in the European Union: learning from experience, The European observatory on health systems and policies; 2006.
6. Mainil T, Van Loon F, Dinnie K, Botterill D, Platenkamp V, Meulemans H. Transnational health care: from a global terminology towards transnational health region development. Health Policy. 2012;108:37–44.
7. Glinos IA, Baeten R, Maarse H. Purchasing health services abroad: practices of cross-border contracting and patient mobility in six European countries. Health Policy. 2010;95:103–12.
8. Gan LL, Frederick JR. Medical tourism facilitators: patterns of service differentiation. J Vacat Mark. 2011;17:165–83.
9. Connell J. Medical tourism: sea, sun, sand and… surgery. Tour Manag. 2006;27:1093–100.
10. Taliaferro JD, Remmers W. Identifying integrated regions for health care delivery. Health Serv Rep. 1973;88:337.
11. Harner EJ, Slater P. Identifying medical regions using hierarchical clustering. Soc Sci Med Part D Med Geogr. 1980;14:3–10.
12. Svensson S. Health policy in cross-border cooperation practices: the role of Euroregions and their local government members. Territ Polit Gov. 2017;5:47–64.
13. Paez A, Mercado RG, Farber S, Morency C, Roorda M. Accessibility to health care facilities in Montreal Island: an application of relative accessibility indicators from the perspective of senior and non-senior residents. Int J Health Geogr. 2010;9:52.
14. Mazumdar S, Feng X, Konings P, McRae I, Girosi F. A brief report on primary care service area catchment geographies in New South Wales Australia. Int J Health Geogr. 2014;13:38.
15. Ray N, Ebener S. AccessMod 3.0: computing geographic coverage and accessibility to health care services using anisotropic movement of patients. Int J Health Geogr. 2008;7:63.
16. Turner LG. Quality in health care and globalization of health services: accreditation and regulatory oversight of medical tourism companies. Int J Qual Health Care. 2010;23:1–7.
17. Lunt N, Carrera P. Advice for prospective medical tourists: systematic review of consumer sites. Tour Rev. 2011;66:57–67.
18. Koylu C, Guo D. Smoothing locational measures in spatial interaction networks. Comput Environ Urban Syst. 2013;41:12–25.
19. Gao P, Kupfer JA, Zhu X, Guo D. Quantifying animal trajectories using spatial aggregation and sequence analysis: a case study of differentiating trajectories of multiple species. Geogr Anal. 2016;48:275–91.
20. Slater PB. The identification of Turkish regions using 1965 lifetime interprovincial migration data. Geoforum. 1975.
21. Pandit K. Differentiating between subsystems and typologies in the analysis of migration regions: a U.S. example. Prof Geogr. 1994;46:331–45.
22. Guo D, Zhu X. Origin–destination flow data smoothing and mapping. IEEE Trans Vis Comput Graph. 2014;20(12):2043–2052. https://doi.org/10.1109/TVCG.2014.2346271

23. Holten D, van Wijk JJ. Force-directed edge bundling for graph visualization. Comput Graph Forum. 2009;28:983–90.
24. Gastner MT, Newman MEJ. The spatial structure of networks. Eur Phys J B Condens Matter Complex Syst. 2006;49:247–52.
25. Barthélemy M. Spatial networks. Phys Rep. 2011;499:1–101.
26. Guo D. Flow mapping and multivariate visualization of large spatial interaction data. IEEE Trans Vis Comput Graph. 2009;15:1041–8.
27. Akinci F, Mollahaliloğlu S, Gürsöz H, Öğücü F. Assessment of the Turkish health care system reforms: a stakeholder analysis. Health Policy. 2012;107:21–30.
28. Delil S, Çelik RN, San S, Dundar M. Clustering patient mobility patterns to assess effectiveness of health-service delivery. BMC Health Serv Res. 2017;17:458.
29. Nicosia V, Tang J, Mascolo C, Musolesi M, Russo G, Latora V. Graph metrics for temporal networks. In: Holme P, Saramäki J, editors. Temporal networks. Berlin, Heidelberg: Springer; 2013. pp. 15–40.
30. Santoro N, Quattrociocchi W, Flocchini P, Casteigts A, Amblard F. Time-varying graphs and social network analysis: temporal indicators and metrics. arXiv preprint arXiv:11020629 (2011).
31. Guo D. Coordinating computational and visual approaches for interactive feature selection and multivariate clustering. Inf Vis. 2003;2:232–46.
32. Hersant J, Toumarkine A. Hometown organisations in Turkey: an overview. Eur J Turk Stud Soc Sci Contemp Turk. (2). 2005.
33. Kurtoğlu A. Mekansal bir olgu olarak hemşehrilik ve bir hemşehrilik mekanı olarak dernekler. Eur J Turk Stud Soc Sci Contemp Turk. 2005.
34. Ayata S. Migrants and changing urban periphery: social relations, cultural diversity and the public space in Istanbul's new neighbourhoods. Int Migr. 2008;46:27–64.
35. Akarca AT, Başlevent C. The region-of-origin effect on voting behavior: the case of Turkey's internal migrants. İktisat İşletme ve Finans. 2010;25:9–36.
36. Akarca AT, Tansel A. Impact of internal migration on political participation in Turkey. IZA J Migr. 2015;4:1.
37. Shneiderman B. The eyes have it: a task by data type taxonomy for information visualizations. In: Proceedings of IEEE symposium on visual languages, 1996. IEEE; 1996. pp. 336–343.
38. Laugesen MJ, Vargas-Bustamante A. A patient mobility framework that travels: European and United States–Mexican comparisons. Health Policy. 2010;97:225–31.
39. Kırdar MG, Saracoğlu DŞ. Migration and regional convergence: an empirical investigation for Turkey. Pap Reg Sci. 2008;87:545–66.
40. Erder S. Urban migration and reconstruction of the Kinship networks: the case of Istanbul. In: Liljeström R, Özdalga, E, editors. Autonomy and dependence in the family. Turkey and Sweden in critical perspective. Istanbul: Swedish Research Institute in Istanbul Transactions, vol. 11; 2005. p. 117–138
41. Akdag R, Tosun N, Cinal A. Türkiye'de özellikli planlama gerektiren sağlık hizmetleri 2011–2023. Sağlık Bakanlığı Tedavi Hizmetleri Genel Müdürlüğü, Sağlık bakanlığı yayın 2011:212–240.
42. Dawson D, Jacobs R, Martin S, Smith P. Is patient choice an effective mechanism to reduce waiting times? Appl Health Econ Health Policy. 2004;3:195–203.
43. Lewer JJ, Van den Berg H. A gravity model of immigration. Econ Lett. 2008;99:164–7.
44. Ringard Å, Hagen TP. Are waiting times for hospital admissions affected by patients' choices and mobility? BMC Health Serv Res. 2011;11:170.
45. Paolella G. Pediatric health mobility: is it only an italian problem? Transl Med @ Unisa. 2012;4:57.

10

Online versus in-person comparison of Microscale Audit of Pedestrian Streetscapes (MAPS) assessments

Christine B. Phillips[1*], Jessa K. Engelberg[2], Carrie M. Geremia[2], Wenfei Zhu[3], Jonathan M. Kurka[1], Kelli L. Cain[2], James F. Sallis[2], Terry L. Conway[2] and Marc A. Adams[1]

Abstract

Background: An online version of the Microscale Audit of Pedestrian Streetscapes (Abbreviated) tool was adapted to virtually audit built environment features supportive of physical activity. The current study assessed inter-rater reliability of MAPS Online between in-person raters and online raters unfamiliar with the regions.

Methods: In-person and online audits were conducted for a total of 120 quarter-mile routes (60 per site) in Phoenix, AZ and San Diego, CA. Routes in each city included 40 residential origins stratified by walkability and SES, and 20 commercial centers. In-person audits were conducted by raters residing in their region. Online audits were conducted by raters in the alternate location using Google Maps (Aerial and Street View) images. The MAPS Abbreviated Online tool consisted of four sections: overall route, street segments, crossings and cul-de-sacs. Items within each section were grouped into subscales, and inter-rater reliability (ICCs) was assessed for subscales at multiple levels of aggregation.

Results: Online and in-person audits showed excellent agreement for overall positive microscale (ICC = 0.86, 95% CI [0.80, 0.90]) and grand scores (ICC = 0.93, 95% CI [0.89, 0.95]). Substantial to near-perfect agreement was found for 21 of 30 (70%) subscales, valence, and subsection scores, with ICCs ranging from 0.62, 95% CI [0.50, 0.72] to 0.95, 95% CI [0.93, 0.97]. Lowest agreement was found for the aesthetics and social characteristics scores, with ICCs ranging from 0.07, 95% CI [−0.12, 0.24] to 0.27, 95% CI [0.10, 0.43].

Conclusions: Results support use of the MAPS Abbreviated Online tool to reliably assess microscale neighborhood features that support physical activity and may be used by raters residing in different geographic regions and unfamiliar with the audit areas.

Keywords: Built environment, Walkability, Direct observation, Measurement, Physical activity, Walking, Virtual observation

Background

Inherent to ecological models is a tenet that the environment affects health behaviors [1]. Supportive features of the built environment may be particularly relevant to physical activity [2–5] and often result in health, social and economic co-benefits [5]. The built environment is frequently characterized by macro-level attributes such as walkability, street connectivity or population density. However, *microscale* level details may be important [6–8]. For example, the presence, quality, designs and features of sidewalks, streets, intersections (e.g., sidewalk buffers, transit stops, crosswalk amenities), and streetscape aesthetics and social characteristics (e.g., public art, landscape upkeep, broken windows, graffiti) may help explain physical activity. Modifying microscale

*Correspondence: cbphill3@asu.edu
[1] School of Nutrition and Health Promotion, Arizona State University, Phoenix, AZ, USA
Full list of author information is available at the end of the article

features to support health behaviors is easier and less costly than modifying macro-level features, and may provide significant public health returns relative to resource investment.

In-person microscale assessments

Several field audit tools have been developed to evaluate microscale features for active living [8–10]. Evidence from field audits suggests that microscale neighborhood characteristics strongly relate to physical activity across the life span [3], even after controlling for macro-level walkability [3]. However, detailed microscale data obtained from in-person audits comes at a high price of time and monetary resources. For example, in-person audits require extensive training of staff, driving time and travel costs, and sometimes lodging costs to assess areas outside of one's city. In-person audits are vulnerable to unfavorable weather conditions and may present potential safety risks for auditors. These elements are likely impediments to advancing research and practical implementation. Thus, a relatively small body of work has examined the relationships between microscale features and physical activity, and studies have generally been constricted in the number and/or size of geographic areas studied [2, 3, 8, 11, 12]. The global consequence of a limited research base and relatively few geographic areas is a lack of understanding about how microscale features in communities throughout the world influence physical activity behaviors.

Online audits

"Virtual audits" address many of the limitations of in-person audits. Virtual audit methods have been developed using widely-available online satellite imagery or omni-directional imagery such as Bing Maps Streetside or Google Maps Street View, to conduct virtual microscale audits. Findings have been mostly promising, with virtual audits largely corresponding to in-person direct observations [13–23]. Though encouraging, the generalizability of existing studies is limited, and several studies were constrained to a single city or had small sample sizes [13, 15–17, 20, 24].

One potential benefit of virtual audits is the ability to conduct large-scale studies encompassing diverse geographic areas. Any geographic area accessible via online mapping services could be audited from a remote location. However, one concern is that centralized raters' interpretations of virtual imagery may differ according to degree of contextual understanding or familiarity with an area [25, 26]. Most previous studies either did not specify the location of virtual raters or used raters from the audit area, creating uncertainty about whether raters' familiarity with an area influenced rater agreement. Only

two studies have addressed the issue of area-familiarity between raters using virtual microscale audit tools. Zhu and colleagues [27] demonstrated mostly substantial to excellent inter-rater reliability between online raters with different familiarities of routes in Phoenix using the MAPS Abbreviated Online audit. Wilson and colleagues [18] directly assessed differences in audit site familiarity between in-person and online raters using the Active Neighborhood Checklist and found high overall agreement between in-person raters familiar with the assessment areas (i.e., St. Louis and Indianapolis) and online raters unfamiliar with the assessment areas. It is unknown whether similar agreement would be found using other audit tools, such as MAPS, and in other geographic locations.

Current study aim

The current study aimed to assess inter-rater reliability between local field raters and online raters with varying degrees of familiarity using an adapted version of the previously-validated MAPS tool [3, 28] across two US regions. Data from San Diego, CA and Phoenix, AZ were used. In-person audits were conducted by raters who resided in their audit region. Raters using the online tool resided in the alternate location, and were unfamiliar with their audit sites. Analyses were conducted for individual-level MAPS items, subscale scores, and overall scores within three sections of the MAPS instrument (i.e., route, street segments, and crossings). High agreement between the site-familiar in-person raters and the site-unfamiliar online raters was hypothesized, thus providing a reliable and less geographically-restricted alternative to in-person audits.

Methods
Sample

In-person and online audits were conducted for a total of 120 routes (60 per site) in Phoenix, AZ and San Diego, CA. Phoenix and San Diego are both major US cities with similar population sizes. Phoenix is located in the southwestern US, in the northeastern portion of the Sonoran Desert. San Diego is on the coast of the Pacific Ocean in southern California. The two cities differ in land area, population density, and built environment, as well as climate, topography, and landscaping. Further differentiating the cities is an extensive network of walkable canals interwoven throughout urban Phoenix neighborhoods. Census block groups in both sites were classified according to macro-level walkability and socioeconomic status (SES), using a 2 (high vs. low walkability) × 2 (high vs. low SES) matrix. Walkability was determined using a block group-level composite of net residential density, land use mix, street connectivity and, for San Diego only, retail floor area ratio, as used previously [29]. SES was classified according to Census block group-level median household income.

MAPS residential routes

Residential routes ($n = 40$ per site) included a residential origin point and a pre-determined minimum quarter-mile route toward a pre-selected non-residential destination (i.e., cluster of commercial land uses). In Phoenix, ten route origins consisted of randomly selected residential parcels for each SES/walkability quadrant. In San Diego, ten route origins were randomly selected among each SES/walkability quadrant from existing participant households from a previous study [30].

MAPS commercial routes

Routes were also pre-selected for 20 commercial clusters near participant households balanced across quadrants in each city (5 clusters × 4 quadrants × 2 cities = total commercial routes, $n = 40$). Commercial cluster was defined as adjacent parcels with three or more commercial land uses. Commercial routes consisted of the street segment in front of a pre-selected commercial cluster and the two crossings on either end.

Measurement

The MAPS Abbreviated Online tool was adapted from existing instruments [12, 28] to virtually assess the microscale environment for physical activity. The 120-item original [3] and 60-item Abbreviated MAPS [12] field audit tools were validated in four age groups from three US regions. Same method inter-rater reliability was established for the original MAPS using in-person raters [28] and for the online MAPS Abbreviated Online using online raters [27]. The MAPS Abbreviated Online was designed for use with Google Earth, a free geographic software program based on the Google Maps service which displays both satellite and street level images of Earth in high resolution. Google Earth's Aerial View and Street View platforms offered a perpendicular or oblique view of streets, buildings, and landscapes (Aerial View), as well as eye-level views collecting pedestrian or driver perspectives of streets and buildings via car-mounted 360° cameras (Street View).

Paralleling the original and Abbreviated MAPS in-person instruments, the MAPS Abbreviated Online consisted of four sections: overall route, street segments, crossings, and cul-de-sacs. A total of 62 items were included in the current analyses. Route-level items (35) incorporated characteristics for the full route that were likely consistent (e.g., speed limit, aesthetics) or occurred infrequently (e.g., street amenities, traffic calming) at the segment level. Segment-level items

(14) assessed each street segment between crossings on the route (e.g., sidewalks, building heights, road widths and setbacks, street buffers, bicycle facilities, and trees). Crossing items (10) included features of intersections along the route (e.g., crosswalk markings/materials, curb cut presence [i.e., ramps], pedestrian signage and traffic circles). Cul-de-sac items (3) were collected when one or more cul-de-sacs were present within 400 feet of the participant's home. The cul-de-sacs section assessed the potential recreational environment within a cul-de-sac (e.g., basketball hoops). The number of crossings, segments and cul-de-sacs varied by route, though all routes had at least one segment. Most individual items and subscale scores in the MAPS original [28], Abbreviated in-person [12] and Abbreviated Online [27] tools have demonstrated moderate to excellent inter-rater reliability.

Data collection

Raters and training

Six raters (three per site) were trained and certified using a standard certification process. The training process included ≥15 h of in-person training and a minimum of four test audits (2 residential, 2 commercial) in which raters were required to achieve at least 95% agreement with the expert trainer. For continuous measures, agreement between expert and trainee ratings was defined as plus or minus 1 measurement unit. More details about the training and certification process can be found at [31].

In-person audits

In-person route audits were randomly assigned to raters residing in their respective sites (i.e., site-familiar). In-person audits were conducted using the MAPS Abbreviated Online from May to July of 2013 following the standard MAPS field audit protocol detailed here [31].

Online audits

Virtual audits replicating the in-person routes were randomly assigned to in-person raters residing in the alternate city (i.e., site-unfamiliar). Aerial and Street View were used to conduct the virtual audits. For Aerial View, assessments were conducted from a zoom-level of approximately 2000 feet above ground level. For Street View, raters virtually traveled the assigned route while rotating perspective 180° approximately every 100 feet and completing the assessment items along the route. Raters used the most recent layer of information on Google Earth and recorded the date of the images. Aerial View image dates for Phoenix ranged from November 2012 to November 2014; Street View images ranged from June 2007 to June 2012. Aerial View images for San Diego were dated March 2013; Street View from December 2008 to July 2013.

MAPS abbreviated online scoring

The scoring system applied to online and in-person audits was based on the method conceptualized for the original MAPS [28] and detailed for the MAPS Abbreviated [12] instruments [31]. When multiple crossings, segments and cul-de-sacs subscales were present within the same route, subscales were created using a mean score. Subscale scores within subsections of each instrument section were computed by summing constituent item scores. Subscales were classified according to the direction of expected effect on physical activity and then used to create valence summary scores, explained in detail in [12]. An "overall positive microscale score" was calculated by summing the positive streetscape, aesthetics, segments and crossings scores. Finally, a grand score was calculated by summing the "positive destinations and land use score" and the "overall positive microscale score." Descriptive statistics for items, subscales, valence, overall and grand scores can be found here: http://sallis.ucsd.edu/Documents/MAPS%20Abb%20Online%20Items_Alt%20Method%20Rel.pdf.

Analyses

Dichotomous (no/yes) items from the online MAPS tool were scored as 0/1. Frequency items (0, 1, 2+) were scored as 0, 1, 2. Continuous and descriptive items were recoded as categorical variables for subscales based on distributions, theoretical relevance, and maintaining scoring consistency with other scale items [12, 28]. Inter-rater reliability for subscale, valence and total scores was assessed using intraclass correlation coefficient (ICC). Item-level reliabilities were examined using Kappa statistic (dichotomous variables), ICC (continuous variables) and percent agreement. ICC values were calculated using one-way random effects models with single measurement form (i.e., ICC ((1,1)). Kappa [32] and ICC [33] statistics were evaluated according to guidelines by Landis and Koch [32]: 0.00–0.20 = poor to slight; 0.21–0.40 = fair; 0.41–0.60 = moderate; 0.61–0.80 = substantial; 0.81–1.00 = almost perfect. A limitation to using Kappa and ICC values is sensitivity to low variability in scores, as occurs when there is a very high or low observed occurrence of an attribute. To assist in interpretation of reliability statistics, we also calculated the percentage of audited routes in which the assessed feature was not observed by each rater (i.e., 'Percent without Feature'). This indicates the potential for adverse influence on Kappa and ICC values due to low variability. For example, the absence of public recreation was noted in 90%

of routes in the current sample, resulting in 108 in-person and 109 online routes being coded with scores of 0. Although rater agreement was over 90%, the public recreation subscale ICC was only 0.66, 95% CI [0.55, 0.75]. All data were analyzed using SPSS version 22.0 (SPSS, Inc., Chicago, IL, USA).

Results

A total of 120 routes with 298 segments, 214 crossings and 18 cul-de-sacs were analyzed. Overall, agreement of individual items between in-person field audits and virtual audits was moderate to near-perfect for approximately 75% of the 120 routes. Item-level descriptive and reliability statistics are provided at http://sallis.ucsd.edu/Documents/MAPS%20Abb%20Online%20Items_Alt%20Method%20Rel.pdf. Subscale, valence and overall scores, scoring components, descriptive statistics and reliability statistics are presented in Tables 1, 2, 3 and 4.

Route reliability
Destinations and land use

Eight positive subscales were analyzed in the destination and land use route section. Seven of eight subscales had substantial to near-perfect agreement, with ICC values ranging from 0.62, 95% CI [0.50, 0.72] (places of worship) to 0.92, 95% CI [0.89, 0.95] (restaurant-entertainment). Moderate agreement was found for the schools subscale (ICC = 0.53, 95% CI [0.39, 0.65]). All five destinations and land use subscales with ICC values <0.70 (residential mix, places of worship, schools, private and public recreation) were infrequent occurrences across routes, which resulted in values of zero for more than 80% of audits. The positive valence score created by summing the eight positive subscales showed near-perfect agreement between site-familiar in-person and site-unfamiliar online raters (ICC = 0.93, 95% CI [0.90, 0.95]). Results for route reliability subscales and valence scores are presented in Table 1.

Streetscape characteristics

A positive subscale score for streetscape characteristics was comprised of five items/subscales. Near perfect inter-rater reliability was found for transit stops (ICC = 0.95, 95% CI [0.93, 0.97]), streetlight presence (ICC = 0.91, 95% CI [0.87, 0.93]) and driveway presence (ICC = 0.87, 95% CI [0.81, 0.91]). Presence of traffic calming characteristics and street amenities both had moderate agreement, with ICC values of 0.57, 95% CI [0.44, 0.68] and 0.58, 95% CI [0.45, 0.69] respectively. The positive valence subscale score demonstrated near-perfect agreement (ICC = 0.81, 95% CI [0.73, 0.86]). Results for streetscape characteristics are presented in Table 1.

Table 1 Route level scales and valence scores (N = 120)

Score name	Possible range	Individual items	Inter-rater agreement (ICC)	Confidence interval (CI)	Rater	Mean	SD	Percent without feature
Destination and land use: Positive characteristics								
Residential mix	0–3	0 = commercial 1 = single family 2 = multi-family only and any other mix 3 = apartments over retail only	ICC: 0.73	(0.63, 0.80)	On the ground Online (St view)	1.29 1.23	0.69 0.65	11.6% 10.8% commercial
Shops	0–8	Presence of (0, 1, 2+) grocery/supermarket, convenience stores, liquor/alcohol store, retail stores	ICC: 0.86	(0.81, 0.90)	On the ground Online (St view)	1.65 1.48	1.93 1.78	44.2% 45%
Restaurant-entertain-ment	0–8	Presence of (0, 1, 2+) fast food restaurant, sit-down restaurant, café/coffee shop, entertainment	ICC: 0.92	(0.89, 0.95)	On the ground Online (St view)	1.73 1.71	1.91 1.96	43.3% 43.3%
Institutional-service	0–6	Presence of (0, 1, 2+) bank, credit union, health-related professional, other service	ICC: 0.85	(0.79, 0.89)	On the ground Online (St view)	1.94 2.01	2.03 1.89	41.7% 37.5%
Public recreation	0–2	Presence of (0, 1, 2+) public park	ICC: 0.66	(0.55, 0.75)	On the ground Online (St view)	0.10 0.11	0.30 0.36	90% 90.8%
Private recreation	0–2	Presence of (0, 1, 2+) private recreation facilities	ICC: 0.70	(0.59, 0.78)	On the ground Online (St view)	0.21 0.24	0.53 0.52	85% 80%
School	0–2	Presence of (0, 1, 2+) school	ICC: 0.53	(0.39, 0.65)	On the ground Online (St view)	0.24 0.20	0.52 0.50	89.2% 92.5%
Place of worship	0–2	Presence of (0, 1, 2+) places of worship (e.g., church, synagogue, mosque)	ICC: 0.62	(0.50, 0.72)	On the ground Online (St view)	0.13 0.09	0.38 0.34	80% 84.2%
Destination and land use: Valence and overall								
Land use positive	0–33	Sum residential mix, shops, restaurant-entertainment, institutional service, public recreation, private recreation, school, place of worship	ICC: 0.93	(0.90, 0.95)	On the ground Online (St view)	7.28 7.08	5.91 5.50	– –
Streetscape characteristics: Positive characteristics								
Transit stops	0–2	Number of stops along route (0–6) and amenities at 1st stop (bench, covered shelter), recoded as no stop (0), 1 or more stops (1) or 1 or more stops with amenities at first stop (2)	ICC: 0.95	(0.93, 0.97)	On the ground Online (St view)	0.69 0.71	0.93 0.94	63.3% 62.5%
Traffic calming	0–1	Traffic calming characteristics (pedestrian signage, speed humps, curb extensions)	ICC: 0.57	(0.44, 0.68)	On the ground Online (St view)	0.32 0.30	0.47 0.46	68.3% 70%

Table 1 continued

Score name	Possible range	Individual items	Inter-rater agreement (ICC)	Confidence interval (CI)	Rater	Mean	SD	Percent without feature
Streetlights	0–1	Presence of street lights (any vs. none)	ICC: 0.91	(0.87, 0.93)	On the ground	0.95	0.22	5%
					Online (St view)	0.96	0.20	4.2%
Driveways	0–1	Presence of less than 6 driveways along route (yes or no)	ICC: 0.87	(0.81, 0.91)	On the ground	0.44	0.50	52.5%
					Online (St view)	0.48	0.50	55.3%
Street amenities	0–4	Presence of street amenities [i.e., trash bins (any vs. none), building overhangs ((any vs. none), bike racks (any vs. none), benches (any vs. none)]	ICC: 0.58	(0.45, 0.69)	On the ground	0.63	0.94	61.7%
					Online (St view)	0.57	0.86	62.5%
Streetscape characteristics: Valence and overall								
Streetscape positive	0–9	Transit stops, traffic calming characteristics, street lights, <6 driveways, street amenities	ICC: 0.81	(0.73, 0.86)	On the ground	3.03	1.89	2.5%
					Online (St view)	3.01	1.71	1.7%
Aesthetics and social characteristics: Valence and overall								
Aesthetics/social positive	0–3	Buildings well-maintained (100%), no presence of any physical disorder and extent	ICC: 0.15	(−0.03, 0.32)	On the ground	2.25	0.87	3.3%
					Online (St view)	2.09	0.73	0.8%
Aesthetics/social negative	0–2	Buildings not well-maintained (>100%), presence of any physical disorder and extent	ICC: 0.07	(−0.12, 0.24)	On the ground	0.90	0.92	46.6%
					Online (St view)	0.40	0.72	72.5%
Aesthetics/social overall	−2 to 3	Aesthetics/social positive score − aesthetics/ social negative scores	ICC: 0.27	(0.10, 0.43)	On the ground	1.38	1.28	17.5%
					Online (St view)	1.70	1.19	8.3%

Table 2 Mean of all segments for each route scale and valence scores (n = 120) and cul-de-sac (n = 16) scale and valence scores

Score name	Possible range	Individual items	Inter-rater agreement (ICC)	Confidence interval (CI)	Rater	Mean	(SD)	Percent without feature (%)
Street segments: Positive characteristics								
Building height-setback	0–6	Mean of average building height (feet) to average setback (feet) ratio	ICC: 0.56	(0.42, 0.67)	On the ground	1.06	0.47	7.5
					Online (St view)	1.01	0.45	8.3
Building height/road width plus setback ratio	0–3	Mean of average building Height (feet) to Average Road Width (feet) + Average Setback (feet) ratio	ICC: 0.05	(−0.13, 0.23)	On the ground	0.00	0.03	98.3
					Online (St view)	0.02	0.12	95.8
Buffer	0–2	Mean of buffer presence and buffer width	ICC: 0.89	(0.84, 0.92)	On the ground	0.60	0.83	60
					Online (St view)	0.67	0.84	54.2
Bike infrastructure	0–2	Mean of presence of a marked bicycle lane	ICC: 0.85	(0.79, 0.89)	On the ground	0.45	0.76	74.2
					Online (St view)	0.37	0.71	69.2
Trees	0–5	Mean of trees along sidewalk, even or irregular spacing, shade coverage	ICC: 0.66	(0.54, 0.75)	On the ground	1.96	1.01	3.3
					Online (St view)	2.11	0.95	0.8
Sidewalk	0–3	Mean of sidewalk presence, width of sidewalk, sidewalk continuous	ICC: 0.85	(0.79, 0.89)	On the ground	2.77	0.93	6.7
					Online (St view)	2.72	0.94	7.5
Shortcut	0–1	Presence of an informal path (shortcut) connecting to something else	ICC: 0.65	(0.58, 0.71)	On the ground	0.10	0.31	89.6
					Online (St view)	0.08	0.28	91.6
Street segments: Valence and overall								
Positive	0–25	Mean of positive subscales (building height-setback, sidewalk, buffers, bike infrastructure, trees, shortcut)	ICC: 0.82	(0.75, 0.87)	On the ground	4.21	1.80	0.8
					Online (St view)	4.26	1.82	1.7

Table 3 Crossings—means of all crossings per route: scales and valence scores (N = 107)

Score name	Possible range	Individual items	Inter-rater agreement (ICC)	Confidence interval (CI)	Rater	Mean	(SD)	Percent without feature (%)
Cul-de-sacs								
Overall	0–4	Closeness of cul-de-sac to home, presence of amenities (e.g., basketball hoops), visibility from home	ICC: 0.43	(−0.05, 0.76)	On the ground	−0.05	0.76	1.7
					Online (St view)	−0.10	0.86	0.8
Crossings: Positive characteristics								
Crosswalk amenities	0–5	Mean: Presence of crossing aids, marked crosswalk, high-visibility striping, different material than road, curb extensions	ICC: 0.81	(0.74, 0.87)	On the ground	0.54	0.50	32.5
					Online (St view)	0.54	0.50	33.3
Curb quality	0–2	Mean: Presence of pre-crossing and/or post-crossing ramp lined up with crossing	ICC: 0.87	(0.82, 0.91)	On the ground	1.71	0.59	5.8
					Online (St view)	1.67	0.64	7.5
Intersection control	0–3	Mean: Presence of traffic circle, pedestrian walk signals, count-down signals	ICC: 0.92	(0.89, 0.95)	On the ground	0.66	0.76	41.7
					On the ground	0.54	0.49	32.5
Crossings: Valence and overall								
Positive	0–10	Mean of positive crossing characteristics scales (amenities, quality, intersection control)	ICC: 0.93	(0.91, 0.95)	On the ground	0.69	0.93	63.3
					Online (St view)	0.71	0.94	62.5

Table 4 Final valences and grand scores (n = 120)

Score name	Possible range	Individual items	Inter-rater agreement (ICC)	Confidence intervals (CI)	Rater	Mean	(SD)	Percent without feature
Grand valence and overall								
Overall micro-scale positive	0–47	Sum of 4 subscales: Positive crossing characteristics, positive segments, positive streetscape, positive aesthetics/social	ICC: 0.86	(0.80, 0.90)	On the ground	12.59	4.23	–
					Online (St view)	12.47	3.97	–
Grand score	0–80	Overall microscale positive + land use positive subscale	ICC: 0.93	(0.89, 0.95)	On the ground	20.22	9.08	–
					Online (St view)	19.90	8.46	–

Aesthetics and social characteristics

Positive and negative valence scores and an overall sub-section score (positive minus negative valence scores) were computed for the aesthetics and social character-istics items. Constituent items assessed the maintenance and disorder of the environment. Similar to the poor to fair agreement found at the item level (see http://sal-lis.ucsd.edu/Documents/MAPS%20Abb%20Online%20 Items_Alt%20Method%20Rel.pdf), agreement was poor to slight for both the positive and negative valence scores (ICCs = 0.15, 95% CI [−0.03, 0.32] and 0.07, 95% CI [−0.12, 0.24], respectively), and fair for the overall aes-thetics and social characteristic score (ICC = 0.27, 95% CI [0.10, 0.43]). Results for aesthetics and social charac-teristics are presented in Table 1.

Segment reliability

Six positive subscales in the street segments section were evaluated (Table 2). Four subscales had substan-tial to near-perfect agreement, with ICC values rang-ing from 0.66, 95% CI [0.54, 0.75] (trees) to 0.89, 95% CI [0.84, 0.92] (buffers). Moderate agreement was found for the building height setback subscale (ICC = 0.56, 95% CI [0.42, 0.67]). The ICC value for the building height to road width plus setback ratio subscale was low (ICC = 0.05, 95% CI [−0.13, 0.23]). However, it should be noted that over 95% of the calculated ratios were zero for both online and in-person audits, helping explain the poor ICC. The segments positive valence score had near-perfect inter-rater agreement (ICC = 0.82, 95% CI [0.75, 0.87]).

Crossing reliability

Three positive subscale scores were evaluated in the crossings section (Table 3). All three had near-perfect inter-rater agreement, with ICCs ranging from 0.81, 95% CI [0.74, 0.87] (crosswalk amenities) to 0.92, 95% CI [0.89, 0.95] (intersection control). Near-perfect agree-ment was also found for the crossings positive valence score (ICC = 0.93, 95% CI [0.91, 0.95]).

Cul-de-sac reliability

One positive valence score analyzed for the cul-de-sacs section demonstrated moderate agreement between in-person field audits and virtual audits (ICC = 0.43, 95% CI [−0.05, 0.76]) (Table 3). It is not included in the overall positive microscale score or the grand score because its relation to physical activity is unclear.

Overall positive microscale and grand scores reliability

An overall positive microscale score was calculated by summing positive valence scores for routes (streetscape characteristics and aesthetics and social characteristics),

segments, and crossings. Agreement was near-perfect between in-person and online auditors (ICC = 0.86, 95% CI [0.80, 0.90]). Similarly, the grand score, created by adding the positive valence score for destinations and land use to the overall positive microscale score, had near-perfect inter-rater agreement (ICC = 0.93, 95% CI [0.89, 0.95]). Results are presented in Table 4.

Discussion

The present study examined alternate-form reliability between in-person and online data collection methods using the MAPS Abbreviated audit tool. Overall, there was substantial to near-perfect agreement between site-familiar in-person raters and site-unfamiliar online raters for 21 of the 30 subscales, valence and subsection scores. Lowest reliability was found with aesthetics and social disorder scales. Inter-rater agreement was also near-per-fect for the total positive microscale and grand summary scores. These results indicated that microscale environ-mental features supporting physical activity can be reli-ably assessed virtually using the MAPS online tool.

The present study was designed to address the ques-tion of whether raters auditing built environment fea-tures with the MAPS Abbreviated measure need to be personally familiar with a city or region. Virtual raters unfamiliar with an environment could differ in degree of understanding or familiarity with a city or its particular built environment features [25, 26]. If online auditing by raters not familiar with the region is supported, central-ized auditing could replace expensive in-person audits for reliable features. Because previous studies used local raters or did not specify whether raters were familiar with an area, it was uncertain whether raters' familiarity influenced agreement. In the current study, agreement was generally near-perfect to moderate between in-per-son and virtual raters for the majority of items and scales. These results are consistent with Wilson et al. [18] who found high agreement between in-person and site-unfa-miliar online auditors in two mid-western cities using another audit tool. Both studies provided consistent evi-dence using different audit tools that centralized virtual audits can be used without regard to auditors' physical locations or familiarities with audit areas in the US.

MAPS Online subscales with the highest agreement (e.g., land use and destinations, transit stops, streetlights, and intersection controls) had several common quali-ties. Constituent items in these subscales were generally more quantitative than qualitative (e.g., presence/absence of street buffers and buffer width). Attributes were usu-ally large or easily distinguishable (e.g., sidewalks, traf-fic circles, pedestrian walk signals) and were likely to remain stable over time. These results are consistent with previous comparisons of online and in-person audits which similarly found highest agreement for objectively-assessed items that were relatively impervious to time effects [21] and were highly visible, regardless of audit method [22, 23, 34]. These results suggest that site-unfamiliar and site-familiar online raters performed similarly for the majority of microscale features.

Similar to other studies [17, 21, 34, 35], cross-method agreement was lowest for the aesthetics and social characteristics subsection (e.g., presence and extent of graffiti or condition of facades). Constituent items in this subsection generally had low kappa values and percent agreement. The only exception was the presence of softscape features (e.g., any landscaping), which had 94.2% agreement. Although the kappa value was low for this item (k = −0.01), this was likely due to the high prevalence of softscapes observed along routes for both rating methods (114/120 in-person, 119/120 online) limiting variance in this item.

It is possible that maintenance and disorder items are more difficult to virtually assess when unfamiliar with an area. Online images likely do not provide the same degree of environmental context as physically walking a route, making qualitative assessments difficult. In addition, some of these indicators may be difficult to see on Google Street View or views may be temporarily or permanently blocked. Maintenance and disorder items are also more susceptible to temporal variability than built environment features for streetscape audits in general (e.g., shade or presence of litter or graffiti vs. presence of street lights), meaning that observed conditions may vary considerably between any two time points. Thus, time lapses between online image collection dates and in-person audits may have resulted in inconsistent rater observations. Despite the low agreement for aesthetics and social characteristics items, the MAPS Abbreviated Online tool includes these items to be consistent with the in-person MAPS Abbreviated tool. Data collected online may still be a useful indicator of overall maintenance and disorder, though with limited precision. It is likely that when online raters can notice graffiti and other signs of disorder using Street View, the extent of the disorder may be substantial and worth differentiating from especially well-maintained neighborhoods. However, some investigators using MAPS Abbreviated online may want to exclude these items from data collection, summary scores, or analyses, due to low reliability.

Strengths and limitations

This study had notable strengths that contribute to the generalizability of findings. First, the sample size was large, consisting of 120 routes with 298 street segments and 214 crossings in two geographically distinct metropolitan areas (i.e., coastal city and desert mountain city).

Similar studies evaluating reliability between in-person and virtual audits have had small sample sizes [13, 15, 17, 20], limited audit neighborhoods to a single metropolitan area [13–15, 20] or been restricted in regional diversity [18]. Additionally, a route selection protocol was used to approximate the built environment as individuals would encounter it in everyday life.

The current study's sampling design equally distributed route origins among neighborhoods with high and low SES and walkability. While several prior studies accounted for neighborhood SES [15, 18], we are not aware of any that also controlled for the influence of macro-level walkability (i.e., using GIS data). The inclusion of diverse neighborhoods also likely maximized the prevalence and variance in audit features. Present results suggested online microscale audits were reliable regardless of neighborhood SES, and in neighborhoods that varied on other macro-level features contributing to walkability [29]. It has been suggested that item reliabilities may differ by location [36], in part due to differences in the prevalence of audit features across sites [36, 37] or low variance in audit answers [34]. Therefore, direct reliability comparisons between sites are difficult because low reliability coefficients may be more indicative of frequency of occurrence than differences in agreement. To overcome this limitation, the present study maximized the prevalence and variability of audit features by combining data collected in two cities. Because each site was not analyzed separately, it is possible that the reliability of some items differed by site. It would be important to disentangle prevalence effects from poor rater agreement to understand whether some items are perceived differently depending on location. This may be addressed in future work by increasing the number and diversity of sampled sites and neighborhoods to ensure sufficient variance in item scores across locations.

Several limitations in the current study were inherent to virtual audits in general. First, auditors were reliant on the images available through Google Maps, which dated as far back as 2007 and possibly did not accurately depict the streetscape at the time of the in-person audits. Differences in the timing of in-person and online data collection could have been a potential source of bias. It is possible that some streetscape characteristics were assessed differently depending on what time of day or year data collection occurred. For instance, raters in Phoenix may have differentially assessed the types of landscape depending on whether images were taken during exceptionally hot and dry desert summer months or during the more temperate winter or spring blooming season. Likewise, features may have been assessed differently depending on when data were collected relative to the time of day of litter/trash removal, pedestrian and automobile activity, or weather occurrence.

Handbook of Health Geography

Additionally, image dates varied within and across audit areas, as well as between different image views for the same areas. For example, Google Street View image dates in the present study ranged from 2007 to 2012 for Phoenix and 2008–2013 for San Diego. Aerial Views (based on satellite imagery) were more recent, ranging from 2012 to late 2014. This temporal difference in views occasionally resulted in image inconsistencies, such as a more recent Aerial View displaying a crosswalk marked with high-visibility striping that appeared as an unmarked crosswalk in older Street View images.

A limitation of Street View was that the images were not always complete for an entire segment, such that there were occasionally missing street sections or intentionally obscured image areas for privacy reasons at the request of a home or business owner. However, these issues occurred infrequently and were noted. Relatedly, sometimes images contained large busses, trucks, foliage or other objects that obstructed views along a segment. Along with image composition, virtual audits were reliant on image resolutions that provided a sufficient level of detail for assessed characteristics. Fine-grained attributes such as trip hazards on sidewalks, which performed poorly in the present study, may have been difficult to discern with available image resolutions.

Based on current and previous findings, microscale aesthetics and social features appeared difficult to assess reliably using currently available virtual tools. It is possible these qualities may be better assessed using alternative data collection methods. Future work may explore opportunities that take advantage of emerging technologies to characterize microscale attributes that are highly subjective and transient in nature. For example, recently-developed geolocation-aware mobile crowdsourcing technology could be used in conjunction with measurement burst designs [38] to collect repeated sequences of perceptual data over different time scales. Such data may complement existing online audit tools to facilitate a better understanding about the temporal dynamics of the perceived environment, and if or how this relates to physical activity behaviors.

Most of the challenges noted above occurred infrequently in the present study and given the high degree of overall agreement, did not seem to adversely affect the reliability and practicality of using the MAPS Abbreviated Online tool. Some limitations may be mitigated by establishing rules that would become part of virtual rater training. For example, a rule could be implemented to use features seen in aerial and Street Views based on the most relevant date or date closest to the time period of interest. If the most recent images are desired, researchers may choose to plan audit timelines around anticipated time frames for Street View image collection,

published for each district within specified regions in each country [39]. Because Google Street View now provides historical images, virtual audits may be conducted retrospectively or longitudinally. This offers the potential to learn more about how features change over time in a way that would not be feasible with field audit methods. However, researchers are limited to the historical images available, which may not necessarily correspond to time periods of interest in all locations.

Implications for applications of MAPS

Results from the present study support the MAPS Abbreviated Online audit tool as a reliable alternative to in-person audits generalizable to similar US cities. From an international standpoint, findings may also extend to comparable mountain, desert or coastal metropolitan areas with relatively warm dry climates. Results from Vanwolleghem and colleagues [34] support the use of MAPS outside of the US. Acceptable inter-rater reliability was found for the majority of items assessed in-person, online and using alternate methods in Belgium using the MAPS Global tool, which was adapted for international use [34]. Similar work is being conducted in several other international locations to ascertain the generalizability of MAPS Global outside of the US.

Among the advantages to implementing the MAPS Abbreviated Online tool in research settings are elimination of travel time and costs, weather-related concerns and potential threats to personal safety associated with in-person audits. Moreover, it would enable centralized audit operations, facilitating procedural standardization and efficient use of personnel time. Conceivably, online auditing could promote growth in the study of microscale environmental influences on physical activity by increasing the number, scale and geographic diversity of investigations, with data collected from the same validated instrument. Thus, future studies would benefit from validating MAPS online scores with physical activity data collected from participants in diverse geographic regions and neighborhood types.

Conclusions and recommendations

Audits conducted using publically available online tools appear to be safe, convenient, efficient and cost-effective alternatives to in-person field audits, even with auditors unfamiliar with the assessed regions. Virtual audits are less resource-intensive than in-person audits and are unrestricted by geographic proximity to the audit location or weather. At the time of writing, Google Street View images were available for over 250 regions/states in more than 25 countries, and are expected to continue expanding into areas not currently covered [39]. The development and validation of reliable online audit tools, such as MAPS Abbreviated Online, can provide a means for understanding microscale features in increasingly diverse environments as more locations become virtually accessible.

Abbreviations

AZ: Arizona; CA: California; GIS: geographic information system; ICC: intraclass correlation coefficient; K: kappa; MAPS: Microscale Audit of Pedestrian Streetscapes; SES: socioeconomic status; US: United States.

Authors' contributions

CBP, JE, CG, JS and MA contributed to the manuscript's conception, design, drafting and revisions. JE, CG, KC, TC, JS and MA contributed to the development of MAPS Abbreviated Online, data scoring and analysis. CG, WZ, JK and MA assisted with data collection. CBP, JE, TC, CG and KC assisted with data interpretation. CG, WZ and JK provided manuscript revisions. All authors read and approved the final manuscript.

Author details

[1] School of Nutrition and Health Promotion, Arizona State University, Phoenix, AZ, USA. [2] Department of Family and Preventive Medicine, University of California, San Diego, San Diego, CA, USA. [3] School of Physical Education, Shaanxi Normal University, Xi'an, Shaanxi, China.

Acknowledgements

The authors thank Justin Martinez for assistance with data collection.

Competing interests

JFS: Santech Inc; SPARK physical activity programs of School Specialty Inc. All other authors declare that they have no competing interests.

Funding sources

National Institutes of Health (HL109222, CA198915, HL111378, HL083454, ES014240).

References

1. McLeroy KR, Bibeau D, Steckler A, Glanz K. An ecological perspective on health promotion programs. Health Educ Q. 1988;15(4):351–77.
2. Alfonzo M, Boarnet MG, Day K, McMillan T, Anderson CL. The relationship of neighbourhood built environment features and adult parents' walking. J Urban Des. 2008;13(1):29–51.
3. Cain KL, Millstein RA, Sallis JF, Conway TL, Gavand KA, Frank LD, Saelens BE, Geremia CM, Chapman J, Adams MA, et al. Contribution of streetscape audits to explanation of physical activity in four age groups based on the Microscale Audit of Pedestrian Streetscapes (MAPS). Soc Sci Med. 2014;116:82–92.
4. Casagrande SS, Whitt-Glover MC, Lancaster KJ, Odoms-Young AM, Gary TL. Built environment and health behaviors among African Americans: a systematic review. Am J Prev Med. 2009;36(2):174–81.
5. Sallis JF, Spoon C, Cavill N, Engelberg JK, Gebel K, Parker M, Thornton CM, Lou D, Wilson AL, Cutter CL, et al. Co-benefits of designing communities for active living: an exploration of literature. Int J Behav Nutr Phys Act. 2015;12(1):1–10.
6. Brownson RC, Hoehner CM, Day K, Forsyth A, Sallis JF. Measuring the built environment for physical activity: state of the science. Am J Prev Med. 2009;36(4S):S99–123.
7. Moudon AV, Lee C. Walking and bicycling: an evaluation of environmental audit instruments. Am J Health Promot. 2003;18(1):21–37.
8. Boarnet MG, Forsyth A, Day K, Oakes JM. The street level built environment and physical activity and walking: Results of a predictive validity study for the Irvine Minnesota Inventory. Environ Behav. 2011;43(6):735–75.
9. Active Living Research. Tools and measures. http://activelivingresearch.org/search/site?f[0]=bundle%3Acontent_tools_and_measure. Accessed 28 Dec 2016.
10. Malecki KC, Engelman CD, Peppard PE, Nieto FJ, Grabow ML, Bernardinello M, Bailey E, Bersch AJ, Walsh MC, Lo JY, et al. The Wisconsin Assessment of the Social and Built Environment (WASABE): a multidimensional objective audit instrument for examining neighborhood effects on health. BMC Public Health. 2014;14(1165):1–15.
11. Sallis JF, Cain KL, Conway TL, Gavand KA, Millstein RA, Geremia CM, Frank LD, Saelens BE, Glanz K, King AC. Is your neighborhood designed to support physical activity? A brief streetscape audit tool. Prev Chronic Dis. 2015;12:150098. doi:10.5888/pcd12.150098.
12. Cain KL, Gavand KA, Conway TL, Geremia CM, Millstein RA, Frank LD, Saelens BE, Adams MA, Glanz K, King AC, Sallis JF. Developing and validating an abbreviated version of the Microscale Audit for Pedestrian Streetscapes (MAPS-Abbreviated). J Transp Health. 2017;5:84–96.
13. Ben-Joseph E, Lee JS, Cromley EK, Laden F, Troped PJ. Virtual and actual: relative accuracy of on-site and web-based instruments in auditing the environment for physical activity. Health Place. 2013;19:138–50.
14. Clarke P, Ailshire J, Melendez R, Bader M, Morenoff J. Using google earth to conduct a neighborhood audit: reliability of a virtual audit instrument. Health Place. 2010;16:1224–9.
15. Rundle AG, Bader MDM, Richards CA, Neckerman KM, Teitler JO. Using Google Street View to audit neighborhood environments. Am J Prev Med. 2011;40(1):94–100.
16. Silva V, Grande A, Rech C, Peccin M. Geoprocessing via Google Maps for assessing obesogenic built environments related to physical activity and chronic noncommunicable diseases: validity and reliability. J Healthc Eng. 2015;6(1):41–54.
17. Vanwolleghem G, Van Dyck D, Ducheyne F, De Bourdeaudhuij I, Cardon G. Assessing the environmental characteristics of cycling routes to school: a study on the reliability and validity of a Google Street View-based audit. Int J Health Geogr. 2014;13:19.
18. Wilson JS, Kelly CM, Schootman M, Baker EA, Banerjee A, Clennin M, Douglas MK. Assessing the built environment using omnidirectional imagery. Am J Prev Med. 2012;42(2):193–9.
19. Wu Y, Nash P, Barnes LE, Minett T, Matthews FE, Jones A, Brayne C. Assessing environmental features related to mental health: a reliability study of visual streetscape images. BMC Public Health. 1094;2014(14):1–10.
20. Badland HM, Opit S, Witten K, Kearns RA, Mavoa S. Can virtual streetscape audits reliably replace physical streetscape audits? J Urban Health. 2010;87(6):1007–16.
21. Charreire H, Mackenbach JD, Ouasti M, Lakerveld J, Compernolle S, Ben-Rebah M, McKee M, Brug J, Rutter H, Oppert JM. Using remote sensing to define environmental characteristics related to physical activity and dietary behaviours: a systematic review (the SPOTLIGHT project). Health Place. 2014;25:1–9.
22. Kurka JM, Adams MA, Geremia C, Zhu W, Cain KL, Conway TL, Sallis JF. Comparison of field online observations for meauring land uses using the Microscale Audit of Pedestrian Streetscapes (MAPS). J Transp Health. 2016;3(3):278–86.
23. Lee S, Talen E. Measuring walkability: a note on auditing methods. J Urban Des. 2014;19(3):368–88.
24. Taylor BT, Fernando P, Bauman AE, Williamson A, Craig JC, Redman S. Measuring the quality of public open space using google earth. Am J Prev Med. 2011;40(2):105–12.
25. Hoehner CM, Ivy A, Ramirez LB, Meriwether B, Brownson RC. How reliably do community members audit the neighborhood environment for its support of physical activity? Implications for participatory research. J Public Health Manag Pract. 2006;12(3):270–7.

26. Mooney SJ, Bader MDM, Lovasi GS, Neckerman KM, Teitler JO, Rundle AG. Validity of an ecometric neighborhood physical disorder measure constructed by virtual street audit. Am J Epidemiol. 2014;180(6):626–35.

27. Zhu W, Sun Y, Kurka J, Sallis JF, Geremia C, Cain K, Hooker S, Conway TL, Adams M. Reliability between online raters with varied familiarites of a region: Microscale Audit of Pedestrian Streetscapes (MAPS) tool. Landsc Urban Plann. 2017;167:240–8.

28. Millstein RA, Cain KL, Sallis JF, Conway TL, Geremia C, Frank LD, Chapman J, Van Dyck D, Dipzinski LR, Kerr J, et al. Development, scoring, and reliability of the Microscale Audit of Pedestrian Streetscapes (MAPS). BMC Public Health. 2013;13(1):1–15.

29. Frank LD, Sallis JF, Saelens BE, Leary L, Cain K, Conway TL, Hess PM. The development of a walkability index: application to the Neighborhood Quality of Life Study. Br J Sports Med. 2010;44(13):924–33.

30. Saelens BE, Sallis JF, Frank LD, Couch SC, Zhou C, Colburn T, Cain KL, Chapman J, Glanz K. Obesogenic neighborhood environments, child and parent obesity: the Neighborhood Impact on Kids study. Am J Prev Med. 2012;42(5):e57–64.

31. Sallis JF. Measures: MAPS. http://sallis.ucsd.edu/measure_maps.html. Accessed 2 Jan 2017.

32. Landis JR, Koch GG. The measurement of observer agreement for categorical data. Biometrics. 1977;33(1):159–74.

33. Shrout PE. Measurement reliability and agreement in psychiatry. Stat Methods Med Res. 1998;7(3):301–17.

34. Vanwolleghem G, Ghekiere A, Cardon G, De Bourdeaudhuij I, D'Haese S, Geremia CM, Lenoir M, Sallis JF, Verhoeven H, Van Dyck D. Using an audit tool (MAPS Global) to assess the characteristics of the physical environment related to walking for transport in youth: reliability of Belgian data. Int J Health Geogr. 2016;15:41.

35. Gullón P, Badland HM, Alfayate S, Bilal U, Escobar F, Cebrecos A, Diez J, Franco M. Assessing walking and cycling environments in the streets of Madrid: comparing on-field and virtual audits. J Urban Health. 2015;92(5):923–39.

36. Bader MDM, Mooney SJ, Lee YJ, Sheehan D, Neckerman KM, Rundle AG, Teitler JO. Development and deployment of the Computer Assisted Neighborhood Visual Assessment System (CANVAS) to measure health-related neighborhood conditions. Health Place. 2015;31:163–72.

37. Bethlehem JR, Mackenbach JD, Ben-Rebah M, Compernolle S, Glonti K, Bárdos H, Rutter HR, Charreire H, Oppert J-M, Brug J, et al. The SPOTLIGHT virtual audit tool: a valid and reliable tool to assess obesogenic characteristics of the built environment. Int J Health Geogr. 2014;13:52.

38. Stawski RS, MacDonald SWS, Sliwinski MJ. Measurement burst design. In: Whitbourne SK, editor. The encyclopedia of adulthood and aging. Wiley; 2015. pp. 1–5.

39. Google. Where we've been and where we're headed next. https://www.google.com/intl/en-CA/streetview/understand/. Accessed 12 Jan 2017.

11

Residential area characteristics and disabilities among Dutch community-dwelling older adults

Astrid Etman[1*], Carlijn B. M. Kamphuis[1,2], Frank H. Pierik[3], Alex Burdorf[1] and Frank J. Van Lenthe[1]

Abstract

Background: Living longer independently may be facilitated by an attractive and safe residential area, which stimulates physical activity. We studied the association between area characteristics and disabilities and whether this association is mediated by transport-related physical activity (TPA).

Methods: Longitudinal data of 271 Dutch community-dwelling adults aged 65 years and older participating in the Elderly And their Neighbourhood (ELANE) study in 2011–2013 were used. Associations between objectively measured aesthetics (range 0–22), functional features (range 0–14), safety (range 0–16), and destinations (range 0–15) within road network buffers surrounding participants' residences, and self-reported disabilities in instrumental activities of daily living (range 0–8; measured twice over a 9 months period) were investigated by using longitudinal tobit regression analyses. Furthermore, it was investigated whether self-reported TPA mediated associations between area characteristics and disabilities.

Results: A one unit increase in aesthetics within the 400 m buffer was associated with 0.86 less disabilities (95% CI −1.47 to −0.25; p < 0.05), but other area characteristics were not related to disabilities. An increase in area aesthetics was associated with more TPA, and more minutes of TPA were associated with less disabilities. TPA however, only partly mediated the associated between area aesthetics and disabilities.

Conclusions: Improving aesthetic features in the close by area around older persons' residences may help to prevent disability.

Keywords: Elderly, Mobility, Functioning, Limitations

Background

In ageing societies, limitations in instrumental activities of daily living (IADL) will become increasingly prevalent among community-dwelling older adults. Studies among European older adults showed that the prevalence of one or more IADL limitations increases from 17 to 54% among adults aged 65 years or older up to >90% among adults aged 90 years or older [1–3]. Such limitations are associated with a loss of independent living and high healthcare costs. Policy aimed at improving independent

living of older persons coincides with the wish of older persons to live independently for as long as possible, in which the built environment may play an important role.

The physical design of older adults' residential areas is suggested to contribute to independent living in several ways [4]. A safe and attractive residential area, and the nearby presence of shops and facilities, may increase independent living, as older adults are more likely to be able to do their daily groceries and to visit a hairdresser or pharmacy, independent of help from others. Current literature indeed shows that aesthetics (e.g. green spaces), destinations (e.g. grocery stores), and safety (e.g. lighting) are associated with less disabilities [5]. Previous studies exploring associations between residential area characteristics and disabilities have shown mixed results [6, 7]. These studies generally used cross-sectional

*Correspondence: a.etman@erasmusmc.nl
[1] Department of Public Health, Erasmus University Medical Centre, P.O. Box 2040, 3000 CA Rotterdam, The Netherlands
Full list of author information is available at the end of the article

designs which may weaken associations with residential area characteristics, since disabilities can fluctuate over time [8]. Including repeatedly measured disabilities in a relatively short period captures this fluctuation, and may therefore provide greater reliability of estimates resulting in more robust associations. Importantly, they should not by definition be interpreted as a "real" change.

Physical activity (PA) has shown to slow the progression of disability by decreasing functional limitations. As older persons spend more time being physically active outside than inside their homes [9], transport-related PA (TPA) may play an important role in the prevention of disabilities. A high 'walkable' residential area may promote walking for recreation and transport, which helps older adults to stay physically fit and live longer independently [6, 7]. Highly aesthetic residential areas and residential areas with many functional features (e.g. benches) or facilities are found to be associated with more minutes of transport-related walking [10]. Because older adults use residential areas for activities in daily life [11], transport-related physical activity (TPA) is thought to play an important role in the pathway between area characteristics and disabilities.

This study adds knowledge by investigating the association between residential area characteristics and repeatedly measured disabilities to better capture random fluctuation, and by investigating whether associations, if any, are mediated by TPA levels.

Methods
Design
Data from the Dutch ELANE study (2011–2013) were used. This longitudinal study aimed at studying associations between residential area characteristics and PA, independent living, and quality of life among adults aged 65 years and older living in Spijkenisse, a middle-sized town in the Rotterdam area. Community-dwelling older adults were randomly selected from the municipal register of Spijkenisse. Of the 430 persons interviewed face-to-face at baseline (T0), 277 (response 64.4%) were again interviewed by telephone 9 months later (T1). Some participants lacked data on residential area characteristics (n = 5) or disabilities at follow-up (n = 1), and therefore data of 271 persons were eligible for analyses. A more extensive description of the ELANE study can be found elsewhere [10].

Disabilities
Disabilities were measured at baseline and follow-up by the Lawton and Brody scale [12], a reliable and moderately strong predictor of functioning [12–14]. Participants were asked whether they needed help with the following eight IADL activities: using the telephone,

travelling (e.g. public transport), grocery shopping, preparing a meal, household tasks, taking medicines, finances, and doing laundry. All items had answering categories no (0) and yes (1), therefore sum scores could range between 0 and 8.

Transport-related physical activity
Three repeatedly measured TPA-outcomes were included in the analyses: walking for transport, cycling for transport, and a combination of the two (further referred to as walking, cycling, and total TPA). These were based on questions from the Physical Activity Questionnaire in the LASA study (LAPAQ), a valid and reliable instrument to measure PA among older adults [15, 16]. We calculated total minutes of walking within the last 2 weeks by multiplying the answers to the following questions: 'On how many days did you walk for transport in the past 2 weeks?', and 'How long did you walk for transport on average per day?' Total minutes cycling were calculated based on similar questions for cycling. Total TPA was derived by summing minutes of walking and minutes of cycling. Because 18.1 and 42.6% of the study sample reported walking or cycling time of 0 min at baseline, and respectively 19.9 and 46.1% at follow-up, total walking time, total cycling time, and total TPA time were logtransformed. To meaningfully interpret the results, coefficients and CIs were retransformed after the statistical analyses.

Residential area characteristics
Table 1 shows the ELANE street audit instrument which was used to collect data on residential area characteristics (carried out between June and October 2012 [10]. Sum scores were calculated for aesthetics, functional features, safety, and the presence of destinations by taking together separate items, as suggested by the framework of Pikora et al. [17].

Since the influence of residential area characteristics on health outcomes depends on the size of the area under study [18], we created road network buffers around each participant's home including all routes from a participant's home to streets up to 400, 800, and 1200 m. Road network buffers provide a more accurate exposure to environmental characteristic than traditional neighbourhood boundaries [19]. Scores for aesthetics, functional features, and safety of all audited streets within a buffer were summed and divided by the total number of streets audited in that buffer, resulting in average street scores for each buffer. For destinations, the number of destinations of all the streets in each buffer were summed [10]. For the analyses, longitudinal data were created assuming that the residential area characteristics remained stable over 9 months.

Table 1 Street audit instrument to assess area characteristics, the ELANE study

Area characteristic	Score		
	0	1	2
Aesthetics (range 0–22)			
Litter	Much	Little	Absent
Dog waste	Much	Little	Absent
Graffiti	Much	Little	Absent
Park	Absent		Present
Maintenance benches	Insufficient/n.a.	Reasonable	Sufficient
Maintenance sidewalk(s)	Insufficient/n.a.	Reasonable	Sufficient
Maintenance street	Insufficient	Reasonable	Sufficient
Trees	None	Few	Many
Gardens	None	Few	Many
Other green	Absent	Partly	Mainly
Water	Absent	Partly	Mainly
Functional (range 0–14)			
Sidewalk side 1	Absent	<2 m	≥2 m
Sidewalk side 2	Absent	<2 m	≥2 m
Obstacles sidewalk(s)	Many/n.a.	Few	None
Flatness walking surface	Insufficient	Reasonable	Sufficient
Curb cuts	Insufficient/n.a.	Reasonable	Sufficient
Bench(es)	None	One	More than one
Wastebin(s)	None	One	More than one
Safety (range 0–16)			
Crossings	Absent	Without traffic light(s)	With traffic light(s)
Speed limiters	None	One	More than one
Lighting	Insufficient	Reasonable	Sufficient
Supervision	Insufficient	Reasonable	Sufficient
Ground-level houses	None	Few	Many
Upper-level houses	None	Few	Many
Bicycle lane(s)	Absent	Not seperated from carlane	Seperated from carlane
Traffic speed limit[a]	Walking path	15 km road	50 km road
Destinations (range 0–15)			
ATM	Absent	Present	
Letterbox	Absent	Present	
Bus stop[b]	Absent	More than one	
Supermarket	Absent	Present	
Bakery	Absent	Present	
Vegetable store	Absent	Present	
Butcher	Absent	Present	
Other shops	Absent	Present	
Shopping center	Absent	Present	
Hairdresser	Absent	Present	
Café	Absent	Present	
Nursing home	Absent	Present	
Pharmacy	Absent	Present	
Community center	Absent	Present	
Sport facility	Absent	Present	

[a] Combined walking/cycle path scored 0.5; a 30 km road scored 1.5

[b] One bus stop scored 0.5

Statistical analyses

Descriptive analyses included Chi square tests and t tests to explore sex and age differences between those included (i.e. those participating at both T0 and T1) and those excluded from the main analyses (i.e. lost to follow-up) in terms of demographics, disabilities, and TPA.

Associations between residential area characteristics (aesthetics, functional features, safety, and destinations) and disabilities were tested, followed by analyses to investigate whether TPA mediated this association following conventional rules of mediation analysis as described by Baron and Kenny [20]. We subsequently tested the pathways A, B, C and A' as shown in Fig. 1.

The proportion of persons reporting to have no disabilities at both T0 and T1 was 56.8%. An additional 9.6% of the participants reported no disabilities at T0 only, and another 6.3% reported no disabilities at T1 only. This suggests that many older adults did not experience any limitations in IADL. While some persons reporting no disabilities are "close" to having disabilities, others may still be far away from becoming functionally limited. As such, disabilities can be seen as an underlying latent variable with an unrestricted range, of which the observed outcome is a truncated version [21]. Tobit regression models are suitable for repeatedly measured data and take into account such censored data. Furthermore, longitudinal tobit regression models take into account correlated observations over time within persons. Therefore, multivariate longitudinal sex- and age adjusted tobit regression analyses were conducted to test associations between residential area characteristics and disabilities (pathway A). Associations between area characteristics and TPA (pathway B) were explored by using Generalized Estimating Equations [22] since it is unlikely that the TPA data was censored. Multivariate longitudinal sex–age and for area characteristics adjusted tobit regression analyses were conducted to test associations between TPA and disabilities (pathway C).

Educational level was excluded from analyses because no association was found with disability level.

The longitudinal tobit model can be formulated mathematically as follows [21]:

$$y_{ij}^*|b_i = x_{ij}'\beta + b_i + e_{ij}, \quad e_{ij} \sim N(0, \sigma^2)$$
$$b_i \sim N(0, D)$$

in which y^* is a random latent variable that is not censored, β is the parameter, b_i is the case-specific random intercept with variance D, i refers to case i, j to the jth measurement within case i.

Finally, mediation of the association between area characteristics and disabilities by TPA was investigated (pathway A'). Analyses were performed by using STATA 14.1. Before the regression analyses were performed, panel data were defined (including 271 cases over 2 time periods, resulting in 271 × 2 observations). P values of 0.05 or lower were considered to be significant.

Results

Sample characteristics

Persons lost during follow-up were more often female, and reported on average more minutes walking than the study sample. No differences were found in the composition of both groups by age, minutes of cycling, and disabilities. At T0, 33.6% of the study sample had one or more disabilities. Although no difference was found between the mean number of disabilities at T0 and T1, after 9 months, 16.2% of the study sample had developed disabilities and 12.9% had recovered from disabilities. Also, total minutes of walking, cycling, and total TPA did not differ significantly between T0 and T1 (Table 2). Table 3 shows the scores for residential area characteristics per street for each buffer size. The average scores for aesthetics, functional features, and safety decreased slightly with increasing buffer size; the accumulated number of destinations within a buffer increased with increasing buffer size.

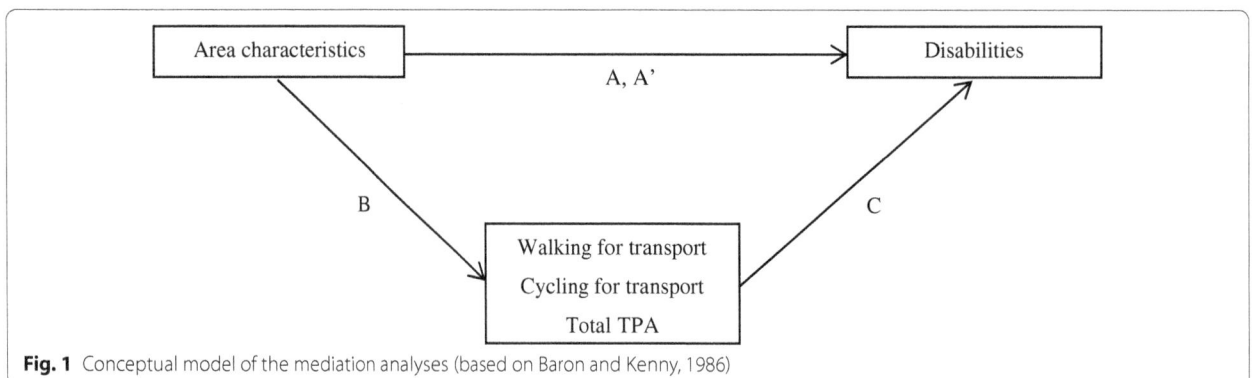

Fig. 1 Conceptual model of the mediation analyses (based on Baron and Kenny, 1986)

Table 2 Descriptive characteristics of the study sample at baseline and 9 months follow-up (N = 271)

		Total (N = 271)
Sex T0	Females	49.1%
Age T0	Mean	74.6 years
Disabilities T0 (range 0–8)	One or more	33.6%
	Mean number of disabilities	0.71 ± 1.35
Disabilities T1 (range 0–8)	One or more	36.9%
	Mean number of disabilities	0.73 ± 1.25
TPA T0 (minutes per 2 weeks)	Walking	344.5 ± 423.8
	Cycling	165.3 ± 248.3
	Total	509.8 ± 517.8
TPA T1 (minutes per 2 weeks)	Walking	349.4 ± 445.7
	Cycling	180.8 ± 357.0
	Total	530.2 ± 601.1

Table 3 Residential area characteristics of the four buffer zones

Area characteristics	Area		
	400 m	800 m	1200 m
Number of observed streets	39 ± 13	138 ± 40	294 ± 86
Aesthetics (range 0–22)	11.9 ± 0.9	11.8 ± 0.7	11.7 ± 0.6
Functional features (range 0–14)	5.8 ± 1.7	5.4 ± 1.1	5.3 ± 0.9
Safety (range 0–16)	6.1 ± 1.0	6.0 ± 0.7	5.9 ± 0.6
Destinations (range 0–∞)	10 ± 9	30 ± 16	57 ± 22

Area characteristics and disabilities

We subsequently tested the pathways A, B, C and A′ (Fig. 1). Within all buffers, area aesthetics showed comparable associations with disabilities, but was only significant in the 400 m buffer in which an increase in the aesthetics score of one point was associated with 0.86 less disabilities (95% CI −1.47 to −0.26; p < 0.05; pathway A) (Table 4). No associations for other area characteristics within the 400 m buffer, or for area characteristics of the 800 and 1200 m buffers with disabilities were found, although the association between aesthetics and disabilities in the 800 m was close to significant.

Area characteristics and TPA

For all three buffer sizes, associations between area characteristics with minutes walking and cycling were found (pathway B). In the 400 and 1200 m buffers, higher safety scores were associated with less cycling and walking respectively. With increasing buffer size, the strength of the association between aesthetics and minutes walking increased which was found significant in the two largest

buffers. Only in the 1200 m buffer, a significant association was found with total TPA: higher scores on aesthetics were associated with more total TPA (Table 5).

TPA and disabilities

Both higher levels of walking and cycling were associated with less disabilities (pathway C; Table 6). An increase of 10 min walking per 2 weeks was associated with 0.01 less disabilities (p < 0.001). An increase of 10 min cycling was associated with 0.02 less disabilities (p < 0.001). An increase of 10 min total TPA was associated with 0.01 less disabilities (p < 0.001).

Mediation

Inclusion of minutes walking and cycling separately to the model in which aesthetics of the 400 m buffer was related to disabilities, resulted in minor attenuations of the coefficient (pathway A′; Table 4). Adding total minutes TPA resulted in the largest attenuation: the regression coefficient changed from −0.86 to −0.69 (95% CI −1.21 to −0.16, p < 0.05). Except for the coefficients for safety in the 800 and 1200 m buffer, all coefficients representing associations between area characteristics and disabilities became closer to zero once TPA outcomes were added to the models.

Discussion

Of the four area characteristics under study, only higher scores on area aesthetics within a 400 m buffer were associated with less disabilities. While transport-related walking and cycling were associated with residential area characteristics and disabilities, only a small part of the association between aesthetics and disabilities was mediated by these factors.

Older adults living in areas with good aesthetics reported less disabilities, which is supported by other studies showing that those residing in areas with more green spaces and better neighbourhood maintenance (e.g. maintenance of streets and pavements) had lower levels of disabilities [5, 23]. We did not find associations with disabilities for the other area characteristics, which is in contrast to literature showing that more functional features (e.g. presence of sidewalks), traffic-related safety, and destinations (e.g. grocery stores) are associated with lower levels of disabilities [5, 24]. Differences in results may be due to different measures of disabilities and area characteristics, but may also reflect that the influence of the built environment on disabilities varies by country. In a sensitivity analysis, area characteristics were linked to the specific IADL-items regarding 'limitations in travelling (e.g. by public transport)' and 'limitations in grocery shopping' which are perhaps more directly related to mobility as compared to some elements of our IADL

Table 4 Age and sex adjusted associations between area characteristics and disabilities (pathway A and A'; N = 271)

Area	Area characteristic[a]	Pathway A			Pathway A'								
		Disabilities			Disabilities adjusted for transport-related walking			Disabilities adjusted for transport-related cycling			Disabilities adjusted for total TPA		
		β	(95% CI)	p	β	(95% CI)	p	β	(95% CI)	p	β	(95% CI)	p
400 m	Aesthetics	−0.86*	(−1.47 to −0.26)	0.01	−0.77*	(−1.34 to −0.19)	0.01	−0.71*	(−1.26 to −0.16)	0.01	−0.69*	(−1.21 to −0.16)	0.01
	Functional features	0.27	(−0.09 to 0.64)	0.14	0.22	(−0.13 to 0.57)	0.22	0.32	(−0.01 to 0.65)	0.06	0.22	(−0.10 to 0.53)	0.17
	Safety	0.22	(−0.35 to 0.78)	0.45	0.22	(−0.32 to 0.76)	0.43	0.06	(−0.46 to 0.57)	0.84	0.17	(−0.32 to 0.66)	0.49
	Destinations	−0.03	(−0.08 to 0.02)	0.21	−0.02	(−0.07 to 0.02)	0.28	−0.03	(−0.07 to 0.01)	0.15	−0.02	(−0.06 to 0.02)	0.26
800 m	Aesthetics	−0.97	(−1.96 to 0.02)	0.05	−0.81	(−1.75 to 0.13)	0.09	−0.83	(−1.72 to 0.07)	0.07	−0.66	(−1.51 to 0.19)	0.13
	Functional features	0.35	(−0.30 to 0.99)	0.29	0.32	(−0.30 to 0.93)	0.31	0.40	(−0.18 to 0.99)	0.18	0.28	(−0.27 to 0.84)	0.31
	Safety	0.04	(−0.78 to 0.86)	0.93	−0.06	(−0.84 to 0.71)	0.88	−0.07	(−0.81 to 0.67)	0.86	−0.13	(−0.84 to 0.57)	0.71
	Destinations	−0.00	(−0.03 to 0.02)	0.74	−0.00	(−0.03 to 0.02)	0.93	−0.01	(−0.03 to 0.02)	0.51	0.00	(−0.02 to 0.02)	0.99
1200 m	Aesthetics	−1.21	(−2.74 to 0.32)	0.12	−0.85	(−2.31 to 0.62)	0.26	−1.18	(−2.66 to 0.30)	0.12	−0.48	(−1.81 to 0.85)	0.48
	Functional features	0.62	(−0.64 to 1.88)	0.34	0.48	(−0.72 to 1.68)	0.43	0.63	(−0.60 to 1.85)	0.32	0.26	(−0.83 to 1.35)	0.64
	Safety	0.01	(−1.05 to 1.08)	0.98	−0.13	(−1.15 to 0.88)	0.80	−0.01	(−1.04 to 1.02)	0.99	−0.21	(−1.13 to 0.71)	0.65
	Destinations	−0.01	(−0.03 to 0.01)	0.50	−0.01	(−0.02 to 0.01)	0.57	−0.01	(−0.03 to 0.01)	0.44	−0.00	(−0.02 to 0.01)	0.70

* $p < 0.05$

[a] Adjustments were made for age, sex, and the other area characteristics

Table 5 Age and sex adjusted associations between area characteristics and TPA (pathway B; N = 271)

Area	Area characteristic[a]	TPA								
		Walking			Cycling			Total TPA		
		β	(95% CI)	p	β	(95% CI)	p	β	(95% CI)	p
400 m	Aesthetics	1.34	(0.86–2.11)	0.19	1.44	(0.85–2.46)	0.17	1.35	(0.91–2.00)	0.13
	Functional features	0.77	(0.60–1.00)	0.05	1.27	(0.93–1.72)	0.13	0.92	(0.73–1.15)	0.44
	Safety	1.09	(0.72–1.65)	0.68	0.56*	(0.34–0.91)	0.02	0.91	(0.63–1.30)	0.59
	Destinations	1.02	(0.98–1.05)	0.32	0.98	(0.95–1.03)	0.45	1.01	(0.98–1.04)	0.59
800 m	Aesthetics	2.06*	(1.00–4.26)	0.05	1.10	(0.46–2.62)	0.82	1.77	(0.94–3.35)	0.08
	Functional features	0.85	(0.54–1.34)	0.47	1.42	(0.82–2.46)	0.21	0.93	(0.62–1.39)	0.72
	Safety	0.58	(0.32–1.05)	0.07	0.70	(0.34–1.42)	0.32	0.62	(0.37–1.05)	0.07
	Destinations	1.02	(1.00–1.04)	0.07	0.98	(0.96–1.00)	0.12	1.01	(0.99–1.03)	0.23
1200 m	Aesthetics	4.53*	(1.49–13.79)	0.01	1.53	(0.53–4.44)	0.43	4.26*	(1.61–11.30)	0.00
	Functional features	0.60	(0.24–1.47)	0.26	0.81	(0.34–1.92)	0.63	0.51	(0.23–1.12)	0.09
	Safety	0.45*	(0.21–0.98)	0.04	0.77	(0.36–1.62)	0.49	0.54	(0.28–1.08)	0.08
	Destinations	1.01	(0.99–1.02)	0.42	1.00	(0.98–1.01)	0.56	1.01	(0.99–1.02)	0.30

Beta coefficients less than 1 represent negative associations, beta coefficients more than 1 represent positive associations

* p < 0.05

[a] Adjustments were made for age, sex, and the other area characteristics

Table 6 Associations between TPA and disabilities adjusted for area characteristics (pathway C; N = 271)

	Disabilities		
	β	(95% CI)	p
Adjusted for area characteristics within 400 m			
Walking	−0.01*	(−0.02 to −0.01)	0.00
Cycling	−0.02*	(−0.03 to −0.01)	0.00
Total TPA	−0.01*	(−0.02 to −0.01)	0.00
Adjusted for area characteristics within 800 m			
Walking	−0.01*	(−0.02 to −0.01)	0.00
Cycling	−0.02*	(−0.03 to −0.01)	0.00
Total TPA	−0.01*	(−0.02 to −0.01)	0.00
Adjusted for area characteristics within 1200 m			
Walking	−0.01*	(−0.02 to −0.01)	0.00
Cycling	−0.02*	(−0.03 to −0.01)	0.00
Total TPA	−0.01*	(−0.02 to −0.01)	0.00

* p < 0.05

scale. Associations with area characteristics were only found for travelling: higher scores on aesthetics within all buffers were associated with less limitations in travelling (beta coefficient up to −0.26 in the 1200 m buffer, CI −0.42 to −0.11; p < 0.05). This beta coefficient showed the highest drop (to −0.20) after total TPA was added to the model ("Appendix"). Based on a systematic review it has been recommended to revise built environment instrument including more disability-specific items [25]. Although the measure for functional features the ELANE neighbourhood scan did include width of side-walks and the presence of curb cuts, the scan for example did not include availability of signage or accessibility of green spaces or facilities [25]. Previous work based on ELANE baseline data showed a positive association between the presence of destinations and walking for transport [10]. We did not find this association in our current study, which may be caused by a lack of power due to the smaller study population.

A negative association was found between safety and transport-related walking in the 1200 m buffer. There is inconsistent evidence for associations between safety and walking which could be attributed to the complexity of measuring safety [26]. In a sensitivity-analysis we split our safety measure into a set of traffic safety items (i.e. presence of crossings, speed limiters, bicycle lanes, and traffic speed limits) and a set of social safety items (i.e. presence of lighting, supervision, houses, and apartments). Within the 400 m buffer, no significant associations were found between both safety measures and cycling (in contrast to the main finding presented in Table 5). Within the 1200 m buffer, higher scores for traffic safety were associated with less cycling. To improve research on safety and PA, Foster and Giles-Corti [26] suggested to combine objective measurement of safety with subjective measures of safety in which besides judgements (e.g. crime is a problem in the neighbourhood), and emotional responses (e.g. being fearful about the crime) should also be taken into account [26].

Although most associations were found non-significant, the results of the mediation analyses indicated the possible role of TPA in the associations between area characteristics and disabilities. TPA only partly explained the association between aesthetics and disabilities which may be due to the small effect size of the association between TPA and disabilities. The finding that an increase of 10 min cycling per 2 weeks was associated with 0.02 less disabilities, implicates that for example an increase of 25 min cycling per week may decrease disabilities (range 0–8) with 0.1. Other studies did also find effects of increasing minutes of physical activity per week. For example, Rist et al. found physical inactivity to be associated with 0.14 more IADL limitations over 2 years [27]. Another study by Boyle et al. showed that among non-disabled persons, the risk to develop IADL disability decreased with 7% for each additional hour of physical activity per week [28]. Despite the mixed findings of studies on the association between PA and disability, as some do not find significant associations, our findings relate to the thought that physical activity is modestly associated with disability [28]. TPA only partly explained the association between aesthetics and disabilities. It is of interest to investigate other possible mediating factors such as other health behaviors (e.g. recreational PA, nutrition), mental health, and social participation, which may be promoted by area characteristics [29, 30] and could potentially prevent disabilities [31, 32].

This study is among the first to study the role of area characteristics for disability among older persons and the role of transport-related physical activity. A main strength of the study was the use of repeatedly measured disabilities which was justified by the finding of substantial variation in disabilities between baseline and follow-up. For this purpose we applied longitudinal logit regression models which are able to capture these random fluctuations. The variation could be due to real differences in disabilities at both moments in time; previous studies also showed that the development of disabilities is a dynamic process [8]. The variation could also result from random measurement error of disabilities. Such measurement error increases the likelihood of bias towards the null in studies using disabilities measured at a single time. Although it is possible to recover from disabilities, older adults who have recovered are at high risk of recurrent disabilities [33].

Several limitations should also be mentioned. Firstly, 153 participants (35.6%) were lost to follow-up because they were not willing to participate (n = 135), unreachable by telephone (n = 11), had health problems (n = 3) or provided other reasons (n = 4). As compared to the overall sample at baseline, those lost to follow up were more often women, and reported more minutes walking at baseline, but did not differ in disability scores. It may limit the generalizability of the study results as those being most physically active may have been underrepresented in the study sample. The effect on the main outcome, pathway A, is expected to be limited as no differences were found in disability scores. Secondly, study participants were interviewed face-to-face at baseline and by telephone at follow-up. Although we cannot exclude the possibility that different methods may have resulted in over- or underestimations, the overall impact may be limited since the same procedure was used for all participants, i.e. both interviews asked for self-reported levels of PA and disabilities. Thirdly, the association between area characteristics and cycling for transport may be underestimated since 23.8% of the data used to measure area characteristics was related to walking only (i.e. characteristics of walking paths). Moreover, it is suggested to use larger longitudinal datasets and to use more accurate measurement of area characteristics related to cycling, in order to get more insight in associations between the built environment and disabilities and the role of TPA.

Fourthly, it should be recognized that causality cannot be proven, since findings presented are based on an observational study. Self-selection may have played a role in the interpretation of associations as active older adults self-selecting themselves into areas conducive for PA. Additional analyses showed that self-selection probably did not affect the results, as only 6.3% (n = 17) had moved to their current residence in the past 5 years. The most prevalent reason for moving was a lower level of maintenance of the house (n = 9). One person reported a reason related to the built environment, i.e. because of a more attractive neighbourhood. Associations between TPA and disability may be confounded by other lifestyle factors such as smoking and BMI [34], and health-related factors such as mental health, as for example depressive persons are more likely to be less physically active and to develop disabilities as compared to non-depressed persons [35, 36]. Finally, to capture the development of disabilities more accurately, it is suggested to study disabilities over a longer time-period.

Conclusions

Better aesthetic features of the area close by the residences of community-dwelling older adults were associated with less disabilities, but only a small part of this association seemed to be mediated by TPA. Higher scores for aesthetics and safety were associated with higher levels of TPA, and TPA was associated with disabilities. Preventive measures to reduce or prevent disabilities may include area characteristic improvements, however more research is needed to strengthen our results.

Author's contributions
AE conducted the analysis and wrote the manuscript while being supervised by FJL. FHP, CBMK, and AB critically reviewed the manuscript. All the authors read and approved the final manuscript.

Author details
[1] Department of Public Health, Erasmus University Medical Centre, P.O. Box 2040, 3000 CA Rotterdam, The Netherlands. [2] Department of Human Geography and Spatial Planning, Utrecht University, Utrecht, The Netherlands. [3] Department of Urban Environment and Safety, TNO, Utrecht, The Netherlands.

Acknowledgements
Special thanks to Sander Schaminee from the Netherlands Organisation for Applied Research TNO for his contribution to the creation of network buffers. Furthermore, thanks to Christa Wortman, Yvonne Roest, Sanne Tamerus, and Daniëlle de Keijzer for their contribution to the data collection.

Competing interests
The authors declare that they have no competing interests.

Ethics approval and consent to participate
At T0, a random sample was informed about the study by letter and an information flyer, and was asked to participate in the study. Through phone calls it was investigated whether persons had received the letter and flyer, whether they fulfilled the inclusion criteria, and it was registered whether they were willing to participate through oral consent (according to the Dutch law). At follow-up, persons who participated at T0 were informed about the goals of the second measurement through phone calls, and again oral consent to participate in a short follow-up interview 9 months after T0 was obtained. The study was approved by the institutional medical ethics committee of Erasmus MC Rotterdam (METC).

Funding
This study was financially supported by the Netherlands Organisation for Health Research and Development (ZonMw), Project Number 314030301.

Appendix: Results of pathway A, A' and C for IADL items grocery shopping and travelling
See Tables 7, 8, 9, and 10.

Table 7 Age and sex adjusted associations between area characteristics and grocery shopping (pathway A and A'; N = 271)

| Area | Area characteristic[a] | Pathway A | | | Pathway A' | | | | | | | | |
| | | Grocery shopping | | | Grocery shopping adjusted for transport-related walking | | | Grocery shopping adjusted for transport-related cycling | | | Grocery shopping adjusted for total TPA | | |
		β	(95% CI)	p	β	(95% CI)	p	β	(95% CI)	p	β	(95% CI)	p
400 m	Aesthetics	−0.05	(−0.10 to 0.01)	0.08	−0.04	(−0.10 to 0.01)	0.12	−0.04	(−0.09 to 0.01)	0.12	−0.04	(−0.09 to 0.01)	0.15
	Functional features	−0.00	(−0.03 to 0.03)	0.88	−0.01	(−0.04 to 0.02)	0.64	0.00	(−0.03 to 0.03)	0.92	−0.01	(−0.03 to 0.02)	0.72
	Safety	0.03	(−0.02 to 0.08)	0.31	0.03	(−0.02 to 0.08)	0.27	0.02	(−0.03 to 0.06)	0.51	0.02	(−0.03 to 0.07)	0.36
	Destinations	−0.00	(−0.01 to 0.00)	0.55	−0.00	(−0.00 to 0.00)	0.66	−0.00	(−0.01 to 0.00)	0.46	−0.00	(−0.00 to 0.00)	0.63
800 m	Aesthetics	−0.01	(−0.10 to 0.07)	0.75	0.00	(−0.09 to 0.09)	0.99	−0.01	(−0.10 to 0.07)	0.78	0.00	(−0.08 to 0.09)	0.88
	Functional features	−0.02	(−0.08 to 0.03)	0.46	−0.02	(−0.08 to 0.03)	0.39	−0.01	(−0.07 to 0.04)	0.59	−0.02	(−0.08 to 0.03)	0.39
	Safety	0.02	(−0.06 to 0.09)	0.66	0.00	(−0.07 to 0.08)	0.88	0.01	(−0.06 to 0.08)	0.78	−0.00	(−0.07 to 0.07)	0.98
	Destinations	0.00	(−0.00 to 0.00)	0.82	0.00	(−0.00 to 0.00)	0.60	−0.00	(−0.00 to 0.00)	0.97	0.00	(−0.00 to 0.00)	0.58
1200 m	Aesthetics	−0.00	(−0.14 to 0.13)	0.97	0.03	(−0.11 to 0.16)	0.69	0.00	(−0.13 to 0.14)	0.99	0.05	(−0.08 to 0.18)	0.45
	Functional features	−0.03	(−0.14 to 0.08)	0.56	−0.04	(−0.15 to 0.07)	0.44	−0.03	(−0.14 to 0.08)	0.55	−0.06	(−0.16 to 0.05)	0.29
	Safety	0.01	(−0.08 to 0.11)	0.79	−0.00	(−0.10 to 0.09)	0.95	0.01	(−0.08 to 0.11)	0.82	−0.01	(−0.10 to 0.08)	0.84
	Destinations	0.00	(−0.00 to 0.00)	0.18	0.00	(−0.00 to 0.00)	0.13	0.00	(−0.00 to 0.00)	0.19	0.00	(−0.00 to 0.00)	0.09

* p < 0.05

[a] Adjustments were made for age, sex, and the other area characteristics

Table 8 Associations between TPA and grocery shopping adjusted for area characteristics (pathway C; N = 271)

	Grocery shopping		
	β	(95% CI)	p
Adjusted for area characteristics within 400 m			
Walking	−0.02*	(−0.03 to −0.01)	0.00
Cycling	−0.02*	(−0.03 to −0.01)	0.00
Total TPA	−0.04*	(−0.05 to −0.02)	0.00
Adjusted for area characteristics within 800 m			
Walking	−0.02*	(−0.03 to −0.01)	0.00
Cycling	−0.02*	(−0.03 to −0.01)	0.00
Total TPA	−0.04*	(−0.05 to −0.02)	0.00
Adjusted for area characteristics within 1200 m			
Walking	−0.02*	(−0.03 to −0.01)	0.00
Cycling	−0.01*	(−0.01 to 0.00)	0.00
Total TPA	−0.04*	(−0.05 to −0.02)	0.00

* p < 0.05

Table 9 Age and sex adjusted associations between area characteristics and travelling (pathway A and A'; N = 271)

Area	Area characteristic[a]	Pathway A — Travelling			Pathway A' — Travelling adjusted for transport-related walking			Travelling adjusted for transport-related cycling			Travelling adjusted for total TPA		
		β	(95% CI)	p	β	(95% CI)	p	β	(95% CI)	p	B	(95% CI)	p
400 m	Aesthetics	−0.11*	(−0.17 to −0.05)	0.00	−0.11*	(−0.17 to −0.05)	0.00	−0.10*	(−0.16 to −0.04)	0.00	−0.10*	(−0.16 to −0.04)	0.00
	Functional features	0.03	(−0.00 to 0.07)	0.07	0.03	(−0.01 to 0.06)	0.10	0.04*	(0.01 to 0.07)	0.02	0.03	(−0.00 to 0.06)	0.08
	Safety	0.03	(−0.02 to 0.09)	0.20	0.04	(−0.02 to 0.09)	0.17	0.02	(−0.04 to 0.07)	0.50	0.03	(−0.02 to 0.09)	0.21
	Destinations	−0.01*	(−0.01 to −0.00)	0.03	−0.01*	(−0.01 to −0.00)	0.04	−0.01*	(−0.01 to −0.00)	0.01	−0.00*	(−0.01 to −0.00)	0.03
800 m	Aesthetics	−0.17*	(−0.27 to −0.07)	0.00	−0.16*	(−0.26 to −0.06)	0.00	−0.17*	(−0.26 to −0.08)	0.00	−0.15*	(−0.24 to −0.06)	0.00
	Functional features	0.03	(−0.03 to 0.09)	0.37	0.03	(−0.04 to 0.09)	0.40	0.04	(−0.02 to 0.10)	0.18	0.03	(−0.03 to 0.08)	0.38
	Safety	0.10*	(0.02 to 0.18)	0.02	0.09*	(0.01 to 0.17)	0.02	0.09*	(0.01 to 0.17)	0.02	0.08*	(0.01 to 0.16)	0.04
	Destinations	−0.00	(−0.00 to 0.00)	0.31	−0.00	(−0.00 to 0.00)	0.41	−0.00	(−0.00 to 0.00)	0.12	−0.00	(−0.00 to 0.00)	0.45
1200 m	Aesthetics	−0.26*	(−0.42 to −0.11)	0.00	−0.24*	(−0.40 to −0.09)	0.00	−0.26*	(−0.41 to −0.10)	0.00	−0.20*	(−0.34 to −0.06)	0.01
	Functional features	0.09	(−0.04 to 0.22)	0.16	0.08	(−0.04 to 0.21)	0.19	0.09	(−0.04 to 0.21)	0.17	0.06	(−0.05 to 0.18)	0.30
	Safety	0.13*	(0.02 to 0.23)	0.02	0.11*	(0.01 to 0.22)	0.04	0.12*	(0.02 to 0.23)	0.03	0.10*	(0.00 to 0.20)	0.04
	Destinations	−0.00	(−0.00 to 0.00)	0.07	−0.00	(−0.00 to 0.00)	0.08	−0.00	(−0.00 to 0.00)	0.06	−0.00	(−0.00 to 0.00)	0.10

* p < 0.05

[a] Adjustments were made for age, sex, and the other area characteristics

Table 10 Associations between TPA and travelling adjusted for area characteristics (pathway C; N = 271)

	Travelling		
	β	(95% CI)	P
Adjusted for area characteristics within 400 m			
Walking	−0.02*	(−0.03 to −0.00)	0.01
Cycling	−0.03*	(−0.04 to −0.02)	0.00
Total TPA	−0.04*	(−0.06 to −0.03)	0.00
Adjusted for area characteristics within 800 m			
Walking	−0.01*	(−0.03 to −0.00)	0.01
Cycling	−0.03*	(−0.04 to −0.02)	0.00
Total TPA	−0.04*	(−0.06 to −0.03)	0.00
Adjusted for area characteristics within 1200 m			
Walking	−0.01*	(−0.03 to −0.00)	0.02
Cycling	−0.02*	(−0.02 to −0.01)	0.00
Total TPA	−0.04*	(−0.06 to −0.03)	0.00

* p < 0.05

References

1. Van Houwelingen AH, Cameron ID, Gussekloo J, et al. Disability transitions in the oldest old in the general population. The Leiden 85-plus study. Age. 2014;36:483–93.
2. Millán-Calent IJC, Tubío J, Pita-Fernández S, et al. Prevalence of functional disability in activities of daily living (ADL), instrumental activities of daily living (IADL) and associated factors, as predictors of morbidity and mortality. Arch Gerontol Geriatr. 2010;50:306–10.
3. Crimmins EM, Kim JK, Solé-Auró A. Gender differences in health: results from SHARE, ELSA and HRS. Eur J Public Health. 2011;21:81–91.
4. WHO. International classification of functioning, disability and health. Geneva: World Health Organization; 2001.
5. Rosso AL, Auchincloss AH, Michael YL. The urban built environment and mobility in older adults: a comprehensive review. J Aging Res 2011;2011:816106. doi:10.4061/2011/816106.
6. Lawrence RH, Jette AM. Disentangling the disablement process. J Gerontol B Psychol Sci Soc Sci. 1996;51:173–82.
7. Verbrugge LM, Jette AM. The disablement process. Soc Sci Med. 1994;38:1–14.
8. Hardy SE, Dubin JA, Holford TR, et al. Transitions between states of disability and independence among older persons. Am J Epidemiol. 2005;161:575–84.
9. Jansen FM, Prins RG, Etman A, et al. Physical activity in non-frail and frail older adults. PLoS ONE. 2015;10(4):e0123168.
10. Etman A, Kamphuis CBM, Prins RG, et al. Characteristics of residential areas and transportational walking among frail and non-frail Dutch elderly: does the size of the area matter? Int J Health Geogr. 2014;4(13):7.
11. Prins RG, Pierik F, Etman A, et al. How many walking and cycling trips made by elderly are beyond commonly used buffer sizes: results from a GPS study. Health Place. 2014;27:127–33.
12. Lawton MP, Brody EM. Assessment of older people: self-maintaining and instrumental activities of daily living. Gerontologist. 1969;9:179–86.
13. McGrory S, Shenkin SD, Austin EJ, et al. Lawton IADL scale in dementia: can item response theory make it more informative? Age Ageing. 2014;43:491–5.
14. Vittengl JR, White CN, McGovern RJ, et al. Comparative validity of seven scoring systems for the instrumental activities of daily living scale in rural elders. Aging Ment Health. 2006;10(1):40–7.
15. Stel VS, Smit JH, Pluijm MF, et al. Comparison of the LASA Physical Activity Questionnaire with a 7-day diary and pedometer. J Clin Epidemiol. 2004;57:252–8.
16. Buurman BM, Parlevliet JL, Van Deelen BAJ, et al. A randomised clinical trial on a comprehensive geriatric assessment and intensive home follow-up after hospital discharge: the Transitional Care Bridge. BMC Health Serv Res. 2010;29:296.
17. Pikora T, Giles-Corti B, Bull F, et al. Developing a framework for assessment of the environmental determinants of walking and cycling. Soc Sci Med. 2003;56:1693–703.
18. Diez Roux AV, Evenson KR, McGinn AP, et al. Availability of recreational resources and physical activity in adults. Am J Public Health. 2007;97:493–9.
19. Perchoux C, Chaix B, Cummins S, et al. Conceptualization and measurement of environmental exposure in epidemiology: accounting for activity space related to daily mobility. Health Place. 2013;21:86–93.
20. Baron RM, Kenny DA. The moderator-mediator variable distinction in social psychological research: conceptual, strategic, and statistical considerations. J Pers Soc Psychol. 1986;51:1173–82.
21. Twisk J, Rijmen F. Longitudinal tobit regression: a new approach to analyze outcome variables with floor or ceiling effects. J Clin Epidemiol. 2009;62:953–8.
22. Hanley JA, Negassa A, Edwardes MD, et al. Statistical analysis of correlated data using generalized estimating equations: an orientation. Am J Epidemiol. 2003;15:364–75.
23. Schootman M, Andresen EM, Wolinsky FD, et al. Neighborhood conditions and risk of incident lower-body functional limitations among middle-aged African Americans. Am J Epidemiol. 2006;1:450–8.
24. Borst HC, Miedema HME, De Vries SI, et al. Relationships between street characteristics and perceived attractiveness for walking reported by elderly people. J Environ Psychol. 2008;28:353–61.
25. Gray JA, Zimmerman JL, Rimmer JH. Built environment instruments for walkability, bikeability, and recreation: disability and universal design relevant? Disabil Health J. 2012;5(2):87–101.
26. Foster S, Giles-Corti B. The built environment, neighborhood crime and constrained physical activity: an exploration of inconsistent findings. Prev Med. 2008;47:241–51.
27. Rist PM, Marden JR, Capistrant BD, et al. Do physical activity, smoking, drinking, or depression modify transitions from cognitive impairment to functional disability? J Alzheimers Dis. 2015;44(4):1171–80.
28. Boyle PA, Buchman AS, Wilson RS, et al. Physical activity is associated with incident disability in community-based older persons. J Am Geriatr Soc. 2007;55(2):195–201.
29. Van Cauwenberg J, De Bourdeaudhuij I, De Meester F, et al. Relationship between the physical environment and physical activity in older adults: a systematic review. Health Place. 2011;17:458–69.
30. Botticello AL, Rohrbach T, Cobbold N. Disability and the built environment: an investigation of community and neighborhood land uses and participation for physically impaired adults. Ann Epidemiol. 2014;24(7):545–50.
31. Pahor M, Guralnik JM, Ambrosius WT, et al. Effect of structured physical activity on prevention of major mobility disability in older adults: the LIFE study randomized clinical trial. JAMA. 2014;18:2387–96.
32. Stuck AE, Walthert JM, Nikolaus T, et al. Risk factors for functional status decline in community-living elderly people: a systematic literature review. Soc Sci Med. 1999;48(4):445–69.
33. Hardy SE, Gill TM. Recovery from disability among community-dwelling older persons. JAMA. 2004;7:1596–602.
34. Van Den Brink CL, Picavet H, Van Den Bos GA, et al. Duration and intensity of physical activity and disability among European elderly men. Disabil Rehabil. 2005;27(6):341–7.
35. Roshanaei-Moghaddam B, Katon WJ, Russo J. The longitudinal effects of depression on physical activity. Gen Hosp Psychiatry. 2009;31(4):306–15.
36. Bruce ML. Depression and disability in late life: directions for future research. Am J Geriatr Psychiatry. 2001;9(2):102–12.

12

Cross-border spatial accessibility of health care in the North-East Department of Haiti

Dominique Mathon[1], Philippe Apparicio[1*] ⓘ and Ugo Lachapelle[2]

Abstract

Background: The geographical accessibility of health services is an important issue especially in developing countries and even more for those sharing a border as for Haiti and the Dominican Republic. During the last 2 decades, numerous studies have explored the potential spatial access to health services within a whole country or metropolitan area. However, the impacts of the border on the access to health resources between two countries have been less explored. The aim of this paper is to measure the impact of the border on the accessibility to health services for Haitian people living close to the Haitian-Dominican border.

Methods: To do this, the widely employed enhanced two-step floating catchment area (E2SFCA) method is applied. Four scenarios simulate different levels of openness of the border. Statistical analysis are conducted to assess the differences and variation in the E2SFCA results. A linear regression model is also used to predict the accessibility to health care services according to the mentioned scenarios.

Results: The results show that the health professional-to-population accessibility ratio is higher for the Haitian side when the border is open than when it is closed, suggesting an important border impact on Haitians' access to health care resources. On the other hand, when the border is closed, the potential accessibility for health services is higher for the Dominicans.

Conclusion: The openness of the border has a great impact on the spatial accessibility to health care for the population living next to the border and those living nearby a road network in good conditions. Those findings therefore point to the need for effective and efficient trans-border cooperation between health authorities and health facilities. Future research is necessary to explore the determinants of cross-border health care and offers an insight on the spatial revealed access which could lead to a better understanding of the patients' behavior.

Keywords: Spatial accessibility, Health care, Enhanced two-step floating catchment area, Border, Haiti, Dominican Republic

Background

The geographical accessibility of health services is an important issue in public health and for improved health outcomes, especially in developing countries [1–6]. During the last two decades, numerous studies have explored the potential spatial access to health services within a whole country or metropolitan area [7–10]. Scholars have also analyzed cross-border mobility for health care

in several diverse contexts [11–24]. But fewer studies address the impact of an international border and its openness on the spatial access to health care resources [25, 26].

The concept of borders has been evolving throughout the years from their being seen as barriers to their being considered as contact zones, but regional integration and border openness have been questioned in several contexts [27–32]. Studies analyzing cross-border mobility for the use of health care services emphasize the uniqueness of the different border contexts and the importance of the direction of flows [16, 24]. Cross-border mobility for health care access may be explained by a variety of factors. It depends on the various individuals' situations

---

*Correspondence: philippe.apparicio@ucs.inrs.ca
[1] Environmental Equity Laboratory, INRS Centre Urbanisation Culture Société, 385, rue Sherbrooke Est, Montréal, Québec H2X 1E3, Canada
Full list of author information is available at the end of the article

and needs. It may be motivated by dissatisfaction with health care provision in the home country or by actual deficiencies there. A lack of coverage (in terms of health care insurance) or a quest for specialized health care may influence individual choice. Glinos et al. [12] indicate that, during the decision-making process, patients balance factors such as proximity, family support and social ties. Affordability, availability and quality of care are also determinants. Analyzing patient mobility between Laos and Thailand, Bochaton [14, 15] demonstrates the importance of well-established mobility practices as well as social networks among border populations in the seeking of cross-border health care. Social networks are also considered by Dione [16] as one of the determinants of patients' cross-border mobility in four African countries sharing a border. Proximity (physical accessibility) is also one of the main determinants of patient mobility in the very different contexts of European [11] and African countries [16].

Access to health care is multidimensional, and most of the studies on patients' cross-border mobility for health care access have used the seminal framework developed by Penchansky and Thomas [33]. These authors consider five dimensions in order to measure "the degree of fit between the clients and the system" [33]. Two of these dimensions are spatial: (1) availability (adequacy between the supply and the demand); and (2) accessibility, or the location of the supply relative to the location of the clients. The other three are aspatial and reflect socioeconomic and cultural factors: (1) accommodation, or the adequate matching of the supply organization with the clients' abilities and perceptions; (2) affordability, or the prices of the services relative to the clients' income or ability to pay; and (3) acceptability (clients' and providers' attitudes toward one another). These dimensions may act as either facilitators or barriers.

Regarding spatial accessibility, scholars define this in terms of the possible use of the services (potential accessibility) and their actual use (realized accessibility) [34, 35]. This differentiation between potential access and realized access makes it possible to better identify the barriers to or facilitators of access. The extent of the spatial separation between supply and demand can therefore be analyzed. In this article, we focus on potential spatial accessibility in a borderland context. The border acts either as a geographical constraint or as a facilitator.

Our hypothesis is that accessibility varies depending on the level of border openness. In addition, the lack of services (push factor) in Haiti and the more attractive supply (pull factor) in the Dominican Republic may lead to polarized flows in a push/pull dynamic.

The aim of this paper is to evaluate the spatial accessibility of health care services for Haitians living along the Haitian-Dominican border, and to measure the impact of this border on their health care access using the well-known E2SFCA method.

The Haitian-Dominican border

The Haitian-Dominican border inherited from the colonial period has given rise to a "double insularity" [36, 37] that has been settled through a long process of social and spatial differentiation as well as ideological distancing [36–38]. Both countries have forged and asserted their particular national identities through their respective histories and struggles to achieve the construction of their own nation state [37, 39]. The discontinuities (territorial, cultural, socioeconomic and political) are therefore quite visible at the Haitian-Dominican border [40, 41]. An entire apparatus (gates, military control on the Dominican side, etc.) is in place to mark and create this distance [41–43]. At the same time, the relative and recent border opening has given rise to a transitioning process which is redefining the function of the border as moving toward a "space of coexistence and cooperation" while sustaining asymmetrical and conflicting interactions along the border line [40, 42, 44, 45].

Officially (since 1987), the border has been opened during the day and closed at night. There are four official entry points and several informal crossing points, the number of which is not precisely known [38]. These informal crossing points underscore the permeability of the border as well as the complexity of the cross-border mobility [43]. The flow of the population may be constrained by different conflictual situations: a national decision (epidemiological surveillance, control of smuggling, etc.) or a particular local situation (protest about Dominican soldiers' aggressive behaviours, protest over national decisions, protests from Haitian or Dominican traders, etc.) [44]. From 2000 to 2016, the border was closed a number of times for varying numbers of hours or days. But the intensity and importance of the commercial exchanges for both countries, at different levels, may act as a leverage for conflict settlement.

Cross-border movements from both sides have existed since the colonial period, but Haitian labour flows started in the early twentieth century with the North American occupation of both countries [38, 43, 46–48]. Various mechanisms are in place in the Dominican Republic to regulate such flows (illegality of the Haitian work force, massive deportations, etc.) [38, 48]. According to the recent survey on migration, more than 80% of immigrants in the Dominican Republic are Haitian [49, 50]. The importance of Haitian labour for the construction industry as well as for the agricultural sector is well documented [38, 43, 46, 47, 49–51]. Some studies [38, 46] have revealed a "feminization of Haitian migration flows." Others [42] have emphasized the difficulty of distinguishing between irregular migration, smuggling and trafficking.

On the other hand, there is some evidence that the percentage of Haitian immigrants using health care facilities is higher than for other immigrants [49]. Furthermore, during the last two decades, the Dominican Republic has been used to channel international aid to Haiti. Montiel et al. [46] emphasize the differential impact of this, including, for example, the reinforcement of the Dominican health care system at the expense of the Haitian one. They consider this to be a factor that could have encouraged a growing number of Haitians to cross the border in search of health care [46]. Their comments are in line with evidence from other studies addressing cross-border health care mobility in different contexts [12, 15, 16]. But beyond the significant and quite systematic health outcome disparities between both countries (Table 1), what are the differences between the two health care systems?

Main characteristics of the public health care systems in Haiti and the Dominican Republic

The health care system in most Latin American and Caribbean countries is segmented, with a variety of financing

Table 1 Basic health indicators for Haiti and the Dominican Republic

Health indicators	Haiti	Dominican Republic
Life expectancy at birth (2016) *	63.3	73.9
Men	61.2	70.8
Women	65.5	77.1
Mortality rate of the under 5 years (probability of death before age of 5 per 1000 live births, 2016)**	67	30.7
Maternal mortality ratio (per 100,000 live births, 2014)***	359	92
New HIV infections among adults 15–49 years old (per 1000 uninfected population, 2015)****	0.21	0.36
Births attended by trained personnel (%)	50.0[a]	68.6[b]
Skill health professionals density (per 10,000 habitants)	6.5[c]	28.2[d]

Sources: *World Development Indicators. World Bank Group at databank.worldbank.org

**Estimates Developed by the UN Inter-agency Group for Child Estimation (UNICEF, WHO, World Bank, UN DESA Population Division) at childmortality.org

***WHO, UNICEF, UNFPA, World Bank Group, and the United Nations Population Division. Trends in Maternal Mortality: 1990–2015. Geneva, World Health Organization, 2015

****2015, Source: UNAIDS/WHO; estimates 2016

[a] 2015

[b] 2014; PAHO/WHO, Health in the Americas—Summary: Regional Outlook and Country Profiles, 2017

[c] Source: MSPP, 2012

[d] Source: 2005–2013, WHO Global Health Workforce Statistics database

structures and affiliation types. It is also fragmented, with a supply offered by many institutions (public and private) and facilities that are not well integrated into the health care network [52]. This fragmentation and segmentation exacerbate inequities in access [52], which is also the case in Haiti [53] and the Dominican Republic [53, 54].

Reforms of the health care system: Access to health care and equity

During the last two decades, both countries—like most Latin American [53, 54] and Caribbean countries [55]—have been involved in an ongoing process of reforming their health care sector. These reforms are intended to improve health outcomes and to reduce health inequities. They are based on the following principles: a regulatory role for public health institutions, multisectoral production of health care, universal access, equity and solidarity, and efficiency and efficacy of the health care system [56–59]. Changes have been made in the structure and organization of the public health care system in both countries in order to improve access to health care and especially to primary care. Nevertheless, the pace and the implementation of such reforms have fluctuated from one side of the border to the other [55].

In the Dominican Republic, the reform has been the starting point for universal access to health care [54]. Catchment areas have been defined to maximize resource allocation for primary care as well as for equity. Citizens must be assigned to or registered in a Primary Care Unit (*Unidad de Atención Primaria*). But the coverage is still deficient (less than 50% of the population was covered in 2012), with disparities found among different socioeconomic groups (the poorest have limited access to health care) and also between rural and urban areas [54].

In Haiti, changes have also been made to improve coherence with administrative boundaries and respect for the equity and universality principles included in the health reform [60]. But the Haitian health system still faces complex organizational and institutional challenges [55]. Moreover, data from the *Enquête Mortalité, Morbidité et Utilisation des Services* (EMMUSV) highlight the lack of coverage: less than 5% of the respondents [61] have health care insurance. As for the Dominican Republic, wealthier and urban people have more access, which means that any form of equity is still largely incomplete [61, 62].

Organization of the health care system

Both countries have a three-tiered health care system [56, 57, 60, 63, 64], but with some specific differences, as shown in Fig. 1. The pyramidal model is organized according to three levels of complexity: primary, secondary and tertiary. It is designed to break away from the

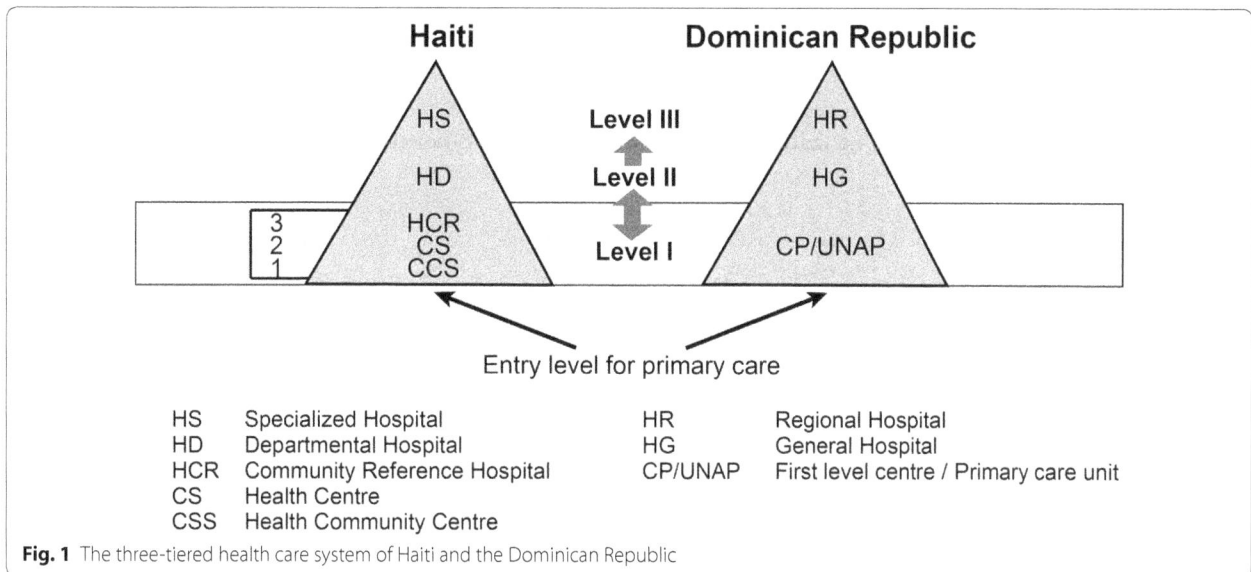

Fig. 1 The three-tiered health care system of Haiti and the Dominican Republic

existing hospital-centred structure in order to improve the population's access to primary care. The reference and counter-reference system allows patients to transit within the system from the entry point to specialized services when required.

The primary level consists of outpatient services and community care. The first level therefore offers basic health care (minimum service package) and prevention and promotion activities. One of the main organizational differences between the Haitian and Dominican health care systems is found at this level. In Haiti, the primary level is subdivided into three parts. It includes different kinds of facilities located in distinct territorial entities: (1) Health community centre located in the *Section communale* (the smallest territorial division) and offering ambulatory care and prevention and promotion activities; (2) Health centre in the *Commune* delivering preventive and curative care, including normal childbirth; and (3) Community Reference Hospital (HCR) in the *Arrondissement* providing a range of care including sensitive interventions requiring specialists in internal medicine, surgery, pediatrics, obstetrics and gynecology. However, the official documents are somewhat confusing, as two of them [57, 65] consider only two subdivisions and others [60] mention three. Either way, the subdivision appears to be the Haitian health authorities' response in order to accommodate the prevailing in terms of primary care facilities and to carry out the transition process toward the mainstream pyramidal model [60, 65].

It is important to emphasize that, in the Dominican Republic, each citizen is assigned a Primary Care Unit near their home (*Unidad de Atención Primaria—UNAP*) regardless of their insurance system [59], which is not the case in Haiti. Moreover, these units offer the same range of services as the first two Haitian first-level subdivisions.

The facilities of the second level (General Hospital in the Dominican Republic, whether administered at the municipal or provincial level, and Departmental Hospital in Haiti) offer basic specialized care in both countries. The services offered by the third level cover all contingencies during hospitalization and attend to the most complex cases.

Binational cooperation in health

The Haitian health master plan (2012–2022) considers reinforcing coordination with the Dominican Republic in order to reduce health issues in the epidemiological field in the borderland regions. It also seeks to develop relevant strategies and partnerships in the management of infectious diseases. There is a binational agreement for the control of tuberculosis aimed at successful coordination of the actions undertaken in the borderland regions and mainly targeting migrants, the populations of the *bateyes* (settlements around sugar mills where Haitian migrant workers live in very precarious conditions) and of the industrial areas, as well as those living in the borderland regions. In the case of natural disasters (floods in 2004 and the earthquake in 2010), the Dominican health facilities have supported the Haitian population by offering medical services to those needing them [44, 66, 67]. There are also coordinated vaccination campaigns in the borderland regions. But, as far as the official documents of both countries indicate, there is no cross-border cooperation in health care involving any hospitals or other facilities.

Data and methods

Study area

The area studied is in the northern part of the island of Haiti/Quisqueya, and focuses on the region along the Haitian-Dominican border, with one official daytime entry point (Ouanaminthe-Dajabón) and several informal crossing points (Fig. 2). Evidence for the last three decades has shown a significant growth in the intensity and diversity of interactions along the border, especially at the entry point, that is, Ouanaminthe-Dajabón [68, 69], the border's second leading entry point.

The cities of Ouanaminthe and Dajabón have played an important role throughout the history of both countries [70]. They have also witnessed violent conflicts such as the massacre of thousands of Haitians in October 1937. This borderland is evolving nowadays from a barrier to a contact zone and an interdependent zone [41, 69, 70]. Several stakeholders (international organizations, the transnational capital, merchants, grassroots organizations, etc.) are engaged in this process [70]. The relocation of a private Dominican industrial free-trade zone in the fertile plain of Maribahoux in Ouanaminthe (a project financed by the International Finance Corporation) however highlights the advantages derived by the Dominican Republic from its different level of development from that of Haiti. It shows how such disparities are helping to widen the gaps and are fostering more asymmetrical interactions [41, 70, 71]. Furthermore, the recent proliferation of binational projects promoted and financed by international organizations is tending to set the framework for a new era of cross-border cooperation [41] in different fields, including health issues.

The level of poverty is globally higher in the borderland regions of both countries [72, 73], but there are still important disparities in terms of infrastructures, services, etc. between the North-East Department and the Province of Dajabón. As shown in Fig. 2, the Haitian side of the border is denser, with more and larger sized cities.

In the health sector, this intense mobility has forced the implementation of binational mechanisms for epidemiological surveillance. Gaps in the supply of social services (health, education) tend to lead to asymmetrical interactions and polarized flows in a push/pull dynamic [68, 69, 74]. On the other hand, few studies [49, 75] have indicated that the ratio of foreigners using health care facilities is higher in the Dominican borderland region compared with the rest of the country.

Statistics from the Dominican public health secretary show that, in 2015, almost 10% of public hospital patients (consultation and emergency) in the Province of Dajabón were foreigners. The rate is even higher for the primary care centres (35%) (Table 2). Information about foreign patients' nationality is not available. The high percentage of Haitian migrants (87.2% of the immigrant population in Dominican Republic was born in Haiti according to the Second National Immigrant Survey held on 2017) and

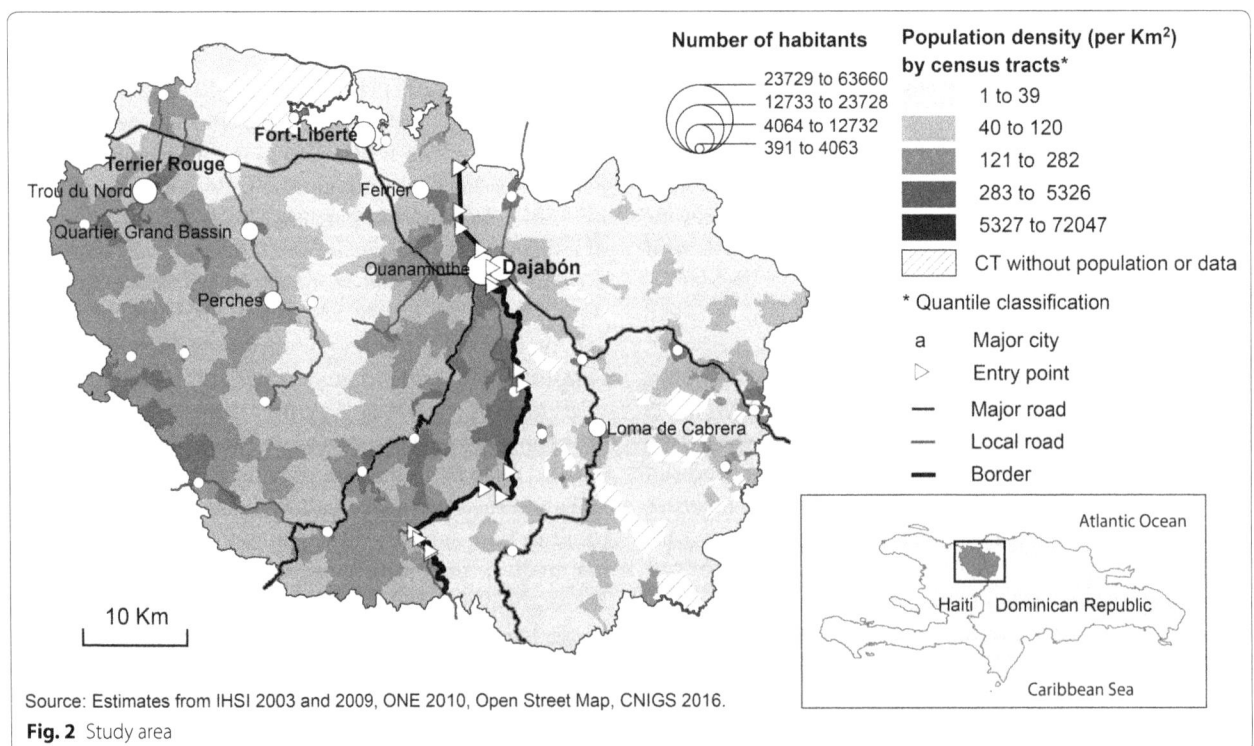

Number of habitants
- 23729 to 63660
- 12733 to 23728
- 4064 to 12732
- 391 to 4063

Population density (per Km²) by census tracts*
- 1 to 39
- 40 to 120
- 121 to 282
- 283 to 5326
- 5327 to 72047
- CT without population or data

* Quantile classification

- a   Major city
- ▷   Entry point
- —   Major road
- —   Local road
- ▬   Border

Source: Estimates from IHSI 2003 and 2009, ONE 2010, Open Street Map, CNIGS 2016.

Fig. 2 Study area

Table 2 Dominican health care facilities use for consultation and Emergency by national and foreign patients, 2015.
Source: **MSP, Vice Ministry of Planning and Development – Department of Health Information (DIS)**

Health care facilities	National patients			Foreign patients		
	Consultation	Emergency	Total	Consultation	Emergency	Total
Hospital Municipal Partido*	6475	7337	13,812	610	380	990
Hospital Dr. Ramon Adriano Villalona*	15,478	4910	20,388	1265	420	1685
Hospital Municipal Restauración*	9881	2332	12,213	2902	472	3374
Hospital Ramon Matias Mella*	15,963	14,502	30,465	555	819	1374
First Level Centers (29) **	45,456	3068	48,524	24,568	1602	26,170

(29) equals to the number of first level centers/primary care units

*Database of monthly records of Hospitals Services (67A) 2015 updated on April 27th 2016

**Monthly reports of services of the centers of first level of attention (R-8) 2015

proximity to the border suggest that most of those foreign patients are Haitian, but there is no direct evidence for this. The condensed version of the Second National Immigrant Survey (ENI-2017) indicates that 77% of the migrants born in Haiti as well as 78% of those born in Dominican Republic of foreigners parents used the public health services [50], Moreover, hundreds of thousands of Haitian descendants [39] are not considered to be Dominicans because of the 2013 judgment TC/0168/13 of the Dominican Constitutional Court and the 169-14 Law [76]. It is thus difficult to estimate the percentage of patients crossing the border to obtain health care and the proportion of Haitians living in the Dominican Republic.

Data

Three types of GIS data are needed to assess the potential accessibility of health care services.

a. *For the supply side*: The geographic locations of public health facilities in each country have been collected from the websites of the health secretaries of Haiti and the Dominican Republic. Data on the number of health professionals for each health facility have been provided by the Department of Information of the Dominican Republic's public health ministry (*Departamento de Información de salud*). For Haiti, such data were available on the health map on the website of the public health ministry (*Ministère de la santé publique et de la population*). According to those respective sources, there is a total of 70 public health facilities (35 on each side) and 932 health professionals (322 on the Haitian side and 610 in the Dominican Republic) (Fig. 3). It is worth noticing on the Haitian side (North-East Department), there is only one public facility of the second level and none at the border city of Ouanaminthe. Meanwhile the Province of Dajabon counts with four public facilities

of the second level (municipal hospitals or general hospital) and one of them located in the border city of Dajabón.

b. *For the demand side*: The demographic data have been extracted from the censuses at the equivalent of the census block level (*Section d'énumération— SDE*) for Haiti (N=422) and at the neighbourhood level (*Barrio*) for the Dominican Republic (N=202). The neighbourhood was the finest spatial unit available. The average population is 868 for the *SDE* and 317 for the *Barrio*. The demographic data for Haiti and the Dominican Republic were provided by the national statistical institutes (*Institut Haïtien de Statistiques et d'Informatique—IHSI* and *Oficina Nacional de Estadística—ONE*, respectively). Because the last census in Haiti was held in 2003, we had to estimate the population for 2010 (the year of the Dominican census). Our estimates are based on those made by the IHSI for 2009, in applying their population growth rate. The use of a centroid considers that the population is evenly distributed within the spatial unit used (*SDE* or *Barrio*), which is not the case, especially for a scattered rural population area. To better reflect the reality of the settlements in the rural areas, we use an adjusted centroid of the spatial unit. The adjustments are based on photo interpretations of Google and Bing imagery.

c. *For the travel distance*: The road network data were retrieved from Open Street Map (OSM) for both countries. Data were also provided by Haiti's National Centre of Geospatial Information (*Centre National d'Information Géospatiale – CNIGS*). The data were validated using Google and Bing imagery. The road classification of the Haitian and Dominican transport secretaries was used. A maximum travel speed was assigned to each class of road as indicated in Table 3 based on various sources and photointerpretation to

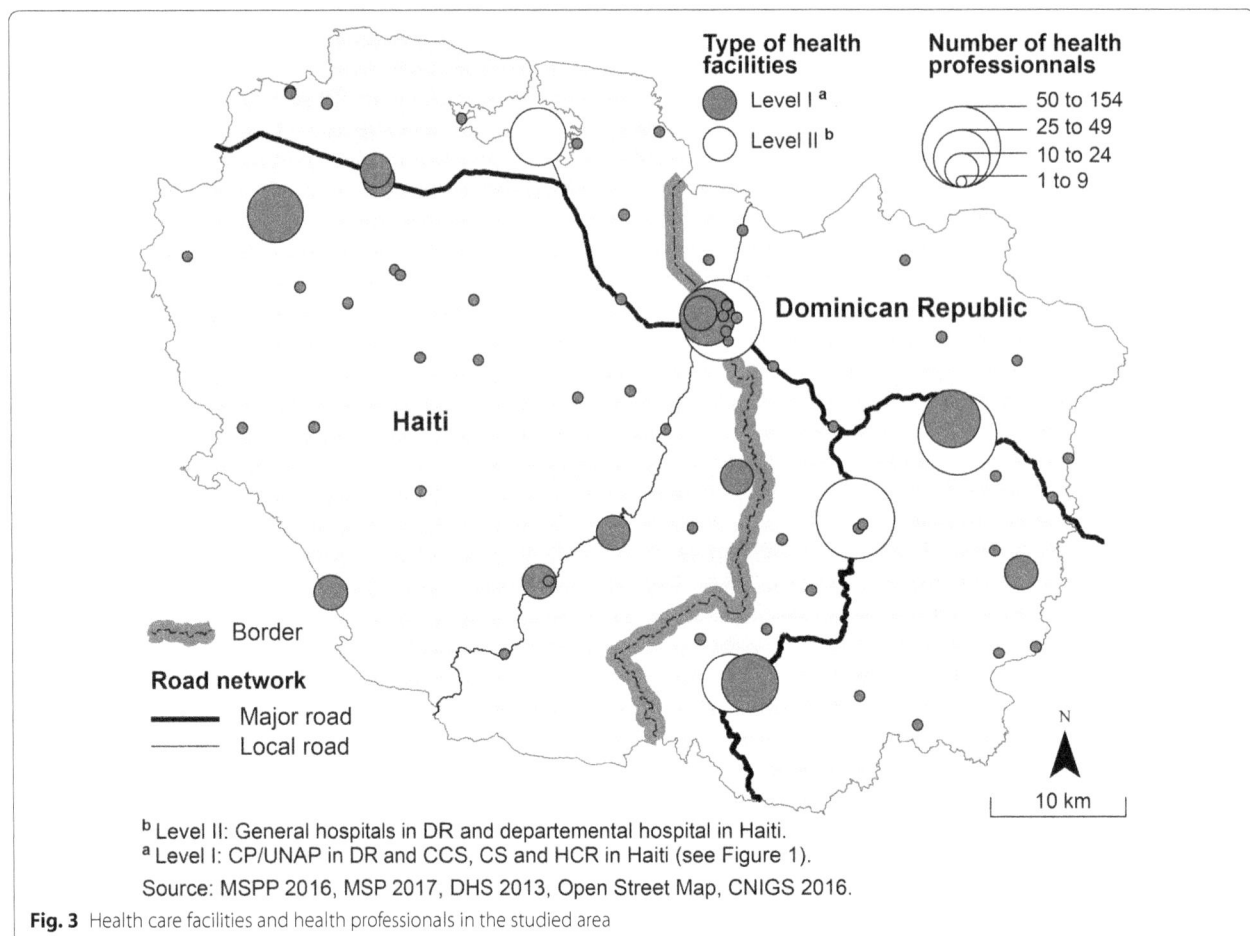

Fig. 3 Health care facilities and health professionals in the studied area

Table 3 Road classification and speed

Country	Road type	Speed
Haiti*	National roads	70 km/h
	Departmental roads and segment of national roads in living areas	50 km/h
	Communal roads, local roads, streets	30 km/h
	Track and others, unclassified roads	15 km/h
	Pathways	3 km/h
Dominican Republic**	Major roads and regional roads	80 km/h
	Local roads	50 km/h
	Streets	35 km/h
	Country roads	30 km/h
	Others, unclassified roads	15 km/h
	Pathways	3 km/h

Sources: *MTPTC 2015; CIAT 2010

**2010 at oisevi.org; DIGESETT, Ley 241-67

assess roads conditions. For pathways, the maximum travel speed is 3 km/h in order to in some way reflect the geographic constraints, since the central part of the area studied is nested in a mountainous chain. The entry points were georeferenced based on aerial photo interpretation.

Methods

To measure the impact of the opening of the border on the spatial access to health care, we consider different scenarios with varying border crossing time impedance: open, semi-open, or closed. These scenarios are hypothetical, since the level of control is not the same along the border or at the informal crossing points or entry points. Furthermore, different factors (objective and subjective) influence the smoothness of the flows of Haitians at the Dominican border.

The estimates of the time spent crossing are based upon: (1) on-site observations in July 2016 and June 2017 at the Ouanaminthe-Dajabón entry point; and (2) informative discussions with key resources in Ouanaminthe and organization members working along the border line.

a. The first scenario is an open border, where there is less control (or almost none) at the Dominican border. The border is open on Friday and Monday when the so-called "binational" market takes place in Dajabón. Haitians are "free" to cross, and no papers are needed. But, due to the intense flows, delays could be observed. A 15-min cost is thus added to the travel time required to cross the border in order to take into account light traffic or migration controls.

b. The second and third scenarios consider the border half closed. In this case, there is more control at the Dominican border. It is a twofold situation: a) a normal border control for migration and light traffic (scenario 2); and b) stricter control and heavy traffic (scenario 3). The cost varies from 30 min for scenario 2–60 min for scenario 3.

c. In the fourth and last scenario, the border is closed. No crossing is permitted. This is, for example, the case during the night or in some other particular contexts such as conflicts, elections, etc.

For all four scenarios, we consider only one direction flow: from Haiti to the Dominican Republic. This choice is based on the hypothesis that, due to the disparities between both countries, a push/pull dynamic polarizes cross-border flows toward the Dominican Republic.

The Enhanced Two-Step Floating Catchment Area (E2SFCA) method

The potential spatial accessibility as described earlier is the distance between the supply (in this case, the number of health professionals) and the demand, defined by the overall population. Numerous studies have demonstrated the importance of the distance (metres or travel time) to access health care in developing countries [1, 2, 4]. Geographic constraints as well as road conditions can trigger low access to health care and impact the use of health care facilities, with important repercussions for health outcomes and public health. Several methods are used to measure spatial accessibility [77, 78]. The approach based on available supply assumes that all users within the same catchment area have equal access regardless of the geographic constraints [9, 77]. The gravity model and its derived two-step floating catchment area (2SFCA) method consider spatial interactions and the mobility of the population [35]. The well-known two-step floating catchment area method computes the ratio between the supply (number of physicians or health professionals) and the demand (population) within a catchment area for each supply point at first and ultimately for each demand point [79, 80]. To overcome the limitations of the 2SFCA, an enhanced method has been developed by Luo and Qi [10] by applying weights to differentiate travel time zones in accounting for distance decay.

This method is used to evaluate the cross-border potential spatial accessibility of the health care services. Since the area studied includes rural areas, the catchment area (within a 60-min driving, motorbiking and walking time) has been divided into four travel time zones, as proposed by some authors [79, 81]: 0–15, 15–30, 30–45 and 45–90 min. The 45–90 min travel zone considers the 60-min cost for a semi-open border with stricter control, as indicated above. The maximum travel speed for each class of road accounts for the assumed mixed transportation mode (walking combined with motorbiking, the most usual transportation mode in the studied area).

The method is implemented in two steps, using the equations below. The first step assigns an initial ratio to each health service within the catchment area. In the second step, for each demand location within the catchment area, we search all supply locations and then sum up the initial ratio R_j at these locations. The resulting A_k represents the accessibility of the population at location k, R_j the supply-to-population ratio at the health service (supply) location j that falls within the catchment area, and d_{kj} the distance (min) between k and j. The same distance weights derived from the Gaussian function used in step 1 are applied to different travel time zones to account for distance decay. A larger value implies better accessibility.

$$R_j = \frac{S_j}{\sum\limits_{k \in \{d_{kj} \in D_r\}} P_k W_{kj}} = \frac{S_j}{\sum\limits_{k \in \{d_{kj} \in d_1\}} P_k W_1 + \sum\limits_{k \in \{d_{kj} \in d_2\}} P_k W_2 + \sum\limits_{k \in \{d_{kj} \in d_3\}} P_k W_3 + \sum\limits_{k \in \{d_{kj} \in d_4\}} P_k W_4}$$

$$A_k = \sum\limits_{k \in \{d_{kj} \in D_r\}} R_j = \sum\limits_{k \in \{d_{kj} \in d_1\}} R_j W_1 + \sum\limits_{k \in \{d_{kj} \in d_2\}} R_j W_2 + \sum\limits_{k \in \{d_{kj} \in d3\}} R_j W_3 + \sum\limits_{k \in \{d_{kj} \in d_4\}} R_j W_4$$

where S_j represents the weight given to service S such as its size (i.e. number of health professionals) ("supply side"), d_{kj} is the distance (travel time) between spatial unit centroid k and health service j, d_0 is the threshold travel time (min), P_k represents the demand at location k that falls within catchment area j and W_1, W_2, W_3, $W_4 = 1.00$, 0.80, 0.55, 0.15 with a slow step-decay function or 1.00, 0.60, 0.25, 0.05 with a fast step-decay function.

The calculations are done using two kinds of software (ArcGIS and SAS). The cost-distance matrix obtained using the Network Analyst extension in ArcGIS has been exported to SAS to compute the E2SFCA. The final results are mapped in ArcGIS.

Statistical analysis was conducted to explore the differences and variation for the E2SFCA calculations. The Wilcoxon test was computed to assess the differences and variation observed in the E2SFCA results for each scenario and country. Finally, linear regression models were used to predict the accessibility of health services (E2SFCA) according to the four scenarios and their variation. All statistical analyses were carried out using SAS software.

Results

As mentioned before, four simulations are considered to measure the impact of the opening of the border on the level of accessibility of public health services for the borderland population of the North-East Department and the Province of Dajabón. To facilitate the comparison between the four scenarios, a quantile classification with five classes has been used and mapped (Fig. 4). Following are the results for each scenario.

Scenario 1: Open border

The first scenario is with an open border. A penalty of 15 min is added to the travel time of Haitians crossing the border. The results show contrasting levels of accessibility in the North-East Department between areas next to the border and more remote locations (Fig. 4a). Two features stand out. First, a large area located mostly in the commune of Ouanaminthe has the highest ratio of accessibility. A smooth gradation is observed to the west (along the national road connecting this region with the North Department and its capital, Cap-Haïtien, the second most important city in Haiti), and to the northwest toward Fort-Liberté (the North-East Department's capital). Second, a sharp drop in the level of accessibility is seen between those two regions (respectively [P60 to P80[and [P80 to Max], the last two quintiles) and the other remote locations (corresponding to the first quintile, [Min to P20[). The areas with the highest level of accessibility are those where hospitals with a larger number of health professionals are located. They are also better connected to a road network in good condition, with higher maximum speeds.

The pattern in the Dominican Republic is quite different: the municipalities at the edge of the Province have the highest level of accessibility, and those next to the border have moderate to low access. There are scattered areas with a very low level of access to health care. Dajabón, the main city of the Province, has a moderate level of accessibility with an open border because of its proximity to Ouanaminthe, a city with a population of 60,000. Therefore, an open border induces potential overload of the Dominican health care services due to an increased demand from Haitians and consequently lowers the health professional-to-population accessibility ratio for the Dominicans. But the overall situation in terms of accessibility in the Dominican Republic remains better than in Haiti, even with an open border.

Scenario 2 and scenario 3: Half-closed border

Scenario 2 is with a half-closed border, with a 30-min cost to cross the border, and the scenario 3 is with a 60-min cost. The map indicates some changes in the pattern compared with the open border (Fig. 4b). First, there is a small drop in the extent of the area with the highest accessibility on the Haitian border side. Second, on the Dominican side, the level of accessibility is globally higher than that observed in the first scenario because of a decrease in the potential demand from Haitians at the Dominican sites.

Scenario 3 is a half-closed border, with a 60-min cost added for crossing the border, indicating more control on the Dominican border (Fig. 4c). The results show a significant reduction in the extent of the area with a higher level of accessibility on the Haitian side of the border. On the Dominican side of the border, there is a noticeable improvement in the overall level of accessibility in the Province of Dajabón. The 60-min cost added causes a significant decrease in the Haitians' potential demand at the Dominican sites which is limited to the 15 min travel zone. Therefore, the Dominicans accessibility level increases beyond the 30–45 min travel zones. The results also emphasize the impact of the low road coverage especially on the Haitian population's access to health resources.

Scenario 4: Closed border

With the border closed, the results show the potential spatial accessibility of health care facilities in each country (Fig. 4d). Globally, the level of accessibility is higher in the Dominican Republic than in Haiti. In fact, the quasitotality of the Haitian spatial units belongs to the first two quintiles (light gray), while those of the Dominican

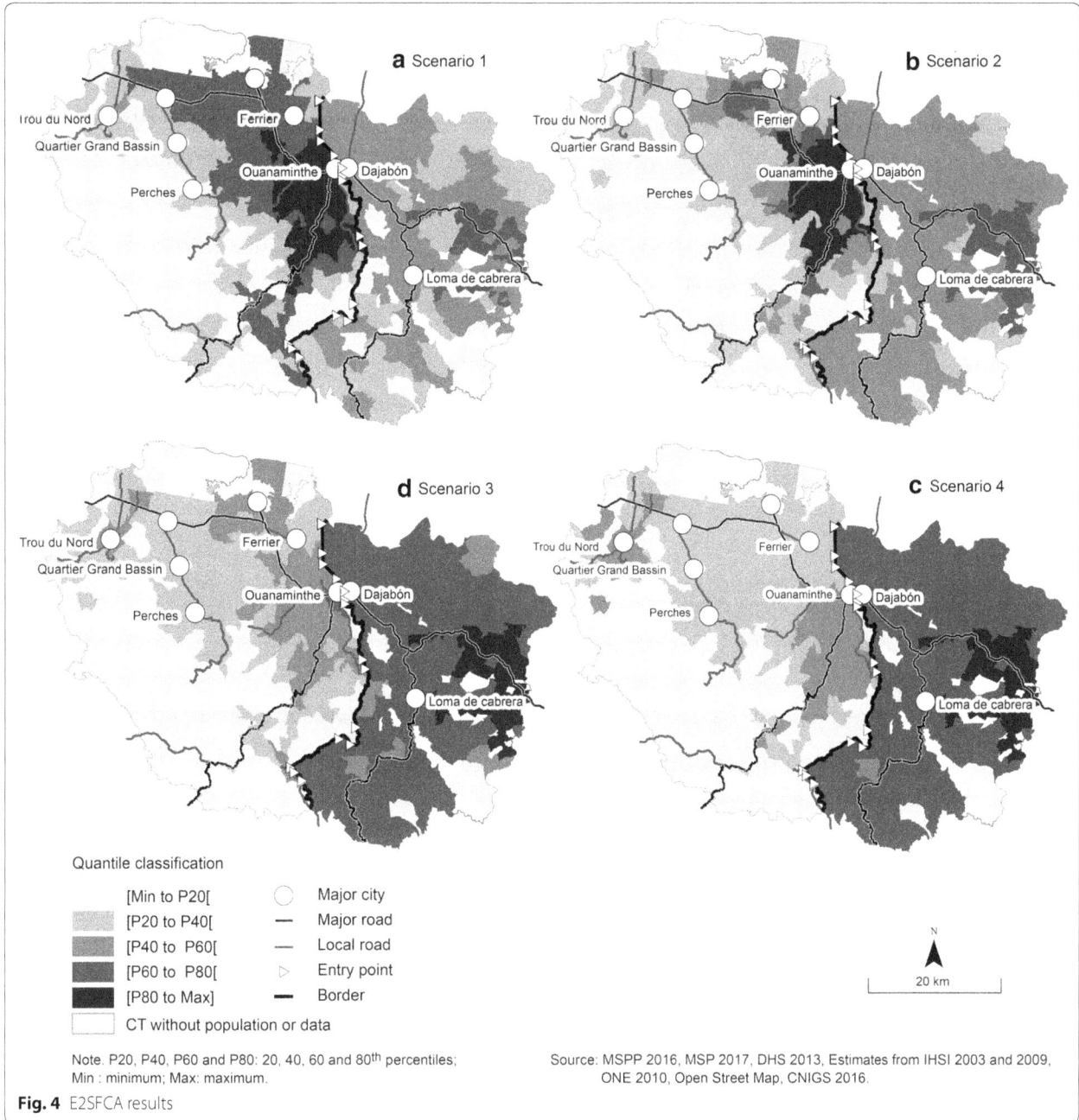

Quantile classification

[Min to P20[○ Major city
[P20 to P40[— Major road
[P40 to P60[— Local road
[P60 to P80[▷ Entry point
[P80 to Max]   ▬ Border
CT without population or data

Note. P20, P40, P60 and P80: 20, 40, 60 and 80th percentiles;   Source: MSPP 2016, MSP 2017, DHS 2013, Estimates from IHSI 2003 and 2009,
Min : minimum; Max: maximum.   ONE 2010, Open Street Map, CNIGS 2016.

Fig. 4 E2SFCA results

Republic belong to the last two quintiles (dark gray), drawing attention to the existing disparities between both countries in terms of potential accessibility to health care. This scenario also confirms the striking gaps within the North-East Department, especially between the remote locations and the urban areas.

Variation between scenario 4 and scenario 1

Figure 5 shows the variation in the level of spatial accessibility between scenario 4 (closed border) and scenario 1 (open border). It highlights the areas most affected by the border's level of openness. As shown in Fig. 5, the solid blue areas are those that benefit from an open border. The red ones are those gaining better access when the border is closed. The border has almost no impact on an extended territory (pale yellow) of the North-East Department where the variation differences are negative but close to zero.

In both countries, the areas next to the border are those that are more sensitive to the impact of the border on

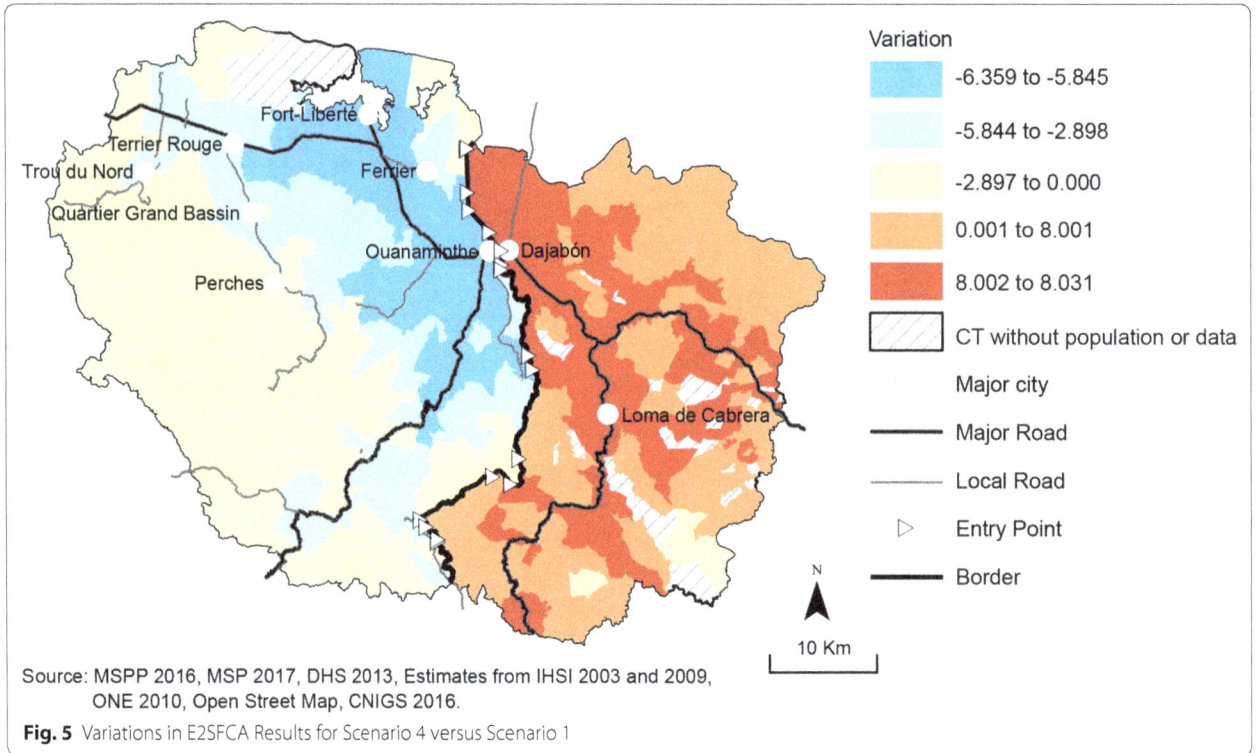

Source: MSPP 2016, MSP 2017, DHS 2013, Estimates from IHSI 2003 and 2009,
        ONE 2010, Open Street Map, CNIGS 2016.

Fig. 5 Variations in E2SFCA Results for Scenario 4 versus Scenario 1

their level of spatial accessibility. Those areas are the ones where an open border induces an increased demand from Haitians at the Dominican health services located near the border (within the 15–45 min travel zone). It is also important to note the importance of the road network in the border effect, as the pattern is aligned with the main road network. For example, borderland areas (southern part of the North-East Department in Haiti) covered with pathways and with geographic constraints don't benefit at the same level as those with a good road network coverage. A similar sensibility pattern is observed in the Province of Dajabón.

Results of nonparametric test and regression models

To explore differences (location and scale) and variation in the E2SFCA results for each country, we conduct a nonparametric test (Wilcoxon test). Figure 6 shows that, scenarios 2 (mean rank = 283 for Haiti vs

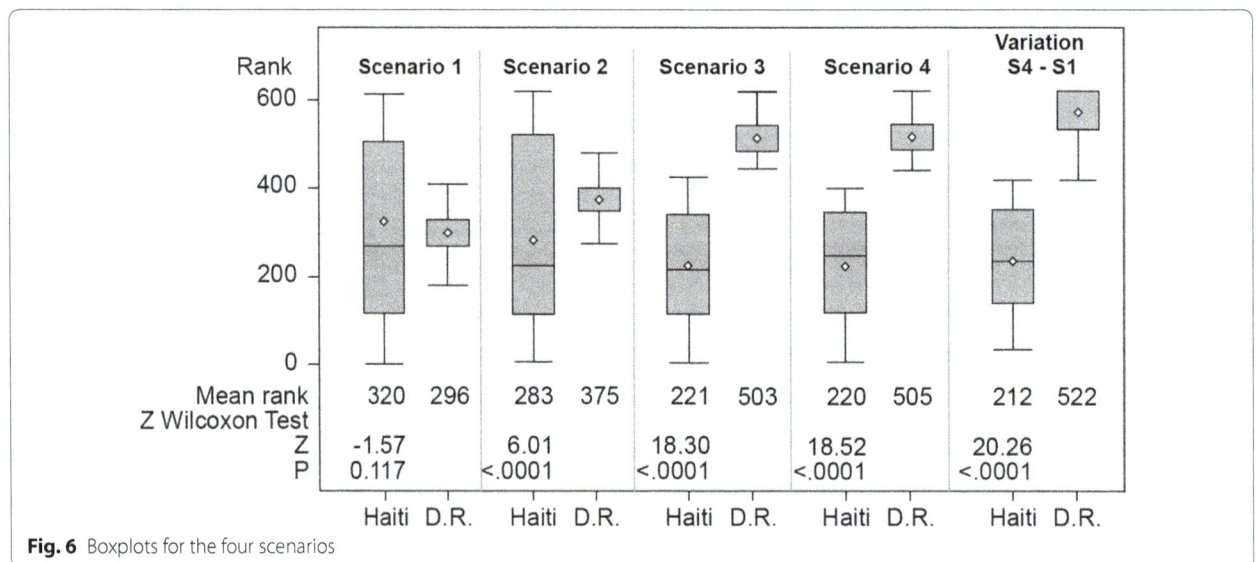

Fig. 6 Boxplots for the four scenarios

375 for Dominican Republic, $z = 6.01$, $p < 0.0001$) to 4 (mean rank $= 220$ for Haiti, 505 vs Dominican Republic, $z = 1.52$, $p < 0.0001$), as well as for the variation (scenario 4–scenario 1) (mean rank $= 212$ for Haiti vs 522 for Dominican Republic, $z = 20.26$, $p < 0.0001$), the results are significant ($p < 0.0001$), but that is not the case for scenario 1 (mean rank $= 320$ for Haiti vs 296 for Dominican Republic, $z = -0.17$, $p = 0.117$). It is relevant to note: a) the dispersion of the scores for Haiti compared to those for the Dominican Republic; and b) the gap in mean rank between Haiti and the Dominican Republic for scenario 3 (border half-closed) and scenario 4 (closed border). The variability and dispersion in the range for Haiti emphasize the disparities within the North-East Department shown in Fig. 4. The results for the variation between an open border and a closed border confirm the impact of the border on the level of spatial accessibility of health care for the Haitian population.

Finally, several linear regression models are conducted to predict the accessibility of health services (E2SFCA results) according to the four scenarios and variation between the two extremes. Two independent variables are introduced in these models: Haiti (D.R. is defined as the reference category), and rural area (versus urban area). The results of these models are shown in Table 4.

First, note that R^2 increases from 0.15 to 0.89 for scenarios 1–4. Next, the degree of border openness has a significant impact on accessibility on both sides of the border, to the detriment of Haiti (with increasingly strong negative regression coefficients). Not surprisingly, the coefficients for rural areas confirm that these areas have poorer accessibility, regardless of the scenario. In addition, the positive and significant coefficient for the variation between scenarios 4 and 3 shows that the closure of the border strongly affects accessibility in urban centres that are close to the border.

Table 4 Linear regression for E2SFCA ($n = 624$)

Scenarios	Coefficient			
	Intercept	Haiti[a]	Rural[b]	R^2
Scenario 1	7.98	−0.68 **	−2.33 ***	0.15
Scenario 2	10.54	−3.03 ***	−2.82 ***	0.24
Scenario 3	13.60	−8.47 ***	−2.37 ***	0.68
Scenario 4	14.10	−11.49 ***	−0.79 ***	0.89
Δ Scenario 4– Scenario 1	6.12	−10.81 ***	1.54 ***	0.85

Signif. codes:: *** 0.001, ** 0.01

[a] Reference: Dominican Republic

[b] Reference: urban

Discussion

The E2SFCA results and statistical analyses clearly highlight the impact of the border on the potential spatial accessibility of public health services for Haitian and Dominican border populations with a peculiar pattern caused by the one directional movement assumed for the model. In fact, the simulations carried out show that Haitian populations in areas close to the border line—particularly near an entry point (formal or informal)—and served by a road network in good condition have higher levels of accessibility when the border is open (scenario 1) or semi-closed (scenario 2), with a 30-min penalty. At the same time, an increased demand from Haitians of those specific areas for the Dominican health services lowers the health professional to population accessibility ratio in Dominican Republic causing striking variations according to the openness of the border. It is therefore interesting to note that, by increasing the cost from 30 to 60 min, the level of accessibility varies widely across the border. Thus, the opening of the border only impacts spatial accessibility for the Haitian population in the vicinity (travel time zones 0–15 min and 15–30 min). These results are not surprising, as these areas have a road network in good condition, confirming the importance of a good road network [4, 82–84] and of the type of distance [78] in potential spatial accessibility. As a result, rural areas are those with the lowest level of accessibility, on the one hand, and, on the other hand, these areas benefit very little from the opening of the border, despite its proximity. A weak road network (absence of roads or roads in poor condition) and topographical constraints associated with a limited offer of services (type of service and number of health professionals) indeed characterize Haitian rural areas. In Dominican Republic, an open border besides creating as mentioned before a decrease in the level of accessibility generates more disparities within the Province of Dajabón, especially for the population at its edges. Introducing a 30 or a 60-min cost for a semi-closed border smoothens the gaps within Dajabón since the Haitians' demand at the Dominican health services decrease.

Scenario 4 highlights the differences in the potential spatial accessibility of health services between the two countries. These differences clearly underline the health and spatial discontinuities due to the border. The disparities in the spatial accessibility of public health services are very low (or almost non-existent) within the Dominican territory, in striking contrast with Haiti, where they are high. Those gaps can lead to a one-directional flow like the one assumed by the model. Furthermore, several empirical studies [16, 85, 86] in different border contexts indicate a pattern of polarized flows because of an unsatisfied demand in one side and a more attracted one on the other side. Nevertheless, this push/pull dynamic could have considerable impact on the health services of the recipient country depending on their public health care capacity, the volume of cross-border patients and the borderland context including the level of cooperation or integration of the countries involved. It is worth noticing that the challenges for both countries regarding those issues are high even more when considering the results of the potential spatial accessibility model.

However, an optimization of the E2SFCA to weight the population according to the real use of health services on both sides of the border would have given a closer insight into the reality of potential spatial accessibility. It would also have been appropriate to assess the impact of the border on potential spatial accessibility by integrating socioeconomic and demographic factors to analyze the correlation between population characteristics and cross-border spatial accessibility.

The results also call for better cooperation and integration of the two countries' health care systems. In this regard, the stakes for Haiti and the Dominican Republic are high, not only because of the instability of relations between the two countries, but also because of the thorny issue of migration. As Alexandre [48] points out, cross-border movements between Haiti and the Dominican Republic, including movements linked to health, cannot be thought of without considering a reform of the migration legislation in both countries.

Conclusion

The results emphasize the impact of a good road network on the spatial accessibility of health care, as discussed in many studies. They also show the impact of the openness of an international border on the potential accessibility of health care in borderland regions, highlighting the importance of distance. Proximity is thus seen as one of the determinants in cross-border mobility and in health care seeking behavior. But other factors such as the attractiveness (quality, cost) of health care services must be considered to analyze individuals' behaviors. In our research, we also assume that all the Haitian population of the North-East Department would potentially choose to cross the border, but this is not actually the case. An optimization of the model would make it possible to better evaluate the impact of the border and to obtain more robust results, with a better appreciation of the reality of the situation. A gender-oriented analysis could also have been of interest considering, inter alia, the high maternal mortality rate in Haiti and the high number of unassisted deliveries, particularly in the rural Haitian areas.

The study also highlights the need for more research so as to better understand the determinants of cross-border health care use. Moreover, the distance thresholds are arbitrary and do not necessarily reflect specific patients' behavior, suggesting the need for qualitative inquiry to assess the therapeutic. In-depth interviews and surveys could therefore offer an insight into revealed spatial access and lead to a better understanding of patients' behavior and how this is related to their practices around the border.

Furthermore, cross-border movements in health are part of bigger issues. They should be addressed not only in shrinking the gaps in health access resources but also in creating the needed legal and institutional environment for them to develop smoothly.

Authors' contributions
DM is the principal investigator of the study. She carried out the GIS, statistical and mapping analyses. PA revised all the statistical and mapping analyses. PA and UL jointly drafted and critically revised the paper. All authors read and approved the final manuscript.

Author details
[1] Environmental Equity Laboratory, INRS Centre Urbanisation Culture Société, 385, rue Sherbrooke Est, Montréal, Québec H2X 1E3, Canada. [2] Département d'études urbaines et touristiques, Université du Québec à Montréal, Case postale 8888, Succursale Centre-Ville, Montréal, Québec H3C 3P8, Canada.

Acknowledgements
The authors would like to thank the anonymous reviewers for their careful reading of our manuscript and their many insightful comments and suggestions.

Competing interests
The author(s) declare that they have no competing interests.

Funding
The authors are grateful for the financial support provided by the Canada Research Chair in Environmental Equity.

References
1. Perry B, Gesler W. Physical access to primary health care in Andean Bolivia. Soc Sci Med. 2000;50(9):1177–88.
2. Rushton G. Use of location-allocation models for improving the geographical accessibility of rural services in developing countries. Int Reg Sci Rev. 1984;9(3):217–40.
3. Tanser F, Gijsbertsen B, Herbst K. Modelling and understanding primary health care accessibility and utilization in rural South Africa: an exploration using a geographical information system. Soc Sci Med. 2006;63(3):691–705.

4. Rosero-Bixby L. Spatial access to health care in Costa Rica and its equity: a GIS-based study. Soc Sci Med. 2004;58(7):1271–84.
5. Barnes-Josiah D, Myntti C, Augustin A. The "three delays" as a framework for examining maternal mortality in Haiti. Soc Sci Med. 1998;46(8):981–93.
6. Schoeps A, Gabrysch S, Niamba L, Sié A, Becher H. The effect of distance to health-care facilities on childhood mortality in rural Burkina Faso. Am J Epidemiol. 2011;173(5):492–8.
7. Luo W, Wang F. Measures of spatial accessibility to health care in a GIS environment: synthesis and a case study in the Chicago region. Environ Plan. 2003;30(6):865–84.
8. Pan J, Liu H, Wang X, Xie H, Delamater PL. Assessing the spatial accessibility of hospital care in Sichuan Province, China. Geospatial Health. 2015;10(2):261–70.
9. Luo W. Using a GIS-based floating catchment method to assess areas with shortage of physicians. Health Place. 2004;10(1):1–11.
10. Luo W, Qi Y. An enhanced two-step floating catchment area (E2SFCA) method for measuring spatial accessibility to primary care physicians. Health Place. 2009;15(4):1100–7.
11. Glinos I, Baeten R: A literature review of cross-border patient mobility in the European Union. In: Observatoire social européen, Europe for patients; 2006. p. 115.
12. Glinos I, Baeten R, Helble M, Maarse H. A typology of cross-border patient mobility. Health Place. 2010;16(6):1145–55.
13. Glinos IA, Doering N, Maarse H. Travelling home for treatment and EU patients' rights to care abroad: results of a survey among German students at Maastricht University. Health Policy. 2012;105(1):38–45.
14. Bochaton A. Cross-border mobility and social networks: Laotians seeking medical treatment along the Thai border. Soc Sci Med. 2015;124:364–73.
15. Bochaton A: La construction de l'espace transfrontalier lao-thaïlandais. Une analyse à travers le recours aux soins. Espace populations sociétés Space populations societies. 2011;(2011/2):337–351.
16. Dione I: Polarisation des structures de soins de la Haute Casamance: entre construction nationale des systèmes de santé et recours aux soins transfrontalier. Université d'Angers; 2013.
17. Brown HS. Do Mexican immigrants substitute health care in Mexico for health insurance in the United States? The role of distance. Soc Sci Med. 2008;67(12):2036–42.
18. Grossman D, Garcia SG, Kingston J, Schweikert S. Mexican Women Seeking Safe Abortion Services in San Diego, California. Health Care Women Int. 2012;33(11):1060–9.
19. Guendelman S. Health care users residing on the Mexican border what factors determine choice of the U.S. or Mexican Health System? Medical Care. 1991;29(5):419–29.
20. Guendelman S, Jasis M. Giving birth across the border: the San Diego-Tijuana connection. Soc Sci Med. 1992;34(4):419–25.
21. Horton S, Cole S. Medical returns: seeking health care in Mexico. Soc Sci Med. 2011;72(11):1846–52.
22. Laugesen MJ, Vargas-Bustamante A. A patient mobility framework that travels: European and United States-Mexican comparisons. Health Policy. 2010;97(2–3):225–31.
23. Su D, Richardson C, Wen M, Pagán JA. Cross-Border Utilization of Health Care: evidence from a Population-Based Study in South Texas. Health Serv Res. 2011;46(3):859–76.
24. Peiter PC: Condiciones de vida, situación de salud y disponibilidad de servicios de salud en la frontera de Brasil: un enfoque geográfico. Cád Saúde Pública; 2007.
25. De Ruffray S, Hamez G. L'accessibilité transfrontalière aux maternités: Enjeux territoriaux d'une coopération sanitaire dans la Grande Région. In: Moullé F, Duhamel S, editors. Frontières et santé: Genèses et maillages des réseaux transfrontaliers. Paris: L'Harmattan; 2010.
26. Perez S, Balli A: L'accessibilité aux soins dans l'espace frontalier des Alpes du Sud. In: Frontières et santé: genèses et maillages des réseaux transfrontaliers. Paris: L'Harmattan; 2010.
27. Arbaret-Schulz C, Beyer A, Piermay J-L, Reitel B, Selimanovski C, Sohn C, Zander P: La frontière, un objet spatial en mutation. EspacesTemps net. 2004; 29(04).
28. Piermay J-L, Reitel B, Zander P: Introduction. In: Reitel B, editor. Villes et frontières, vol. Collections: Collection Villes (Paris, France). Paris: Paris: Anthropos: Economica; 2002. p. 2–9.
29. Herzog LA. The transfrontier organization of space along the US-Mexico

border. Geoforum. 1991;22(3):255–69.
30. Herzog LA, Sohn C. The cross-border metropolis in a global age: a conceptual model and empirical evidence from the US–Mexico and European border regions. Glob Soc. 2014;28(4):441–61.
31. Anderson J, O'Dowd L. Borders, border regions and territoriality: contradictory meanings, changing significance. Reg Stud. 1999;33(7):593–604.
32. Paasi A. Borders and border-crossings. In: Johnson NC, Schein RH, Winders J, editors. Cultural geography. Chichester: Wiley; 2013. p. 478–93.
33. Penchansky R, Thomas JW. The concept of access. Definition and relationship to consumer satisfaction. Med Care. 1981;19:127–40.
34. Wang F. Quantitative methods and applications in GIS. London: Taylor & Francis Group; 2006.
35. Guagliardo MF. Spatial accessibility of primary care: concepts, methods and challenges. Int J Health Geogr. 2004;3:3.
36. Théodat J-M. Haïti-République Dominicaine: une île pour deux, 1804–1916. Paris: Éditions Karthala; 2003.
37. Théodat J-M, Mathon D, Mathelier R, Casséus M. Quisqueya: un papillon d'envol. In: Mathelier R, Mathon D, Casséus M, editors. Entreprise, Territoire et Développement: Compilation 2002–2003. Port-au-Prince: INESA/Le Nouvelliste; 2003.
38. Wooding B, Mosely-Williams R, Flores C. Les immigrants haïtiens et leurs descendants en République Dominicaine. Haïti: Institut catholique pour les relations internationles, ISPOS; 2005.
39. Silié R. Haïti et la République dominicaine, pays en conflit ou en construction d'une nouvelle amitié? Conjonction La revue franco-haïtienne de l'Institut Français d'Haïti. 2014;2226:98–110.
40. Dilla Alfonso H, Alexis S, Antoine MI, Carmona C, de Jesús Cedano S, Murray GF, Espejo JEN, O'neil DJ, Rapilly M, Sánchez N: La frontera dominico-haitiana: Grupo de Estudios Multidisciplinarios Ciudades y Fronteras; 2010.
41. Redon M. Frontière poreuse, État faible: les relations Haïti/République dominicaine à l'aune de la frontière. Bulletin de l'Association de géographes français. 2010;87:308–23.
42. Petrozziello AJ, Wooding B: Fanm nan Fwontyè, Fanm toupatou: Éclairage sur la violence exercée sur les Immigrantes d'origine haïtienne, celles en transit migratoire et sur les déplacés internes le long de la frontière Dominicano-Haïtienne. Santo Domingo: Colectiva Mujer y Salud, Mujeres del Mundo, Observatoire sur la migration et la Caraïbe; 2011.
43. Jolivet V. Les Haïtiens à Santo Domingo: une masse invisible? Bulletin de l'Association de géographes français. 2010;87:324–35.
44. Wooding B. Women fight for their safety in the Dominican-Haitian border. Migr Dev. 2012;10(18):37–58.
45. Murray GF: Sources of Conflict along and across the Haitian–Dominican border. In: Fwontyè nou—Nuestra Frontera. Santo Domingo Dominican Republic: Pan American Development Foundation; 2010.
46. Montiel Armas I, Canales Cerón AI, Vargas Becerra PN: Migración y salud en zonas fronterizas: Haití y la República Dominicana: CEPAL; 2010.
47. Ministerio del Trabajo, Observatorio del Mercado Laboral Dominicano: Inmigrantes Haitianos y Mercado Laboral, Estudio Sobre los Trabajadores de la Construcción y de la Producción del Guineo en la República Dominicana. In: República Dominicana: Ministerio del Trabajo; 2011.
48. Alexandre G. Vers une gestion ordonnée de la migration entre la République dominicaine et Haïti. Conjonction La revue franco-haïtienne de l'Institut Français d'Haïti. Les realtions Haïti—République dominicaine. 2014;226:132–56.
49. Oficina Nacional de Estadística: Primera Encuesta Nacional de Inmigrantes en la República Dominicana (ENI-2012). In: Santo Domingo, República Dominicana: Oficina Nacional de Estadística; 2013. p. 345.
50. Oficina Nacional de Estadística: Segunda Encuesta Nacional de Inmigrantes en la República Dominicana—ENI-2017—Version resumida del informe general. In: Santo Domingo: Oficina Nacional de Estadística; 2018.
51. Silié R, Segura C, Dore Cabral C. La nueva inmigración haitiana. Santo Domingo: Flacso; 2002.
52. Organización Panamericana de la Salud: Haití. In: Salud OPdl, editor. Salud en las Américas, Edición de 2012: Volumen de países. Washington: Organización Panamericana de la Salud; 2012.
53. Organización Panamericana de la Salud: República Dominicana In. vol. Salud en las Américas. Edición 2012: Volumen de países. Washington: Organización Panamericana de la Salud; 2012.

54. Lavigne M, Vargas LH: Sistemas de protección social en América Latina y el Caribe: República Dominicana. In: (CEPAL) CEpALyeC, editor. *Documento de Proyecto.* . Santiago de Chile: Comisión Económica para América Latina y el Caribe (CEPAL); 2013. p. 40.

55. Cercone JA. Análisis de situación y estado de los sistemas de salud de países del Caribe, vol. 185. Santiago de Chile: United Nations Publications; 2007.

56. Secretaría de Estado de Salud Pública y Asistencia Social: Modelos de Red de los Servicios Regionales de Salud. In: Social SdEdSPyA, editor. 1a edición edn. Santo Domingo: Secretaría de Estado de Salud Pública y Asistencia Social; 2005. p. 199.

57. Ministère de la santé publique et de la population: Politique Nationale de Santé. In: Edited by population MdIspedl. Port-au-Prince; 2012.

58. Bitrán R: Reformas recientes en el sector salud en Centroamérica, vol. 177: United Nations Publications; 2006.

59. Ministerio de Salud Pública: Modelo de atención en salud en el sistema nacional de salud de la República Dominicana. In: (DDEI) DdDEI, editor. vol. 3. Santo Domingo: Ministerio de Salud Pública; 2012.

60. Institut Haïtien de l'Enfance, ICF International: Évaluation de Prestation des Services de Soins de Santé, Haïti, 2013. In: Rockville Maryland: Ministère de la Santé Publique et de la Population (MSPP); 2014.

61. Cayemittes M, Busangu MF, Bizimana JdD, Barrère B, Sévère B, Cayemittes V, Charles E: Enquête Mortalité, Morbidité et Utilisation des Services, Haïti, 2012. In: Haiti: MSPP, IHE et ICF International; 2013.

62. Lamaute-Brisson N: Sistemas de protección social en América Latina y el Caribe: Haití. In: (CEPAL) CEpALyeC, editor. Documento de Proyecto. Santiago de Chile: Comisión Económica para América Latina y el Caribe (CEPAL); 2013. p. 40.

63. Secretaría de Estado de Salud Pública y Asistencia Social: Manual de Sectorización/Zonificación de las UNAP. In Salud CEpIRdS, editor. Santo Domingo: Secretaría de Estado de Salud Pública y Asistencia Social; 2008. p. 78.

64. Secretaría de Estado de Salud Pública y Asistencia Social: Perfil del sistema de salud de la República dominicana. In: Salud SdEdSPyASCEpIRdS, editor. Santo Domingo: Secretaría de Estado de Salud Pública y Asistencia Social/Comisión Ejecutiva para la Reforma del Sector Salud/Organización Panamericana de la Salud; 2007. p. 44.

65. Ministère de la santé publique et de la population: Plan directeur de santé 2012–2022. In: population MdIspedl, editor. Port-au-Prince; 2013.

66. Wooding B. El impacto del terremoto en Haití sobre la inmigración haitiana en república dominicana. América Latina Hoy. 2010;56:111–29.

67. Organización Panamericana de la Salud: Cooperación binacional entre Haití y la República Dominicana. In: Salud OPdl, editor. Organización Panamericana de la Salud; 2011.

68. Dilla Alfonso H. Transborder Urban Complex in Latin America. Estudios Fronterizos. 2015;16(31):4–19.

69. Dilla Alfonso H. Los complejos urbanos transfronterizos en América Latina. Estudios fronterizos. 2015;16(31):15–38.

70. Dilla Alfonso H, de Jesús Cedano S. De problemas y oportunidades: intermediación urbana fronteriza en República Dominicana. Revista mexicana de sociología. 2005;67:99–126.

71. Buzenot L: Les zones franches industrielles d'exportation dans la Caraïbe. Les causes économiques de leur émergence. Études Caribéennes 2010(13).

72. INESA, FLACSO: Inventario de los conocimientos e intervenciones sobre la zona transfronteriza Haití-República Dominicana. In: Santo Domingo/Haití: PNUD/ACDI; 2003.

73. Observatorio Binacional sobre Medio Ambiente M, Educación y Comercio,: Diagnóstico comercio bilateral República Dominicana y República de Haití. In. República Dominicana/Haiti: Observatorio Binacional sobre Medio Ambiente, Migración, Educación y Comercio (OBMEC); 2016.

74. Dilla Alfonso H. República Dominicana: La nueva cartografía transfronteriza. Caribbean Studies. 2007;35(1):181–205.

75. Dilla Alfonso H: La migración transfronteriza urbana en la República Dominicana. In: Santo Domingo: Fundación Friedrich Ebert en República Dominicana; 2011.

76. Icart J-C. Cela ne se fait pas! Développements récents dans le dossier des migrations et de l'apatridie en République dominicaine. Conjonction La revue franco-haïtienne de l'Institut Français d'Haïti. 2014;226:160–82.

77. Higgs G. A literature review of the use of GIS-based measures of access to health care services. Health Serv Outcomes Res Methodol. 2004;5(2):119–39.

78. Apparicio P, Gelb J, Dubé A-S, Kingham S, Gauvin L, Robitaille É. The approaches to measuring the potential spatial access to urban health services revisited: distance types and aggregation-error issues. Int J Health Geogr. 2017;16(1):32.

79. McGrail MR, Humphreys JS. Measuring spatial accessibility to primary care in rural areas: improving the effectiveness of the two-step floating catchment area method. Appl Geogr. 2009;29(4):533–41.

80. Luo W, Wang F. Measures of spatial accessibility to health care in a GIS environment: synthesis and a case study in the Chicago region. Environ Plan B Plan Des. 2003;30:865–84.

81. Wan N, Zou B, Sternberg T. A three-step floating catchment area method for analyzing spatial access to health services. Int J Geogr Inf Sci. 2012;26(6):1073–89.

82. Oppong JR, Hodgson MJ. Spatial accessibility to health care facilities in Suhum District, Ghana. Prof Geogr. 1994;46(2):199–209.

83. Murawski L, Church RL. Improving accessibility to rural health services: the maximal covering network improvement problem. Socio-Econ Plan Sci. 2009;43(2):102–10.

84. Querriau X, Peeters D, Thomas I, Kissiyar M: Localisation optimale d'unités de soins dans un pays en voie de développement: Analyse de sensibilité. CyberGeo. 2004.

85. Bochaton A: " Païï Thaï, païï fang nan":" Aller en Thaïlande, aller de l'autre côté". Construction d'un espace sanitaire transfrontalier: le recours aux soins des Laotiens en Thaïlande. Paris 10; 2009.

86. Tapia Ladino M, Liberona Concha N, Contreras Gatica Y. El surgimiento de un territorio circulatorio en la frontera chileno-peruana: estudio de las prácticas socio-espaciales fronterizas. Revista de Geografía Norte Grande. 2017;66:117–41.

13

Mobility assessment of a rural population in the Netherlands using GPS measurements

Gijs Klous[1,2]* ⓘ, Lidwien A. M. Smit[2], Floor Borlée[2,4], Roel A. Coutinho[1,5], Mirjam E. E. Kretzschmar[1,3], Dick J. J. Heederik[1,2] and Anke Huss[2]

Abstract

Background: The home address is a common spatial proxy for exposure assessment in epidemiological studies but mobility may introduce exposure misclassification. Mobility can be assessed using self-reports or objectively measured using GPS logging but self-reports may not assess the same information as measured mobility. We aimed to assess mobility patterns of a rural population in the Netherlands using GPS measurements and self-reports and to compare GPS measured to self-reported data, and to evaluate correlates of differences in mobility patterns.

Method: In total 870 participants filled in a questionnaire regarding their transport modes and carried a GPS-logger for 7 consecutive days. Transport modes were assigned to GPS-tracks based on speed patterns. Correlates of measured mobility data were evaluated using multiple linear regression. We calculated walking, biking and motorised transport durations based on GPS and self-reported data and compared outcomes. We used Cohen's kappa analyses to compare categorised self-reported and GPS measured data for time spent outdoors.

Results: Self-reported time spent walking and biking was strongly overestimated when compared to GPS measurements. Participants estimated their time spent in motorised transport accurately. Several variables were associated with differences in mobility patterns, we found for instance that obese people (BMI > 30 kg/m^2) spent less time in non-motorised transport (GMR 0.69–0.74) and people with COPD tended to travel longer distances from home in motorised transport (GMR 1.42–1.51).

Conclusions: If time spent walking outdoors and biking is relevant for the exposure to environmental factors, then relying on the home address as a proxy for exposure location may introduce misclassification. In addition, this misclassification is potentially differential, and specific groups of people will show stronger misclassification of exposure than others. Performing GPS measurements and identifying explanatory factors of mobility patterns may assist in regression calibration of self-reports in other studies.

Background

Environmental epidemiological studies aim at evaluating risks to human health from environmental exposures. Human mobility may affect exposure of persons to different environmental substances, especially if exposure levels display strong spatial, or spatio-temporal variation. Examples of such exposures are ultrafine particles of air pollution [1], electromagnetic fields [2] or livestock-associated exposures, such as zoonotic micro-organisms and endotoxins [3–6]. Personal exposure is often approximated by assigning exposure levels on a single location—usually the home address—to study participants, although this may lead to misclassification of exposure. Exposure misclassification can bias risk estimates, and this bias is often towards the null, in particular when misclassification is non-differential [7–10]. This essentially means that health effects from environmental exposures may remain undetected.

*Correspondence: g.klous@umcutrecht.nl
[2] Institute for Risk Assessment Sciences (IRAS), Division Environmental Epidemiology and Veterinary Public Health (EEPI-VPH), Utrecht University, Yalelaan 2, 3584 CM Utrecht, The Netherlands
Full list of author information is available at the end of the article

In this study we assessed modes of transport, in particular the duration people spent in motorised or non-motorised transport, and the distance from home for these movements. Mobility patterns can be assessed in multiple ways, using e.g. questionnaire data [11–14] or time activity diaries [14, 15]. Since the 1990s, Global Positioning Systems (GPS) are available that allow for objective measurement of a persons' movements [16–18]. Measurements with GPS devices and activity diaries are time consuming and thus, questionnaires to assess mobility are often still the method of choice when studying large groups of people. However, self-reports of mobility assessed with questionnaires may be subject to bias and misclassification [11–14], especially if participants answer in a socially desirable way [19, 20]. In addition, the majority of studies addressing mobility are performed among city dwellers [14]. Living in a rural area is likely associated with different mobility patterns [21] and also with different exposures to area-specific emissions, e.g. from livestock farms in the vicinity (Fig. 1). Furthermore, people living in rural areas might spend more time outdoors [21].

In the present study, the main aim was to assess the different modes of transport of a rural population in the Netherlands using GPS measurements. Secondary aims were to explore if we could identify characteristics that explained differences in patterns of transport modes between participants, and to compare self-reported mobility to GPS measured mobility patterns.

Methods
Study population
The current study was embedded in the Dutch "Livestock Farming and Neighbouring Residents' Health Study" (Dutch acronym; VGO). The VGO study focusses on the health of non-farmer residents living in an area with a high density of livestock farms in the Netherlands. In a population-based cohort of 2494 participants (farmers were excluded a priori) [22], a medical examination was conducted by trained fieldworkers (March 2014–February 2015) [23] General Practitioners' (GPs) Electronic Medical Records (EMRs) were available for 2426 participants (97%) via the Netherlands Institute for Health Services Research (NIVEL, see also http://www.nivel.nl/en), one of the partners in the VGO study. Assessment included a questionnaire (VGO questionnaire) on health, lifestyle factors and the participants' occupational and residential history. NIVEL provided, when VGO participants gave permission, information regarding asthma, history of heart diseases and beta-blocker usage. VGO cohort members who agreed to be invited for follow-up research were eligible to participate in the GPS study. Medical Ethical approval was obtained for the VGO

study from the Medical Ethical Committee of the University Medical Centre Utrecht (protocol number 13/533).

Study design
From September 2014 to January 2016, eligible subjects were invited to participate in the GPS study. This means that while some participants used GPS loggers in the winter, others used it in the summer. Our dataset therefore pertains to a whole year sample across all seasons. Participants filled in a questionnaire (Q1, see Additional file 1: 11. Questionnaire (Q1)) that inquired about participants' usual mobility habits regarding different transport modes and time spent outdoors during a regular week. Upon return of Q1, GPS trackers and a second questionnaire (Q2) were sent to participants, including instructions on how to carry the GPS logger for 7 consecutive days. Participants were asked to put the GPS logger next to their keys, in their bag or jacket, so they would not forget it when they left the house. After the GPS-measurement week, Q2 about study adherence and start and end dates of GPS tracker carriage was filled in and GPS loggers were returned to the study centre.

GPS data
We used TracKing Key Pro GPS loggers (Land Air Sea systems Woodstock IL, USA). These devices enable continuous logging at 1-s intervals. GPS loggers are equipped with a motion sensor, providing data logging only when a participant is moving, thus reducing battery depletion. We set our measurements to 1 s measurement intervals, and the median total logging duration was 187 h (IQR 143–235 h). Data obtained from GPS loggers were date, time, X and Y coordinate and speed (km/h). These GPS loggers were previously tested and showed a high positional accuracy when being outdoors [18].

Questionnaire data
Q1 included items regarding usual duration of time spent outdoors (hours per day) during the week and weekend, occupational status (being employed/self-employed: yes/no), working from home (yes/no), working days (number), having an outdoor occupation (yes/no), number of outdoor working hours (hours per workday) and outdoor activities during leisure time (walking, biking, sports, spending time close to home, other, in hours per week). Furthermore, transport modes for commuting were asked separately for transport during work hours and during leisure time. Transport modes were stratified by spring/summer, autumn/winter and additionally divided into the sub-categories public transport, car, moped/motorcycle, electric bike, bicycle, on foot and other transport modes. Duration of these transport times was provided in minutes per day for commuting

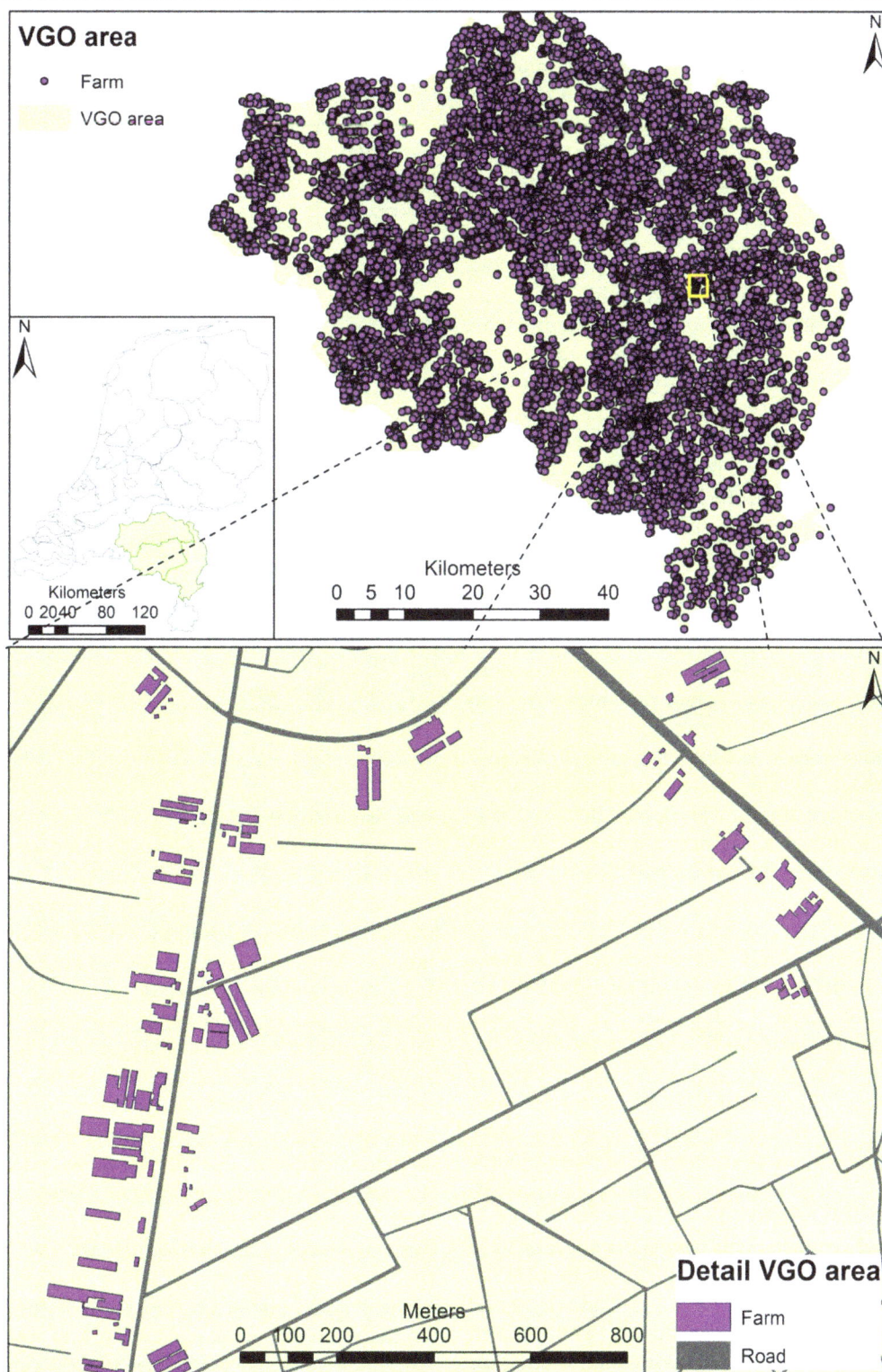

Fig. 1 The research area, this map illustrates the rural situation within our research area. Not only are there many farms present in our research area ('VGO area' map) these farms are also very close together, with multiple farms per kilometre close to roads <50 m ('Detail VGO area' map)

and work-related transport, and in minutes per week for leisure–time transport, participants could report multiple travel modes per trip, therefore alternating mobility patterns should have been captured (Additional file 1: 11. Questionnaire (Q1), an English translation of Q1).

Q2 inquired whether and when participants had left the GPS logger at home during the measuring period and if people had deviated from their normal weekly movement patterns.

Additional participant characteristics and potential explanatory factors for differences in mobility patterns (gender, age, educational level, job status, dog and live-stock ownership, hay fever, BMI (measured), smoking status, asthma status, COPD status (self-reporting combined with spirometry data from VGO health survey) and cardiovascular health (recent heart attacks, arrhythmia, ill heart functioning and beta-blocker usage) were obtained from the VGO health assessment and the VGO baseline questionnaire completed at the time of the health assessment (March 2014–February 2015) [22, 23].

Meteorological data
Meteorological data on precipitation and temperature over the whole measurement period were retrieved from the Royal Netherlands Meteorological Institute. Data from the weather station Eindhoven was used, because this was the most centrally located station of the study area [24]. Percentage of time with rainfall (between 6.00 and 22.00 h) and the average temperature were calculated for the measurement period of each participant.

Data cleaning
We received GPS files from 940 participants. Of these, 34 had to be excluded due to device failure. Two participants did not adhere to the study protocol in that they either did not carry the GPS or did not fill in Q2. In addition, we applied two exclusion criteria: First we excluded persons who had carried the GPS for less than 24 h (N = 19) and second, we excluded persons where the self-reported outdoor time exceeded 3SD of the study population (N = 16). Excluded people reported >64% of their time as being outdoors, which we considered as unrealistic extreme values. One person did not return Q2 and was therefore excluded as well (Fig. 2). In addition, if a participant indicated in Q2 that they had not carried the GPS logger for a specific day, this day was removed from the analyses. More detailed information is provided in Fig. 3. Note that excluded participants did not differ strongly regarding general characteristics (age, sex, education level), compared to participants who remained in the analyses.

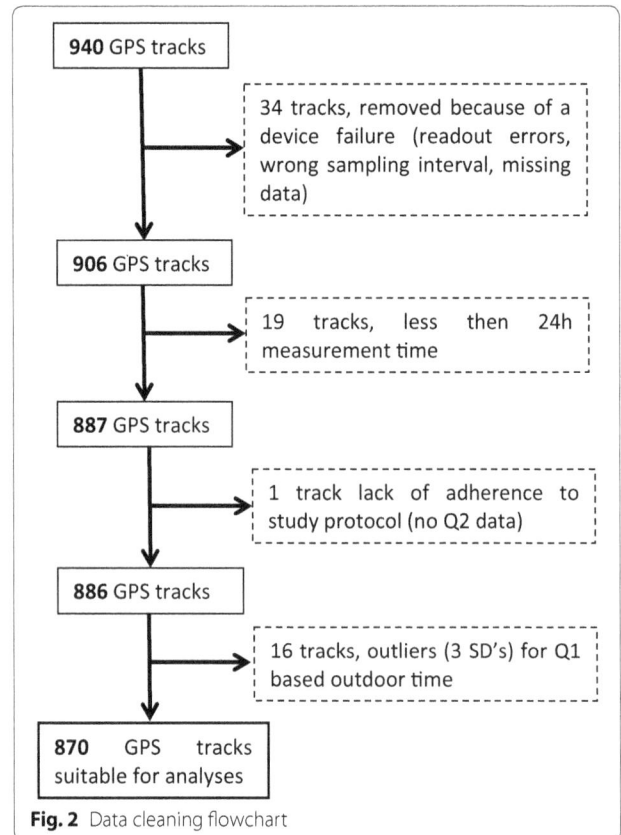

Fig. 2 Data cleaning flowchart

Processing of spatial data
Home addresses (street, postal code, address) were geo-coded using Dutch cadastral data (BAG data). A drawback of GPS-tracking is loss of accuracy when a GPS tracker has no clear view of the sky, especially when being indoors [18] resulting in a point cloud (Additional file 1: 1. Example pictures for spatial analysis, Supp. Figure 1). Therefore, point clouds around the home were filtered by excluding all coordinates logged within a 60 m radius around a home location; this distance was based on visual inspection of point clouds around a range of home addresses. Other GPS measurements were classified as indoors when at least 45 points were located within the outline of a building polygon. These polygons were then supplied with a 20 m buffer and all points within this buffer were classified as indoors for further analyses. Again, this cut-off was based on visual inspection: Fewer than 45 indoor points were more likely to appear as linearly-ordered points, indicating smaller spatial inaccuracies when passing a building (Additional file 1: 1. Example pictures for spatial analysis, Supp. Figure 2), while cloud patterns of coordinates were more likely indicating indoor locations, and were often located in public buildings such as sports facilities or supermarkets.

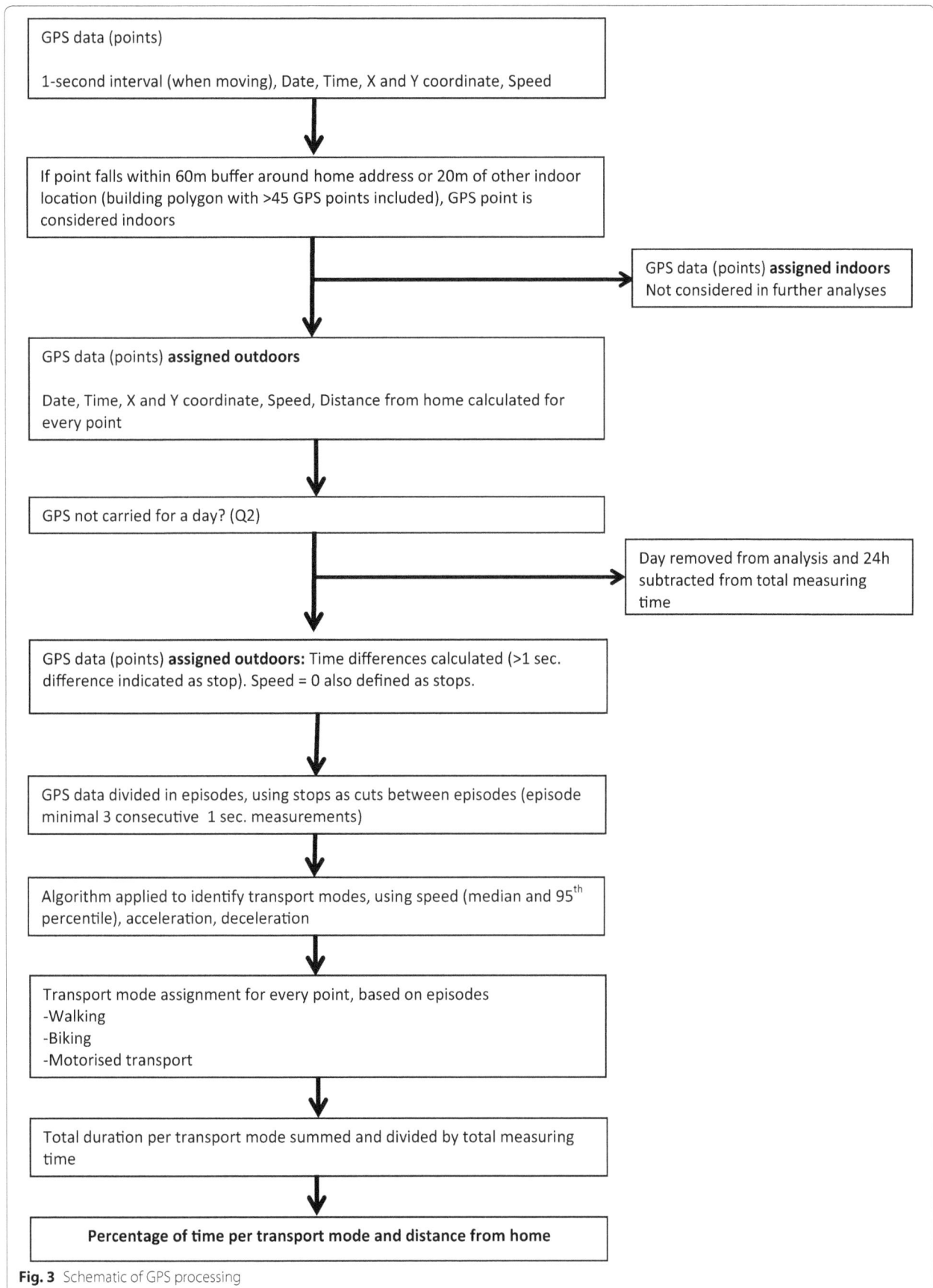

Fig. 3 Schematic of GPS processing

For every point the time differences with the previous point was calculated, if the difference was more than 1 s or speed was 0 km/h, then the point was indicated as a stop. These stops were then used to separate individual mobility episodes. The speed profile of each episode was analysed using a previously developed algorithm that assigns type of transport mode to speed patterns, based on a combination of speed, acceleration and deceleration [25]. Three types of transport modes were assigned to speed profiles: walking, biking or motorised transport. For each transport mode, total duration was assessed and was divided by the total tracking time, resulting in the percentage of time spent per specific transport mode. We analysed our data on a 24 h scale, this means we aimed to evaluate on average 168 h (24×7) per participant. Distances from the home address were calculated for each GPS coordinate, by calculating the distance between the GPS coordinate and the border of the 60 m buffer around the home address. Figure 3 shows a schematic of GPS processing.

Processing of Questionnaire data
In Q1 we asked for mobility per season (spring/summer and autumn/winter), the reported durations for these seasons were linked to the seasons in which participants performed the GPS measurement, the months October–March were considered as autumn/winter and April–September as spring/summer. We expressed data from Q1 pertaining to self-reported transport modes in percentages of time spent per week. Time spent outdoors was calculated by adding the durations for all reported transport modes (commuting, work-related and leisure time) together with time involved in outdoor activities. To compare questionnaire and GPS datasets, time spent outdoors close to home (e.g. gardening, house hold duties, child care, etc.) was subtracted from the total reported time outdoors, as by removing all points within 60 m around a place of residence, we were not able to differentiate erroneous GPS locations from time spent outdoors in close proximity to the home.

Statistical analysis
Participants were first assigned to an outdoors group based on tertiles of time spent outdoors as provided from their Q1 responses and GPS data ['little' (Q1 $\leq 9.5\%$, GPS $\leq 2.4\%$ of time), 'sometimes' (Q1 9.5–17.5%, GPS 2.4–4.2% of time) and 'often' outdoors (Q1 >17.5%, GPS >4.2% of time)], see Additional file 1: 5. Percentages of time spent outdoors, for distributions of time spent outdoors. They were subsequently assigned to an outdoors group based on identical cut-off values using the tertiles derived from GPS measurements. Cohen's kappa analyses were then used to compare self-reported data with GPS measured categories of time spent outdoors.

We evaluated six different models with the following dependent variables: percentage of time spent outdoors, percentage of time spent in non-motorised and in motorised transport, mean distance from home while walking, biking and in motorised transport. We chose these outcome variables because they might be interesting for exposure assessment in future studies and differences in exposure due to walking, biking and motorised transport have been analysed extensively before [26].

The following factors were used in the models as independent variables, these were a priori expected to influence time spent outdoors in active transport modes negatively: Chronic Obstructive Pulmonary Disease (COPD) [27], asthma [28], previous heart diseases [29, 30], higher Body Mass Index (BMI) [classified as being overweight (>25–30 kg/m^2) or obese (>30 kg/m^2)] [31–33], current smoking [32] and having any symptom in a broad spectrum of health symptoms (Additional file 1: 2. Data used for explanatory variable analysis, Supp. Table 1, and 12. Items from VGO study questionnaire (VGO questionnaire)), attributed to the presence of livestock in the vicinity [34]. In contrast, we expected former and never smokers and people using beta-blockers to be more physically active, the latter on doctors' advice [35]. We also evaluated whether age (<45, 45–55, 55–65 and >65 years, see Additional file 1: 3. Age distribution of participants in VGO GPS study, Supp. Figure 3, for an age distribution), gender, educational level (low, medium, high) [30], working status (job: yes/no), having an outdoors occupation and the number of workdays per week, were associated with mobility patterns [36]. Furthermore, we expected that people were more frequently outdoors if they reported more time spent outdoors close to home (hours per week) [37], owning a dog (yes/no) [38, 39] or keeping hobby farm animals (yes/no) [37]. The influence of weather conditions, namely average temperature during the measuring period (<5, 5–10, 10–15 (reference group), 15–20, 20–25, >25, all in °C, see Additional file 1: 4. Distribution of avarage temperature during GPS measuring period, Supp. Figure 4, for a temperature distribution) and average rainfall during the measuring period (percentage of time with rainfall between 6.00 and 22.00 h, during measurement) were also evaluated.

Univariate linear regression analyses were performed, followed by multiple linear regression with full models that included all possible explanatory factors for differences in time spent outdoors and distances from home, we used log-transformed data, since data was log normally distributed (data not shown). Supervised stepwise backwards selection (SSBS) models, always including age, gender and educational level, were performed in R. Final SSBS models were selected on the basis of the lowest Akaike's Information Criterion (AIC). Additional file 1: 6.

Supplementary Table 2 (percentage of time) and 7. Supplementary Table 3 (distances from home address) display model outcomes with back transformed coefficients and associated 95% Confidence Intervals (CI), which can be interpreted as Geometric Mean Ratios (GMR) [40]. Finally, we performed sensitivity analyses (Additional file 1: 8. Buffer sizes around the home address, 60 m buffer versus 20 m buffer, Supp Figure 6 and Supp. Table 4) on indoor buffer sizes, using 20 m instead of 60 m buffers around the home address. No substantial differences were observed for measured times spent outdoors (Additional file 1: Supp. Table 4) and therefore, the initial 60 m buffers were retained for all analyses. In Q2 we asked whether people had deviated from their normal weekly movement patterns since this can affect our SSBS model estimates. We ran a sensitivity analyses of our SSBS models by running the models using only participants that indicated to have had a 'normal week'. Overall we found no material effects on our model estimates (Additional file 1: 9. Supplementary Table 5 and 10. Supplementary Table 6) and therefore preferred to report on our full study population.

Spatial data was processed using ArcGIS ArcMap 10.2 (ESRI, Redlands, CA, USA), statistical analyses were performed using R 3.2.3. (R Foundation, Vienna, Austria).

Results

From September 2014 to January 2016, 1517 individuals were invited, 1001 (66.0%) agreed to participate in the VGO GPS study and were sent a GPS tracker. A total of 940 GPS tracks contributed to the current analyses, since not all GPS trackers were returned, and 870 tracks remained after data cleaning steps (Fig. 2). The median total GPS measurement duration of all participants was 187 h (IQR 143–235 h), no movement was detected for median 180 h (IQR 136–228 h) and movement was registered for median 6 h (IQR 4–8 h).

Mean age of the participants was 57 years (range 20–72 years), 45% were male and 68% were employed or self-employed. Characteristics of participants are provided in Table 1. Based on GPS data, participants spent a median of 5.5 h/week outdoors: 0.3 h/week walking, 1.1 h/week biking and 3.0 h/week in motorised transport. Median distance from home was 2.0 km for walking (IQR 0.7–7.0), 2.0 km for biking (IQR 0.8–4.4) and 7.4 km for motorised transport (IQR 4.1–14.3) (Table 2).

The (Q1) reported time spent outside was considerably longer compared to GPS measured time spent outside, indicating substantial overestimation (median 4.0 times longer). Especially walking and biking durations were longer based on self-reported compared to GPS measured durations (median 13.7 and 2.8 times overestimated, respectively), while time spent in motorised transport was similar (median 1.2 times higher), see Table 2 and Fig. 4.

Table 1 General characteristics of study population

Variable	Participants
Total respondents in data analysis (N)	870
Age[b] [mean, (range)]	57.0 (20.4–72.0)
Sex[b] [N males, (%)]	391 (44.9)
Education level[b]: low [N (%)]	217 (24.9)
Medium [N (%)]	391 (44.9)
High [N (%)]	262 (30.1)
Job status[a] [N, working (%)]	592 (68.0)
Number of workdays per week[a] (mean, range)	2.1 (0-7)
Working from home[a] [N (% of people with job)]	144 (24.3)
Outdoor occupation[a] [N (% of people with job)]	70 (11.8)
Outdoor occupation[a] [Hours per day(mean, range)]	4.6 (1–16)

Data obtained from Q1 (a) and VGO baseline questionnaire (b) [22, 23]

The Cohen's kappa analyses showed a very low agreement between self-reported and measured time spent outdoors (kappa of 0.09 and 0.01, based on tertiles in GPS and Q1 data, and for using the same cut-off values of GPS data to categorise self-reported data, respectively).

Results of our models evaluating individual characteristics on GPS measured mobility patterns are provided in the Additional file 1: Supplementary Tables 2 (percentages of time) and 3 (distances from the home address). Given the discrepancy of self-reports and GPS-measured information, we refrained from evaluating correlates of self-reports.

For the overall percentage of time spent outdoors, cold average temperatures during the measurement period (below 5 °C) was associated with spending less time outdoors (GMR 0.80–0.81), women spent less time outdoors compared to men (GMR 0.85–0.87). People owning a dog spent more time outdoors compared to non-dog-owners (GMR 1.15–1.16).

Compared to study participants with a low educational level, participants with medium or high educational level tended to use motorised over non-motorised transport. We found that obese people (BMI > 30 kg/m^2) spent less time in non-motorised transport (GMR 0.69–0.74) and people with more workdays spent more time in motorised transport (GMR 1.06–1.12).

Regarding distances from home while walking we observed that higher educated people tended to walk further away from their home (medium educational level GMR 1.31–1.51, high educational level GMR 1.54–1.93), while owning a dog decreased the distance walked from home (GMR 0.51–0.58).

People using beta-blockers walked and biked less far from home than people not using these drugs (walking GMR 0.60–0.71, biking GMR 0.60–0.63). Dog-owners also remained closer to the home while biking, compared with non-dog-owners (GMR 0.73–0.76).

Table 2 Data obtained from the GPS track and Q1

Variable	Time in hours/week, distances in km	
	GPS	Questionnaire
Time indoors [Median (IQR)]	162.5 (159.8–164.5)	146.0 (133.9–154.2)
Time outdoors [Median (IQR)]	5.5 (3.5–8.2)	22.0 (13.8–34.1)
Time walking [Median (IQR)]	0.3 (0.1–0.8)	4.0 (2.0–9.0)
Time biking [Median (IQR)]	1.1 (0.3–2.4)	3.0 (1.0–8.0)
Time in motorised transport [Median (IQR)]	3.0 (1.4–5.2)	3.5 (1.8–6.6)
Distances from home while walking [Median (IQR)]	2.0 (0.7–7.0)	
Distances from home while biking [Median (IQR)]	2.0 (0.8–4.1)	
Distances from home motorised transport [Median (IQR)]	7.4 (4.1–14.3)	

Time values are transformed into hours per week, distances are in km from the home address, distance values were only available from the GPS measurements. Time outdoors is a combination of time walking, time biking, time in motorised transport and other time outdoors

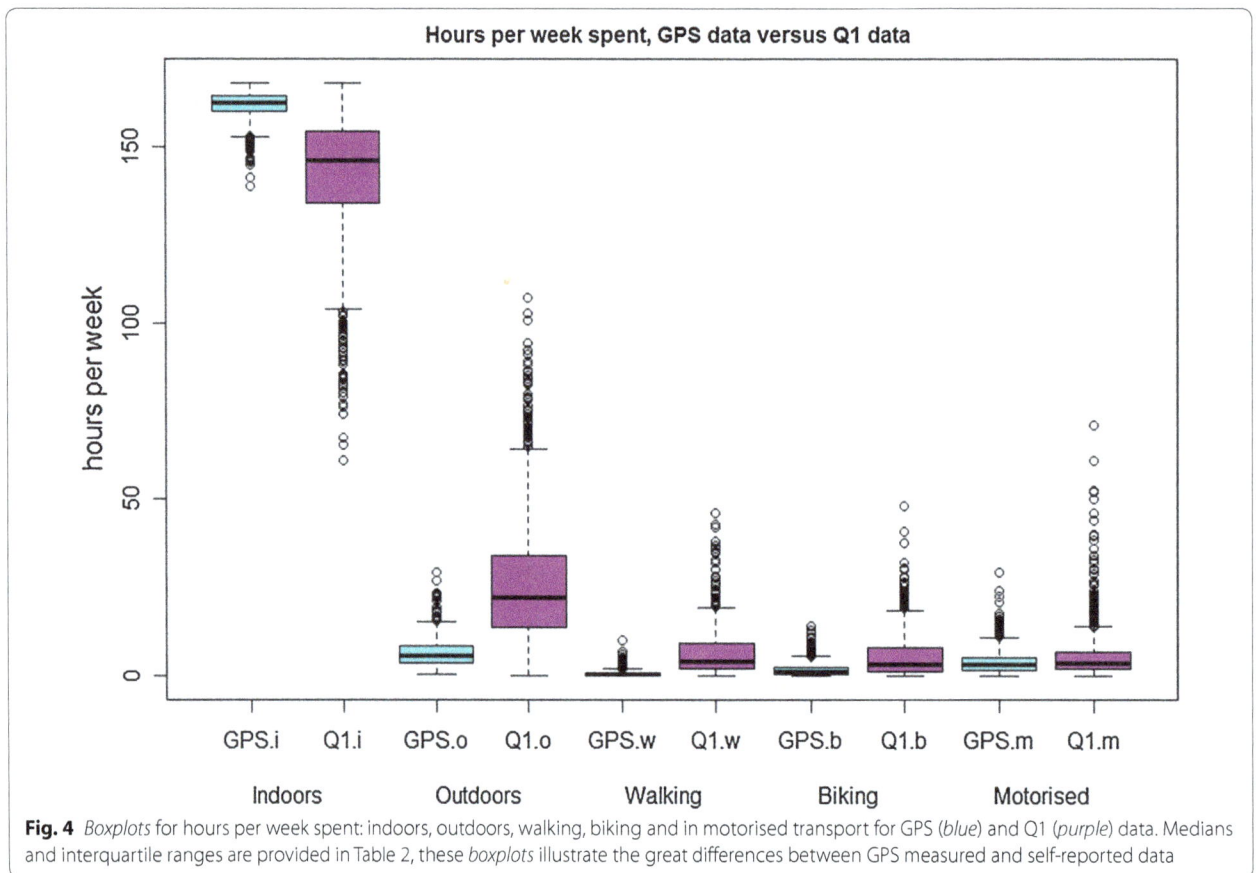

Fig. 4 *Boxplots* for hours per week spent: indoors, outdoors, walking, biking and in motorised transport for GPS (*blue*) and Q1 (*purple*) data. Medians and interquartile ranges are provided in Table 2, these *boxplots* illustrate the great differences between GPS measured and self-reported data

People with COPD and people with more workdays tended to travel longer distances from home in motorised transport (GMR 1.42–1.51 for people with COPD and GMR 1.06–1.09 for each workday). Higher outdoor temperatures (20–25 °C) were associated with shorter distances travelled in motorised transport.

Discussion

We assessed mobility of a rural population of 870 persons in the Netherlands and found that participants significantly overestimated their time spent outdoors in active transport when self-reported data pertaining to "usual mobility patterns" was compared to GPS measured data. In addition, there was low agreement between self-reported and measured categories of low, medium or high amount of time spent outdoors in active transport (kappa of 0.09). Finally, we identified a range of (participant) characteristics that were associated with differences in mobility patterns of our study population.

Strengths

Strengths of our study include the large dataset of GPS-measured as well as self-reported mobility patterns. To the best of our knowledge, there are few previous studies with such extensive datasets. Most studies that focus on GPS measurements included fewer than 300 participants [14, 41]. Few larger studies with GPS measurements (Schuessler and Axhausen 2008 N = 4882 and Bohte and Maat 2009 N = 1104) [42, 43], did not evaluate characteristics that explain observed differences in mobility patterns. Our study was embedded in a larger ongoing cohort study, providing additional information for all participants including health data, work and leisure time activities and data about the socio-economic situation of all participants. This extensive dataset enabled us to explore correlates of a range of individual characteristics with mobility patterns of our rural study population.

Limitations

GPS data has been suggested to add to environmental epidemiological studies, because exposures with a high spatial variability may be more accurately assessed [18]. This is certainly true in the case of GPS logging while in clear view of the sky; in this case, spatial accuracy has been reported to be very high ($\sim$2.5 m) [18, 44]. However, when a GPS is used indoors, the spatial accuracy of the measurements is strongly reduced [45]. Therefore, we used buffers around indoor locations to assign these points as being indoors. This procedure thus clearly does not capture all aspects of mobility, but mobility close to home may have gone undetected. Note, however, that applying differently sized home buffers to differentiate indoor from outdoor points did not strongly affect our results. We used GPS measurements as a 'gold standard', although GPS measured locations can also have errors. However, we knew from previous work that in general, the accuracy is very high (<10 m) in 85% of the time even when used in an urban area [18]. Since we performed our study in a rural area, with less high-rise buildings, we expected that GPS positional error would not have a significant effect on our findings. Nevertheless, our inability to correctly differentiate measured locations to being either inside or in close proximity to the home likely misclassifies time spent in gardens as indoors. Other researchers have attempted to avoid this spatial accuracy problem by combining GPS measurements with other

measurements, such as temperature [46] or a combination of accelerometer, magnetometers and light and temperature sensors [47]. Such a procedure may however increase problems with study adherence if participants have to carry multiple devices, in addition to generating further data analysis complexity.

Another limitation of our study is that we do not have repeated GPS measurements and that participants were only monitored for 1 week. Mobility patterns may change over time, and vary especially with season and weather conditions, as found across our study group. However, we were unable to evaluate whether there are individual differences in the adaptation of mobility patterns to weather or season.

Finally, in our study protocol, we inquired about "usual" daily mobility and not about the actual mobility patterns that participants had followed during our measurement week. We tried to improve match of self-reported and measured data by additionally asking whether participants had deviated from their "usual" weekly mobility patterns in Q2. We found no material differences in the correlates of mobility patterns in a sensitivity analysis of participants who had not deviated from a usual week compared to the full population. Nevertheless, this temporal mismatch may have further contributed to observed variance between self-reports and measured values.

Comparison self-reported and GPS measured mobility

We observed a striking overestimation in self-reported compared to measured time spent outdoors. Total time spent outdoors might be underestimated since we filtered out GPS locations in a 60 m buffer around the place of residence and 20 m of other indoor locations. In particular time spent walking was significantly overestimated. While overestimation of self-reported time spent walking as such is in line with previous reports, the amount of overestimation is not [14]. Kelly et al. performed a systematic review quantifying differences between self-reported and GPS-measured journey durations. Fourteen publications were included in the meta-analysis and self-reported trip durations were overestimated in all included studies when compared to GPS measurements, overestimations ranged from 9.2 to 75.4% [14]. In our analysis we found an overestimation of 13.7 times for walking, 2.8 times for biking and 1.2 times for motorised transport, which means that only overestimation for motorised transport is in line with what was reported by Kelly et al. [14]. There are three underlying reasons that may be driving this strong observed overestimation for time spent walking. First, in our questionnaire, we inquired about walking durations across different activities, but we did not clearly ask for walking that was performed exclusively outdoors, but asked instead for walking that was done "travelling for work". This could have resulted in a conceptual mismatch of self-reported and measured data, especially if a considerable part of daily walking is done indoors, e.g. during shopping for work-related purposes or if walking for work indoors (e.g. as a waiter or cleaner) is perceived as "travelling for work". However, the contribution of walking time of this question to overall walking time had a median below 1%, and only 9.2% of all participants reported any walking for "travelling for work". Second, the algorithm we used to assign transport modes used the 95th percentile of speed, acceleration and deceleration. This algorithm described in Huss et al. [25] was the best performing algorithm to assign transport modes to GPS data, with a kappa agreement of 0.95 for assigned versus actual mode of transport. The results reported by these authors were based on mobility of 12 participants, but speed patterns used to assign mobility in our dataset might have had a wider variation. However, the speed patterns while walking, biking or in motorised transport are so distinct that we still expect the algorithm to be able to assign transport modes correctly in the majority of the cases. In addition, our algorithm assigned "stops" when the GPS device was not moving, if these stops occurred outdoors, transport modes were not assigned, further contributing to an underestimation of measured outdoor time. We checked the cumulative duration of outdoor stops for each participant, and encountered a maximum of 3 min over the whole study population. Therefore, we do not expect that the use of the algorithm would have introduced the difference in reported and measured mobility patterns. Third, our rural population walked only very little outdoors, across the whole group we measured a median of just 15 min outdoor walking per week. Very short durations, however, are easily misreported and several of our participants also commented that average weekly durations per activity were difficult to estimate. Over-reporting of walking times in our dataset was indeed much less pronounced in persons who walked more (median 4.6 times over-reporting in the highest tertile of walking duration), compared to persons who walked less. Reasons for our rural population to walk so little may be that in general, distances in rural areas tend to be large and many people may thus choose not to walk at all for their mobility needs. Misreporting walking duration may introduce exposure misclassification in studies that attempt to assign outdoor exposures to these durations and/or locations. However, given the very short durations of walking outdoors, the absolute error in exposure assignment may still be limited. Also duration of biking was over-reported by our participants, which highlights that in general, participants overestimate their own amount of active transport

outdoors. Motorised transport may be easier to estimate, especially if linked to a fixed schedule in public transport, or if a large part of motorised transport is regular commuting. In studies with a focus on potentially differential concordance/discordance of reported and logged activity locations this disagreement between self-reported and GPS measured spatial data is not present [48, 49]. However, in the current study our focus was on mobility and activity locations were not evaluated as such.

In several previous studies regarding GPS measurements for assessment of physical activity, the authors have not solely relied on GPS measurements, but have combined these with activity diaries or recall interviews [14, 16–18]. Oliver et al. tested the usage of GPS and accelerometry tools to assess transport-related physical activity (i.e. walking, biking); the comparative standard in this study were questionnaire travel logs. They included 37 participants into their study and concluded that GPS and accelerometry were good tools to assess walking and biking activity, although performance of the questionnaire data was not assessed [19]. Sallis et al. compared interviewer-administered and self-reported questionnaires, heart-rate monitors, and accelerometers for activity patterns of fifth graders. Both questionnaire approaches correlated quite well (Pearson's r = 0.76) but correlation between questionnaires and objective measurements (heart-rate monitor and accelerometer) was lower (r = 0.50 and r = 0.30, respectively) [50]. These effects can partially be explained with a tendency to answer in a socially desirable way, resulting in over-reporting of activity durations, as shown by Adams et al. [20]. This means that regression calibration using measurements (GPS or mobile phone data) performed in a subsample of study participants may represent a way to calibrate self-reports [51], although this approach has not been validated in different populations.

Explanatory variables analyses

To the best of our knowledge we are the first to identify several correlates of mobility patterns, which may be especially relevant when assessing exposure to agents with a high spatial variability. For example, certain emissions from livestock farms are only detectable at a short distance: detectable levels of viable organisms have been found between 150 and 160 m from pig stables [4, 52] and at 330 m from poultry stables [3]. Even higher spatial variability can be observed for other environmental exposures, such as particulate matter [53] or electromagnetic fields [2]. This means that if mobility is relevant for personal exposure levels, using a general approach such as assigning exposure to the home address, will misclassify specific groups of people more than others. The identified individual explanatory factors for differences in mobility patterns may thus further assist in regression calibration efforts for other studies, or in the interpretation of previous studies that did not take such explanatory factors into account.

Future perspectives

Until very recently, due to financial, logistic and data management limitations, GPS measurements were only used in a limited way for data collection in mobility assessment. When GPS measurements were collected, this was generally done in small samples of people. Self-reporting with all its disadvantages including recall bias [11–14] was the default method to collect movement data on large cohorts of people [14]. With the increasing capabilities of smartphones [1, 54–57], new opportunities exist to gather objectively measured data regarding spatial positions of people. Dewulf et al. illustrated this by combining location data from mobile phone network providers with air pollution data from a monitoring network in Belgium [1]. Using smartphones for location assessment in studies may thus help in reducing the amount of measurement devices a participant has to carry around. It may further assist in upscaling objective measurements to large cohort study collectives. Epidemiological studies relying on self-reports of usual mobility patterns should be aware of possible over-reporting of active transport patterns. Ways to mitigate this include improving temporal matching by using detailed activity diaries instead of asking for "usual" mobility, or possibly to improve reporting by regression calibration methods [58, 59].

Conclusions

We evaluated mobility of a rural population and found that participants significantly overestimated their time spent outdoors in active transport when self-reported data was compared to GPS measured data. We identified several correlates of mobility patterns, which may be especially relevant when assessing exposure to agents with a high spatial variability. If active transport outdoors is relevant for personal exposure levels, then using a general approach such as assigning exposure to the home address will introduce exposure misclassification that will be stronger in some groups of people than in others. Regression calibration using measurements or these identified explanatory variables may represent a way to calibrate self-reports in future studies.

Authors' contributions
GK, LAMS and FB collected the data. GK performed the analysis and drafted the first version of the manuscript. RAC, DJJH and AH conceived of the study. All authors read and approved the final manuscript.

Author details
[1] Julius Centre for Health Sciences and Primary Care, University Medical Centre Utrecht, Utrecht, The Netherlands. [2] Institute for Risk Assessment Sciences (IRAS), Division Environmental Epidemiology and Veterinary Public Health (EEPI-VPH), Utrecht University, Yalelaan 2, 3584 CM Utrecht, The Netherlands. [3] National Institute for Public Health and the Environment (RIVM), Bilthoven, The Netherlands. [4] Netherlands Institute for Health Services Research (NIVEL), Utrecht, The Netherlands. [5] Faculty of Veterinary Medicine, Utrecht University, Utrecht, The Netherlands.

Acknowledgements
We would like to thank all our participants, Lützen Portengen and Astrid Martens for statistical input and Daisy de Vries for textual input.

Competing interests
All authors report that they have competing interests.

Funding
The VGO-GPS Study is funded by UMC Utrecht. The Livestock Farming and Neighboring Residents' Health (VGO) study was funded by the Ministry of Health, Welfare and Sports and the Ministry of Economic Affairs of the Netherlands, and supported by a grant from the Lung Foundation Netherlands (Grant No. 3.2.11.022).

References
1. Dewulf B, Neutens T, Lefebvre W, Seynaeve G, Vanpoucke C, Beckx C, et al. Dynamic assessment of exposure to air pollution using mobile phone data. Int J Health Geogr [Internet]. 2016;15(1):14.
2. Beekhuizen J, Vermeulen R, Kromhout H, Bürgi A, Huss A. Science of the total environment geospatial modelling of electromagnetic fields from mobile phone base stations. Sci Total Environ [Internet]. 2013;445–446:202–9. doi:10.1016/j.scitotenv.2012.12.020.
3. Schulz J, Formosa L, Seedorf J, Hartung J. Measurement of culturable airborne staphylococci downwind from a naturally ventilated broiler house. Aerobiologia (Bologna). 2011;27(4):311–8.
4. Schulz J, Friese A, Klees S, Tenhagen BA, Fetsch A, Rösler U, et al. Longitudinal study of the contamination of air and of soil surfaces in the vicinity of pig barns by livestock-associated methicillin-resistant *Staphylococcus aureus*. Appl Environ Microbiol. 2012;78(16):5666–71.
5. Schulze A, Römmelt H, Ehrenstein V, van Strien R, Praml G, Küchenhoff H, et al. Effects on pulmonary health of neighboring residents of concentrated animal feeding operations: exposure assessed using optimized estimation technique. Arch Environ Occup Health. 2011;66(3):146–54.

6. Klous G, Huss A, Heederik DJJ, Coutinho RA. Human–livestock contacts and their relationship to transmission of zoonotic pathogens, a systematic review of literature. One Health [Internet]. 2016;2:65–76. doi:10.1016/j.onehlt.2016.03.001.

7. Kersh GJ, Fitzpatrick KA, Self JS, Priestley RA, Kelly AJ, Ryan Lash R, et al. Presence and persistence of *Coxiella burnetii* in the environments of goat farms associated with a Q fever outbreak. Appl Environ Microbiol. 2013;79(5):1697–703.

8. Perchoux C, Chaix B, Cummins S, Kestens Y. Conceptualization and measurement of environmental exposure in epidemiology: accounting for activity space related to daily mobility. Heal Place [Internet]. 2013;21:86–93. doi:10.1016/j.healthplace.2013.01.005.

9. Chaix B, Méline J, Duncan S, Merrien C, Karusisi N, Perchoux C, et al. GPS tracking in neighborhood and health studies: A step forward for environmental exposure assessment, a step backward for causal inference? Heal Place. 2013;21:46–51.

10. Rytkönen MJ. Not all maps are equal: GIS and spatial analysis in epidemiology. Int J Circumpolar Health. 2004;63(1):9–24.

11. Stalvey BT, Owsley C, Sloane ME, Ball K. The life space questionnaire: a measure of the extent of mobility of older adults. J Appl Gerontol. 1999;18(4):460–78.

12. O'Brien M, Jones D, Sloan D, Rustin, M. From the SAGE Social Science Collections. All Rights Reserved. 2016.

13. Meurs H, Haaijer R. Spatial structure and mobility. Transp Res Part D Transp Environ. 2001;6(6):429–46.

14. Kelly P, Krenn P, Titze S, Stopher P, Foster C. Quantifying the difference between self-reported and global positioning systems-measured journey durations: a systematic review. Transp Rev A Transnatl Transdiscipl J [Internet]. 2013;33(4):443–59.

15. Deffner V, Kuchenhoff H, Maier V, Pitz M, Cyrys J, Breitner S, et al. Personal exposure to ultrafine particles: Two-level statistical modeling of background exposure and time-activity patterns during three seasons. J Expo Sci Environ Epidemiol [Internet]. 2016;26(1):17–25.

16. Elgethun K, Fenske RA, Yost MG, Palcisko GJ. Time-location analysis for exposure assessment studies of children using a novel global positioning system instrument. Environ Health Perspect. 2003;111(1):115–22.

17. Dias D, Tchepel O. Modelling of human exposure to air pollution in the urban environment: a GPS-based approach. Environ Sci Pollut Res. 2014;21(5):3558–71.

18. Beekhuizen J, Kromhout H, Huss A, Vermeulen R. Performance of GPS-devices for environmental exposure assessment. J Expo Sci Environ Epidemiol [Internet]. 2013;23(5):498–505.

19. Oliver M, Badland H, Mavoa S, Duncan MJ, Duncan S. Combining GPS, GIS, and accelerometry: methodological issues in the assessment of location and intensity of travel behaviors. J Phys Act Health. 2010;7(1):102–8.

20. Adams SA, Matthews CE, Ebbeling CB, Moore CG, Joan E, Fulton J, et al. The effect of social desirability and social approval on self-reports of physical activity. Am J Epidemiol. 2005;161(4):389–98.

21. Matz CJ, Stieb DM, Brion O. Urban-rural differences in daily time-activity patterns, occupational activity and housing characteristics. Environ Health [Internet]. 2015;14(1):88.

22. Borlée F, Yzermans CJ, Van Dijk CE, Heederik D, Smit LAM. Increased respiratory symptoms in COPD patients living in the vicinity of livestock farms. Eur Respir J [Internet]. 2015;46(6):1605–14. doi:10.1183/13993003.00265-2015.

23. Borlée F, Yzermans CJ, Krop E, Aalders B, Rooijackers J, Zock JP, van Dijk CE, Maassen K, Schellevis F, Heederik D, Smit LAM. Spirometry, questionnaire and Electronic Medical Record based COPD in a population survey: comparing prevalence, level of agreement and associations with potential risk factors. PLoS ONE. 2017;12:e0171494.

24. KNMI website [Internet]. https://www.knmi.nl/Nederland-nu/klimatologie/uurgegevens. Accessed 4 April 2016.

25. Huss A, Beekhuizen J, Kromhout H, Vermeulen R. Using GPS-derived speed patterns for recognition of transport modes in adults. Int J Health Geogr [Internet]. 2014;13(1):40.

26. De Hartog JJ, Boogaard H, Nijland H, Hoek G. Do the health benefits of cycling outweigh the risks? Environ Health Perspect. 2010;118(8):1109–16.

27. Pitta F, Troosters T, Spruit MA, Probst VS, Decramer M, Gosselink R. Characteristics of physical activities in daily life in chronic obstructive pulmonary disease. Am J Respir Crit Care Med. 2005;171(9):972–7.

28. Williams B, Powell A, Hoskins G, Neville R. Exploring and explaining low participation in physical activity among children and young people with asthma: a review. BMC Fam Pract [Internet]. 2008;9(1):40.

29. Giallauria F, Cirillo P, D'agostino M, Petrillo G, Vitelli A, Pacileo M, et al. Effects of exercise training on high-mobility group box-1 levels after acute myocardial infarction. J Card Fail [Internet]. 2011;17(2):108–14.

30. Allman RM, Baker PS, Maisiak RM, Sims RV, Roseman JM. Racial similarities and differences in predictors of mobility change over eighteen months. J Gen Intern Med. 2004;19(11):1118–26.

31. Kyttä AM, Broberg AK, Kahila MH. Urban environment and children's active lifestyle: SoftGIS revealing children's behavioral patterns and meaningful places. Am J Health Promot. 2012;26(5):e137–48.

32. Stuck AE, Walthert JM, Nikolaus T, Büla CJ, Hohmann C, Beck JC. Risk factors for functional status decline in community-living elderly people: a systematic literature review. Soc Sci Med. 1999;48(4):445–69.

33. BMI [Internet]. http://www.nhlbi.nih.gov/health/educational/lose_wt/BMI/bmi-m.htm.

34. Neuberg SL, Kenrick DT, Schaller M. Human threat management systems: self-protection and disease avoidance. Neurosci Biobehav Rev [Internet]. 2011;35(4):1042–51. doi:10.1016/j.neubiorev.2010.08.011.

35. Graham I, Atar D, Borch-Johnsen K, Boysen G, Burell G, Cifkova R et al. European guidelines on cardiovascular disease prevention in clinical practice: executive summary: fourth joint task force of the European Society of Cardiology and other societies on cardiovascular disease prevention in clinical practice (Constituted by representatives of nine societies and by invited experts). Eur Heart J 2007;28(19):2375–414.

36. Stopher P, Zhang Y. Is travel behaviour repetitive from day to day? [Internet]. http://atrf.info/papers/2010/2010_Stopher_Zhang_B.pdf, 33rd Australasian Transport Research Forum (ATRF) 2010, Canberra, ACT, Australia.

37. Bellows AC, Brown K, Smit J. Health benefits of urban agriculture. New York: Community Food; 2003.

38. Brown JD, Stallknecht DE, Valeika S, Swayne DE. Susceptibility of wood ducks to H5N1 highly pathogenic avian influenza virus. J Wildl Dis. 2007;43(4):660–7.

39. Cutt H, Giles-Corti B, Knuiman M, Burke V. Dog ownership, health and physical activity: a critical review of the literature. Health Place. 2007;13:261–72.

40. Kytariolos J, Karalis V, Macheras P, Symillides M. Novel scaled bioequivalence limits with leveling-off properties. Pharm Res. 2006;23(11):2657–64.

41. Chaix B, Kestens Y, Duncan DT, Brondeel R, Méline J, El Aarbaoui T, et al. A GPS-based methodology to analyze environment-health associations at the trip level: case-crossover analyses of built environments and walking. Am J Epidemiol [Internet]. 2016; kww071. http://www.ncbi.nlm.nih.gov/pubmed/27659779.

42. Schuessler N, Axhausen KW. Processing raw data from global positioning systems without additional information. Transp Res Rec J Transp Res Board. 2009;2105(1):28–36.

43. Bohte W, Maat K. Deriving and validating trip purposes and travel modes for multi-day GPS-based travel surveys: a large-scale application in the Netherlands. Transp Res Part C Emerg Technol [Internet]. 2009;17(3):285–97. doi:10.1016/j.trc.2008.11.004.

44. Krenn PJ, Titze S, Oja P, Jones A, Ogilvie D. Use of global positioning systems to study physical activity and the environment a systematic review. Am J Prev Med. 2011;41(5):508–15.

45. Kerr J, Duncan S, Schipperjin J. Using global positioning systems in health research a practical approach to data collection and processing. Am J Prev Med. 2011;41(5):532–40.

46. Nethery E, Mallach G, Rainham D, Goldberg MSMS, Wheeler AJAJ. Using Global Positioning Systems (GPS) and temperature data to generate time-activity classifications for estimating personal exposure in air monitoring studies: an automated method. Environ Health. 2014;13(1):33.

47. Matthews CE, Moore SC, George SM, Sampson J, Bowles HR. Improving self-reports of active and sedentary behaviors in large epidemiologic studies. Exerc Sport Sci Rev. 2012;40(3):118–26.

48. Shareck M, Kestens Y, Gauvin L. Examining the spatial congruence between data obtained with novel activity location questionnaire, continuos GPS tracking, and prompted recall surveys. Int J Health Geogr [Internet]. 2013;12(1):40.

49. Paz-Soldan VA, Reiner RC, Morrison AC, Stoddard ST, et al. Strenghts and weaknesses of Global Positioning System (GPS) data-loggers and semi-structured interviews for capturing fine-scale human mobility: findings from Iquitos, Peru. PLoS Negl Trop Dis. 2014;8(6):e2888.

50. Sallis JF, Strikmiller PK, Harsha DW, Feldman HA, Ehlinger S, Stone EJ, Williston J, Woods S. Validation of interviewer- and self-administered physical activity checklists for fifth grade students. Med Sci Sports Exerc. 1996;28(7):840–51.

51. Matthews CE, Moore C, George SM, Sampson J, Bowles HR. NIH Public Access. 2013;40(3):118–26.

52. Thorne PS. Industrial livestock production facilities: airborne emissions. Encycl Environ Heal [Internet]. 2011;218–26. http://www.sciencedirect.com/science/article/pii/B9780444522726004232.

53. Li J, Jin M, Xu Z. Spatiotemporal variability of remotely sensed PM 2. 5 Concentrations in China from 1998 to 2014 Based on a Bayesian Hierarchy Model. 2014.

54. Gonzalez MC, Hidalgo CA, Barabasi A-L. Understanding individual human mobility patterns. Nature [Internet]. 2008;453(7196):779–82.

55. Ahas R, Silm S, Järv O, Saluveer E, Tiru M. Using mobile positioning data to model locations meaningful to users of mobile phones. J Urban Technol. 2010;17(1):3–27.

56. Glasgow ML, Rudra CB, Yoo E-H, Demirbas M, Merriman J, Nayak P, et al. Using smartphones to collect time–activity data for long-term personal-level air pollution exposure assessment. J Expo Sci Environ Epidemiol [Internet]. 2014;26(September):1–9.

57. Palmer JRB, Espenshade TJ. New approaches to human mobility: using mobile phones for demographic Research. Demography. 2013;50:1105–28.

58. Lim S, Wyker B, Bartley K, Eisenhower D. Measurement error of self-reported physical activity in New York City: assessement and correction. Am J Epidemiol. 2015;181(9):648–55.

59. Saint-Maurice PF, Welk GJ, Beyler NK, Bartee RT, Heelan KA. Calibration of self-report tools for physical activity research: the Physical Activity Questionnaire (PAQ). BMC Public Health. 2014;14:461.

14

Spatial identification of potential health hazards

Alina Svechkina, Marina Zusman, Natalya Rybnikova and Boris A. Portnov*

Abstract

Background and aims: Large metropolitan areas often exhibit multiple morbidity hotspots. However, the identification of specific health hazards, associated with the observed morbidity patterns, is not always straightforward. In this study, we suggest an empirical approach to the identification of specific health hazards, which have the highest probability of association with the observed morbidity patterns.

Methods: The morbidity effect of a particular health hazard is expected to weaken with distance. To account for this effect, we estimate distance decay gradients for alternative locations and then rank these locations based on the strength of association between the observed morbidity and wind-direction weighted proximities to these locations. To validate this approach, we use both theoretical examples and a case study of the Greater Haifa Metropolitan Area (GHMA) in Israel, which is characterized by multiple health hazards.

Results: In our theoretical examples, the proposed approach helped to identify correctly the predefined locations of health hazards, while in the real-world case study, the main health hazard was identified as a spot in the industrial zone, which hosts several petrochemical facilities.

Conclusion: The proposed approach does not require extensive input information and can be used as a preliminary risk assessment tool in a wide range of environmental settings, helping to identify potential environmental risk factors behind the observed population morbidity patterns.

Keywords: Source-oriented models, Receptor-oriented models, Systematic search approach, Disease hotspots, Wind adjustment, Multivariate regression analysis

Background

Air pollution from motor traffic and industrial facilities is known to be linked to respiratory, cardiovascular and cancer morbidity [1–9]. However, since urban areas are often characterized by multiple sources of air pollution, the identification of specific environmental hazards associated with the observed morbidity patterns is not always straightforward [10–13].

Traditional methods, used to identify the specific sources of air pollution, include the residence time analysis (RTA) and the chemical mass balance (CMB) method [14–22]. The former method is based on measurements of different air pollutants at the receptor sites [15, 18, 20, 23], while the CMB method investigates the chemical composition of air particles, by comparing them with particles emitted from different emission sources [14, 16, 22]. However, the empirical implementation of these methods requires a considerable amount of information on the concentration of specific particles, detailed wind regime assessments and topographic attributes, which are not always available to researchers [14, 24–26].

In this study, we suggest an empirical approach to the identification of specific health hazards, which have the highest probability of being associated with the observed morbidity patterns. The proposed approach does not require extensive input information and can be implemented at a *preliminary* risk assessment stage, using basic geo-statistical tools. The proposed method is based on an expectation that the morbidity effect of a particular health hazard weakens with distance [9, 27–29]. As a

*Correspondence: portnov@research.haifa.ac.il
Department of Natural Resources and Environmental Management,
Faculty of Management, University of Haifa, 3498838 Mount Carmel,
Haifa, Israel

result, people living in a close proximity to a morbidity source, are expected to exhibit, *ceteris paribus*, a higher rate of morbidity than those living at a distance from that source [11, 30]. To account for this effect, we estimate distance decay gradients of morbidity for alternative potential "source" locations and then rank these locations based on the strength of association between the observed morbidity patterns and wind-direction weighted proximities to these locations.

Spatial identification of pollution sources and morbidity hotspots

Empirical implementations of morbidity source assessments can be classified into two groups: *source-oriented* approaches and *receptor-oriented* methods [14, 15, 20, 23, 24, 26, 31–33]. The first group of methodologies uses data from different pollution sources and then computes the concentrations of different air pollutants in a given point of space, by taking into account local meteorological conditions and topography [32, 34]. By contrast, the second group of methods uses data on air pollution measured at the pollution receptors' sites and then estimates probable pollution sources, by taking into account the backward wind trajectory and other relevant meteorological conditions (see *inter alia* [14, 20, 35]).

In an early study [15], an identification method of potential emission sources of sulphur dioxide (SO_2) was developed. The method uses SO_2 concentrations measured at the receptor site and then calculates a backward trajectory leading to the potential emission source. In a separate study, [36] discuss the results produced by a chemical transport modeling of particulate matter ($PM_{2.5}$), using data available for Northern Italy. According to the proposed method, ambient air pollution is partitioned between road transport, industries and domestic heating.

In several health geography studies, distances from residential locations to pre-identified environmental hazards are commonly used as proxies for unknown (or unidentified) exposures [37–40]. Potential health hazards, to which this exposure assessment method was applied, included highways, industrial sites, nuclear power plants and gas wells.

Thus, in a recent study, McKenzie et al. [6] estimated the health risk associated with areal proximity to natural gas wells in the Garfield County, Colorado. In a separate study, Sermage-Faure et al. [38] investigated the risk of childhood leukemia around nuclear power plants. The total of 32,753 study subjects were subdivided into groups, according to their residential proximity to the existing power plants, and the observed cancers incidence rates across different proximity bands were mutually compared. The results suggested an excess of leukemia in close proximity to nuclear power plants.

Zusman et al. [11] used proximity to an oil storage site, as a proxy for residential exposure to unknown levels of emissions of volatile and semi-volatile organic compounds from the site. As the study revealed, the rates of lung and non-Hodgkin lymphoma (NHL) cancers declined in line with distance from the storage site, especially among the elderly (P < 0.01). A similar methodological approach was used by [30], who investigated the link between NHL morbidity and residence near heavy roads. In the study, the geographic distribution of NHL patients was adjusted by the overall density of population residing in the study area. The analysis indicated a steady decline in the density of NHL patients as a function of distance from main thoroughfare roads.

Although in the above mentioned and other studies (see *inter alia* [6, 41–43]), areal proximities were used for assessing the adverse effects of different health hazards on human morbidity, this method was mostly applied to *pre-identified* health risk sources, that is, health hazards found at *known* locations—such as roads, industrial sites, etc.

In the past decades, several geo-statistical tests have been also developed to assess disease clusters around predefined sources of environmental hazards. These tests include Stone's Maximum Likelihood Ratio Test [44], Tango's Focused Test [45], Bithell's Linear Risk Score Test [46], and the Lawson-Waller Score Test [47], also known as the "focused tests". Although these tests can be used to identify cluster of events around a single or several *pre-specified* locations, they cannot be used effectively if the source (or sources) of exposure is unknown, the task which the proposed identification method, based on a systematic areal comparison of alternative risk-source locations controlled for confounders, is designed to achieve.

Methods
Identification methodology
Assuming that the rate of morbidity observed in the *i*th point of space ($morb_i$) depends on the distance from the potential source of exposure, *j*, the relationship between $morb_i$ and $dist_{ji}$ can be expressed by the following linear function, reflecting a monotonic decline in $morb_i$ as a function of $dist_{ji}$:

$$morb_i = b_0 + b_1 \cdot dist_{ji} + \varepsilon_i. \tag{1}$$

where b_0, b_1 are coefficients, ε_i = random error term.

As long as the relationship between $morb_i$ and $dist_{ji}$ follows (1) and the locations of specific sources of exposure (e.g., roads, industrial facilities, etc.) are a priori known, the calculation of the strength of association between $morb_i$ and $dist_{ji}$ is technically simple. However, if actual sources of exposure for $morb_i$ for are *unknown*, alternative locations, j, can be assessed, one by one, as potential exposure sources. Such alternative locations can then be ranked by their "probability" of being the exposure source (P_{ji}) for $morb_i$ using the coefficient of determination, R_{ji}^2, between $morb_i$ and $dist_{ji}$:[1]

$$P_{ji} \to R_{ji}^2\left(morb_i, dist_{ji}\right), \quad \forall b_1 \in (-\infty, 0). \tag{2}$$

The interpretation of (2) is relatively simple: values of R_{ji}^2 close to 1 (when b_1 is negative) would indicate a high "probability" that exposure originating from point j is associated with morbidity observed in i, while values of R_{ji}^2 close to 1, when b_1 is positive, would indicate a "protective" effect, and values of R_{ji}^2 close to *zero* will point out at the absence of any significant association between the two variables.

Since the dispersion of air pollutants from a potential risk source is likely to be affected by the wind frequency of from j to i [48, 49], the pairwise Euclidian distances ($dist_{ji}$) can be adjusted:

$$\widetilde{dist}_{ji} = T\left(dist_{ji} \mid W_{ji}\right), \tag{3}$$

where $\widetilde{dist}_{ji}$ = distance between i and j adjusted by wind frequency (W_{ji}) between the points (measured as e.g., annual or seasonal averages of directional wind frequencies), and $T\left(dist_{ji} \mid W_{ji}\right)$ is a distance transformation function (e.g., linear, quadratic and exponential transformations can be used; see "Appendix 2").

To account for the above wind-adjustment effect, (1) can be rewritten as follows:

$$morb_i = f\left(\widetilde{dist}_{ji}\right). \tag{4}$$

Considering that the association between the observed health effect and proximity to a given health hazard can be confounded by other factors (such as e.g., socio-economic status of the local population, residential densities, ethnicity, etc. [5, 13, 50–52]), the *confound* relationship between the rate of morbidity observed in i and $\widetilde{dist}_{ji}$ can be adjusted as follows:

$$morb_i = b_0 + b_1 \cdot \widetilde{dist}_{ji} + b_2 \cdot \mathbf{GEO} + b_3 \cdot \mathbf{SES} + b_4 \cdot \mathbf{POL} + \varepsilon_i, \tag{5}$$

where $b_0, ..., b_4$ are regression coefficients; GEO = vector of geographical attributes of i (e.g., distance to main roads, elevation above the sea level, etc.); SES = vector of socio-economic attributes of i, including e.g., socio-economic status and ethnic makeup of the local

population; POL = vector of air pollution levels measured at the ith point, and ε_i = random error term.

As with (1), the coefficient of determination obtained for (5) can be considered as a measure of probability that morbidity observed in i and originated from j:

$$P_{ji} \to R_{ji}^2\left(morb_i, \widetilde{dist}_{ji}, \mathbf{GEO}, \mathbf{SES}, \mathbf{POL}\right), \quad \forall b_1 < 0. \tag{6}$$

The interpretation of (6) is similar to that of (2): in particular, values of R_{ji}^2 close to 1 (when b_1 is negative) indicate a high "probability" that exposure originating from point j is associated with morbidity observed in i, while values of R_{ji}^2 close to 1 (when b_1 is positive) would indicate a "protective" effect, and values of R_{ji}^2 close to *zero* will point out at the absence of any significant association between the variables. The essential difference between (2) and (6) is that the former equation is uncontrolled for potential confounders, while the latter Eq. (6) takes such confounders into account.

Empirical validation

We tested the proposed identification approach in two stages. During the first stage, we designed several theoretical examples in which *loci* of morbidity rates were positioned around pre-defined sources of exposure. In particular, we generated two identical, regularly spaced arrays of 100 "reference" point each, surrounding two pre-defined sources of exposure—either a point or a line (see Fig. 1; left panel). These arrays of "reference" points served in our tests as both disease observations and points from which potential exposure could have been generated. The rates of morbidity were arbitrarily assigned to each reference point using one simple rule: in line with the expected distance decay relationship, reference points with higher morbidity rates were positioned closer to the pre-defined sources of exposure, while places with lower morbidity rates were positioned farther away from these sources (see Fig. 1; left panel). Then, we estimated bivariate regressions to assess the strength of association between $morb_i$ and $dist_{ji}$ for each "reference" point (a total of 100 equations, one for each reference point).

We also incorporated a stochastic element into our analysis. In particular, in order to test the sensitivity of the models under varying levels of inputs, we used a random number generator to generate stochastic noise around the input morbidity rates in our "point" and "line" examples (see Fig. 1). Next, we ran 100 regressions for each of the simulated samples. The test did not change the regression results substantially. In particular, in the case of the "point" source (see Fig. 1b), the estimates for the distance variable were as follows: B = −11.17 (95% CI −11.71, −10.63), t-stat = −40.84, (95% CI −41.163, −40.76), and

---

[1] For explanation of mathematical symbols used in the paper, see "Appendix 3".

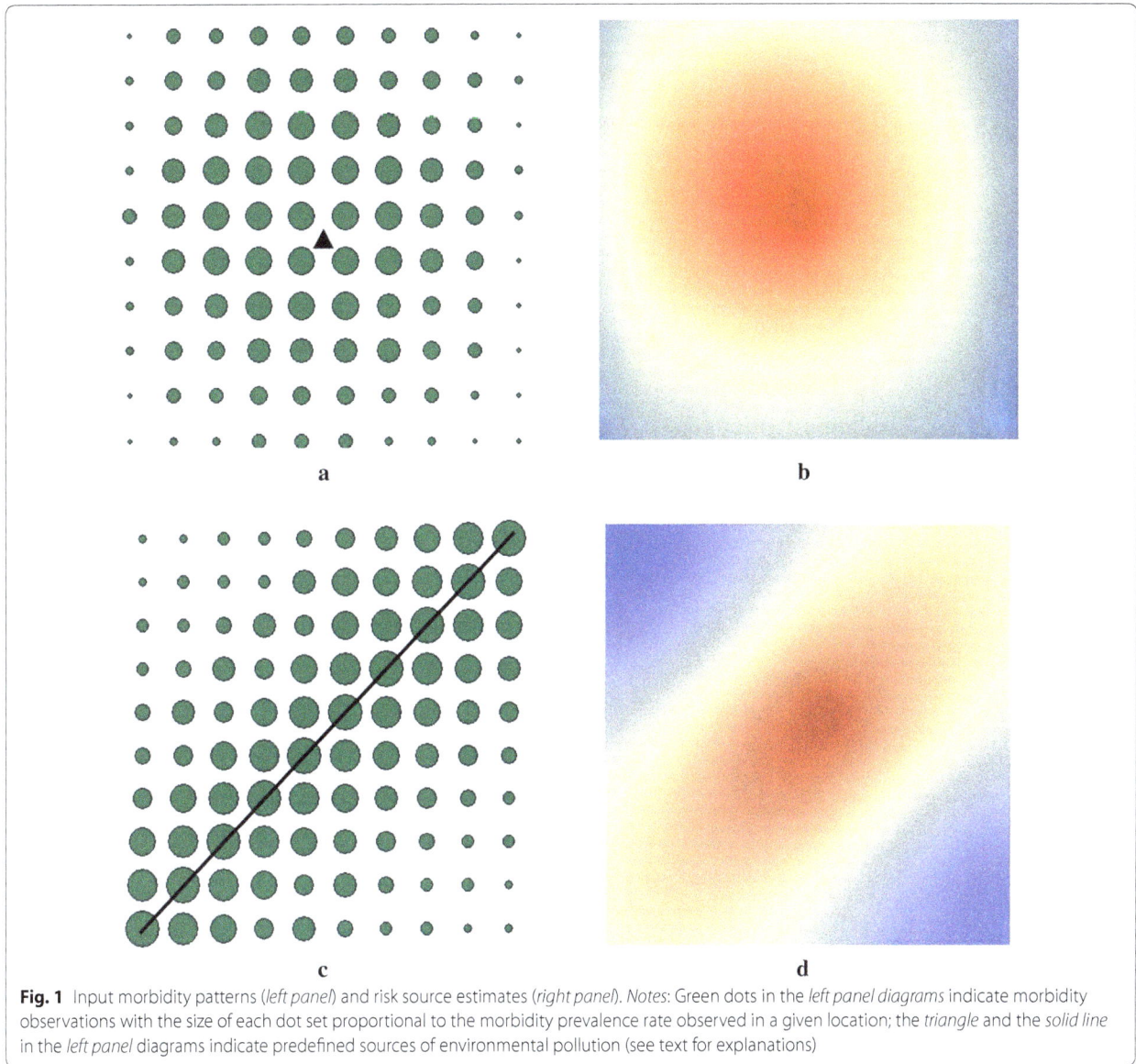

Fig. 1 Input morbidity patterns (*left panel*) and risk source estimates (*right panel*). *Notes*: Green dots in the *left panel diagrams* indicate morbidity observations with the size of each dot set proportional to the morbidity prevalence rate observed in a given location; the *triangle* and the *solid line* in the *left panel* diagrams indicate predefined sources of environmental pollution (see text for explanations)

for the "line" source (Fig. 1d): B $=$ -5.90 (95% CI -7.98, -3.82), and t-stat $=$ -5.47 (95% CI -5.63, -5.36). This confirms that our estimates are essentially robust.

Lastly, we interpolated the R_{ji}^2 values, to create continuous "probability" surfaces, differentiating between areas with high and low values of the coefficients of determination (see Fig. 1; right panel). To this end, we used the Empirical Bayesian Kriging (EBK) method, a kriging interpolation technique, which differs from classical kriging methods by accounting for the error introduced by estimating the semivariogram model [17, 53]. The EBK parameters were set to the default values used by the ArcGIS^{TM}10.x software [54].

At the next step, we applied the proposed identification method to the real world case of the Greater Haifa Metropolitan Area (GHMA) in Israel (Fig. 2), characterized by multiple health hazards. Background information on the study area, its location and geographic attributes is reported in the Additional file 1.

We started our analysis of morbidity patterns in GHMA by geocoding residential addresses of lung and NHL cancer patients, obtained from the Israel National Cancer registry for the year 2012 [55], which are the latest annual records available in the database at the time of the study initiation.[2] Next, we calculated cancer rates in different areas of the GHMA, using the Double Kernel Density (DKD) tools (see Additional file 2).

---

[2] Geocoding is a process of converting street addresses into geographic (X, Y) coordinates suitable for mapping [56].

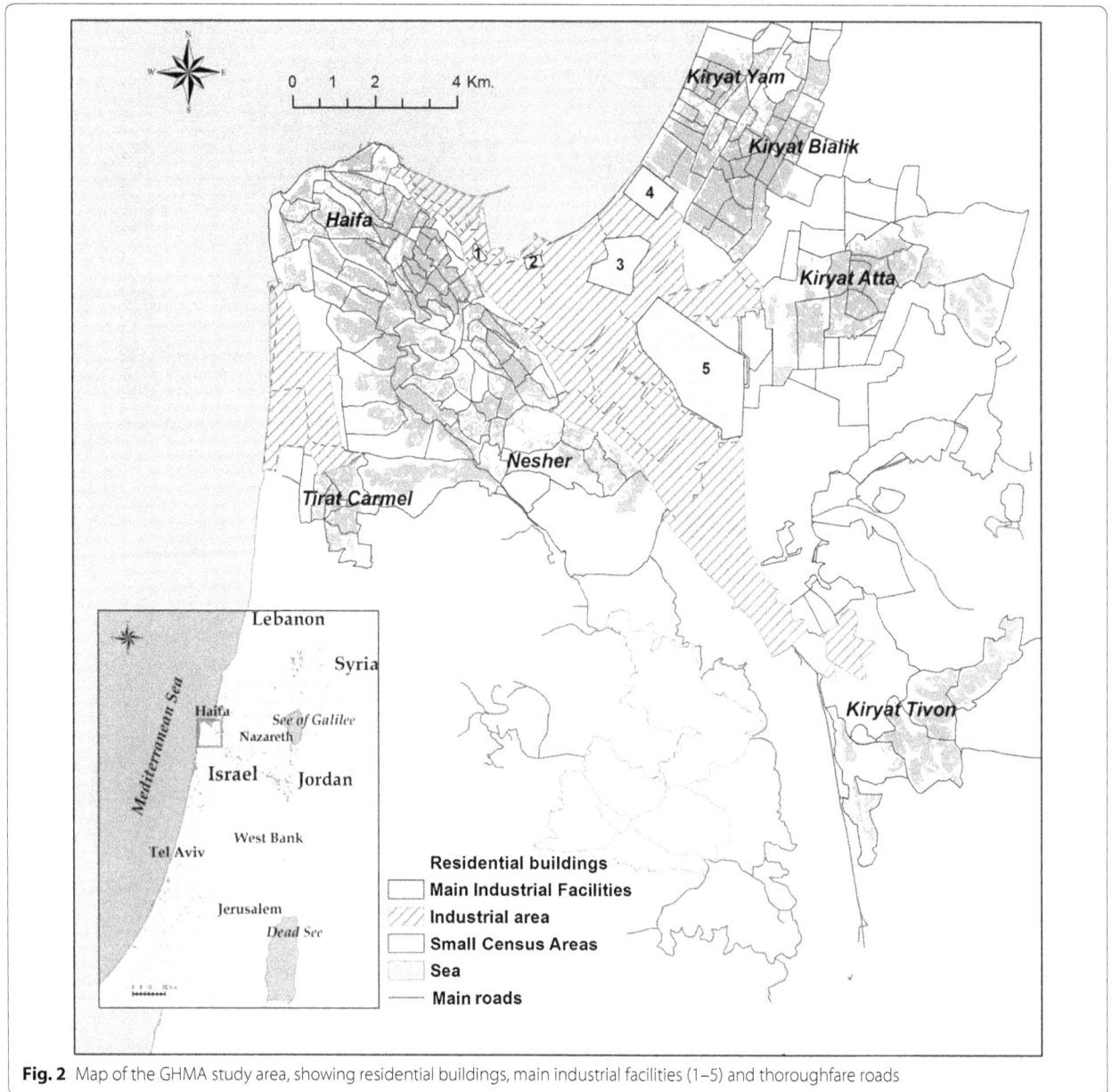

Fig. 2 Map of the GHMA study area, showing residential buildings, main industrial facilities (1–5) and thoroughfare roads

In order to convert the obtained continuous DKD surfaces of cancer density into discrete observations, suitable for a multivariate analysis, we generated 1000 randomly distributed "reference" points covering the entire study area (*i* points). Following the analysis procedure suggested in [11], the reference points created thereby were "spatially joined" with DKD surfaces of both types of cancer under study, enabling us to estimate the cancer morbidity rate for each "reference" point. Using the "spatial join" tool in ArcGIS™10.x software [54], we next assigned the values of several variables, either drawn from small census areas (SCAs) data

(such as socio-economic status, percent of residents employed in manufacturing, the share of total population over 65yo and neighborhood level smoking rates) or generated from NO_x and $PM_{2.5}$ air pollution surfaces, to each reference point.

The air pollution surfaces were interpolated by kriging using annual averages of air pollution obtained from air quality monitoring stations. According to previous studies, cancer latency period can vary substantially, ranging from several years to several decades [57]. To account for this effect, annual averages of NO_x and $PM_{2.5}$, obtained from 20 Air Quality Monitoring

Stations (AQMSs) [58], were lagged by 10 years, which is a temporal lag, commonly used in epidemiological studies of cancer [59–61]. That is, cancer DKD rates estimated for the year 2013 were mutually compared with air pollution data for the year 2003 (see Appendix 1).

We considered the above mentioned variables as potential confounders for the observed cancer rates, as commonly done in epidemiological studies of cancer morbidity [5, 13, 51, 52]. Descriptive statistics of the variables used in the analysis are reported in "Appendix 1".

At the next step, we generated a map (layer) of 1000 evenly distributed points, representing locations of potential environmental hazards (j points). For the arrays of i and j, we next calculated Euclidian distances ($dist_{ji}$), from each morbidity point (i) to each source points (j). After these distance pairs were calculated, we introduced them into regression models as potential explanatory variables, in addition to the above mentioned socio-demographic and geographic attributes, considered as controls. To address the issue of multicollinearity, individual $dist_{ji}$ were introduced into the models separately, one by one, in addition to the constant set of controls, and changes in the coefficient of determinations were traced. The models were estimated separately for two dependent variables—NHL and lung cancer DKD rates.

Because simple Euclidian distances may not be a truly accurate proximity matrix, considering wind frequency and direction, we adjusted these distances by applying a wind frequency transformation discussed in "Appendix 2". By way of this transformation, we calculated wind weighted distances between each pair of i and j $\left(\widetilde{dist_{ji}} \right)$ and then used these wind-adjusted distances in the regression analysis as alternatives to simple Euclidean distances, used during the initial phase of the analysis.

Next, for each morbidity reference point (i), we ran multivariate regressions for both types of cancer under study (that is, lung and NHL cancer separately), using the constant set of the above mentioned socio-demographic explanatory and adding one $\widetilde{dist_{ji}}$ at a time. For 1000 multivariate regressions obtained for each type of cancer (that is, one regression equation for each j point), we used the coefficient of determination (R^2_{ji}) to generate the "probability" surface, covering the entire study area and estimating how well the constant set of socio-demographic variables and wind weighted distance from each potential source point j, to the disease observation point i explain cancer rates observed at i's.

In the initial stage of the analysis, $\widetilde{dist_{ji}}$ were introduced by their linear terms. However, as our analysis revealed, the relationship between the observed cancer morbidity and industrial proximities was best captured by a non-linear (parabolic) function (see Fig. 3), apparently due

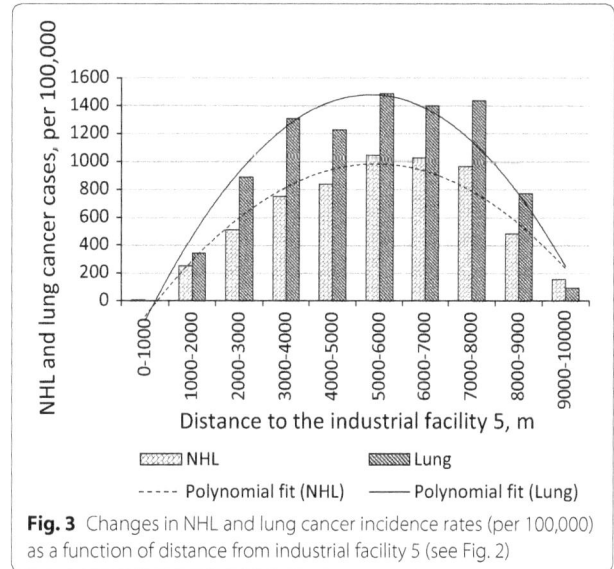

Fig. 3 Changes in NHL and lung cancer incidence rates (per 100,000) as a function of distance from industrial facility 5 (see Fig. 2)

to the fact that plumes of air pollution from tall industrial smokestacks land at some distances from the emission sources. To take this non-linear effect into account, we introduced a quadratic term of $\widetilde{dist_{ji}}$ into the models, in addition to its linear term, and repeated the analysis. To estimate parameters in Eq. (5) multivariate regression models, incorporating linear and non-linear terms, were used. In the following discussion, *only* non-linear models, providing better fits and generality compared to ordinary linear models, are reported.

The probability surfaces were generated using the EBK interpolation technique in the ArcGIS™10.x Software [54], while the multivariate regression analysis was performed using the SPSSv.23™ software [62]. The probability level of less than 0.01 (<1%) was set as the accepted statistical significance level.

Results

Theoretical examples

Figure 1 features morbidity rates, marked by dots surrounding two *pre-defined* sources of exposure—a triangle (Fig. 1a) and a line (Fig. 1c). As mentioned previously, in these diagrams, dots, marking morbidity observations, are sized proportionally to the predefined morbidity rates: the higher the morbidity rate: the bigger the dot that marks it. In line with the expected distance decay relationship, larger dots are positioned closer to the pre-defined sources of exposure, while smaller dots are placed farther away from these sources (see Fig. 1a, c). Concurrently, maps in the right panel (Fig. 1b, d) feature morbidity source estimates, calculated using the estimation approach described in "Empirical validation" section. As Fig. 1b, d show, the spots of high probability of being the source of exposure, marked by orange and red colours in the right panel, correspond, fairly accurately, to the actual locations of the pre-defined health hazards (Fig. 1a, c).

GHMA study

Figure 4a, b shows raster surfaces based on the determination coefficients (R^2_{ji}), obtained from *bivariate* regression models, estimated separately for lung (Fig. 4a) and NHL cancers (Fig. 4b). Concurrently, Fig. 4c, d shows source identification surfaces based on the determination coefficients obtained from *multivariate* regression models. The best performing regression models (both controlled and uncontrolled), are reported in Tables 1 and 2.[3]

Figure 4 has similar coloring such as that used in the theoretical examples, discussed in "Theoretical examples" section and shown in Fig. 1. In particular, warm-coloured pixels in these diagrams correspond to the highest improvements in the models' determination coefficients, observed by adding wind-adjusted distances from these pixels to the models, containing a constant "pre-set" of socio-demographic variables, discussed in the "Empirical validation" section. Concurrently, blue and green colours in these maps mark pixels adding proximity to which result in relatively small changes in the models' determination coefficients.

As Fig. 4 shows, there are two most probable *loci* associated with the observed morbidity—the central business district saturated with traffic routes located in the northeastern part of the study area (for lung cancer cases) and a spot located in the central part of the study area (for both cancer cases under the study) (see Figs. 1, 4a, b). Adding proximities to these spots results in increases in the models' determination coefficients by up to 14–29% in bivariate models and by up to 7–13% in multivariate models, depending on the cancer type under analysis (see Tables 1, 2).

Several interaction effects were also tested. Among them, two effects (i.e., the side of the Carmel mountain vs. elevation above the sea level and the side of the Carmel mountain vs. distance to the identified hotspot), were found to be statistically significant. Regression models incorporating these interaction effects are reported in Table 3.

Discussion

Empirical studies use several methods for the spatial identification of potential health hazards. Such methods are mostly based on the measurements of air pollutants at the receptor sites, followed by a comparison of the results of such measurements with the chemical composition of particles emitted from different emission sources [14, 15, 20, 23, 24, 26, 31, 32, 35]. However, the empirical implementation of these methods requires a considerable amount of information on the concentration of specific particles, detailed wind regime assessments and topographic attributes, which are not always available to researchers [14, 20, 26].

As an alternative approach, proximities of various health hazards, such as roadways, industrial sites, nuclear power plants and gas wells, are commonly used in epidemiological and health geography studies as *proxies* for unknown exposures (see *inter alia* [11, 27, 28, 30].

In the present study, we extend this *distance gradient* method to the spatial identification of a priori *unidentified* hazards. The underlying assumption behind the proposed identification approach is that people living in a close proximity to a morbidity source, tend to exhibit, *ceteris paribus*, a higher rate of morbidity than those living at a distance from that source [11, 30]. To account for this effect, we estimated distance decay gradients of morbidity for alternative potential "risk source" locations and then ranked these locations based on the strength of association between the observed morbidity patterns and wind-direction weighted proximities to these locations.

In empirical studies, several measures are commonly used to estimate the improvement of regression models attributed to changes in the predictors' set. Such measures include the log-likelihood criterion, the Akaike information criterion (AIC), the Bayesian information criterion (BIC), the Schwarz criterion (SBC), Mallow's C_p statistic, and several others. These criteria monitor changes in the regression residuals and thus help to select the combination of explanatory variables and the functional form of the model best fitted to the data under analysis [63]. In this study, we used R^2, a commonly used measure of model fit, also known as the coefficient of determination. Our preference for this measure was motivated by the fact that this measure does not depend on the order of variables, has a specific interval of change (0; 1); it also does not depend on the functional form of the regression equation used [64]. Using this measure and applying it to the constant set of control variables, we monitored changes in the regression fit attributed to changes in wind adjusted distances to alternative hazard locations, which were introduced into the models one by one. Since the set of control variables used in the study included main factors known to affect cancer incidence rates in urban areas [51, 61, 65, 66], we did not consider it feasible to alter this predetermined set of controls. In other words, according to the proposed identification approach, the coefficient of determination, R^2, was considered a likelihood criterion, using which we compared several combinations of input parameters. These

---

[3] The models reported in Tables 1 and 2 feature distances to the pixels adding which resulted in the largest changes in the models' determination coefficients. Such pixels are marked by deep red colors in Fig. 4.

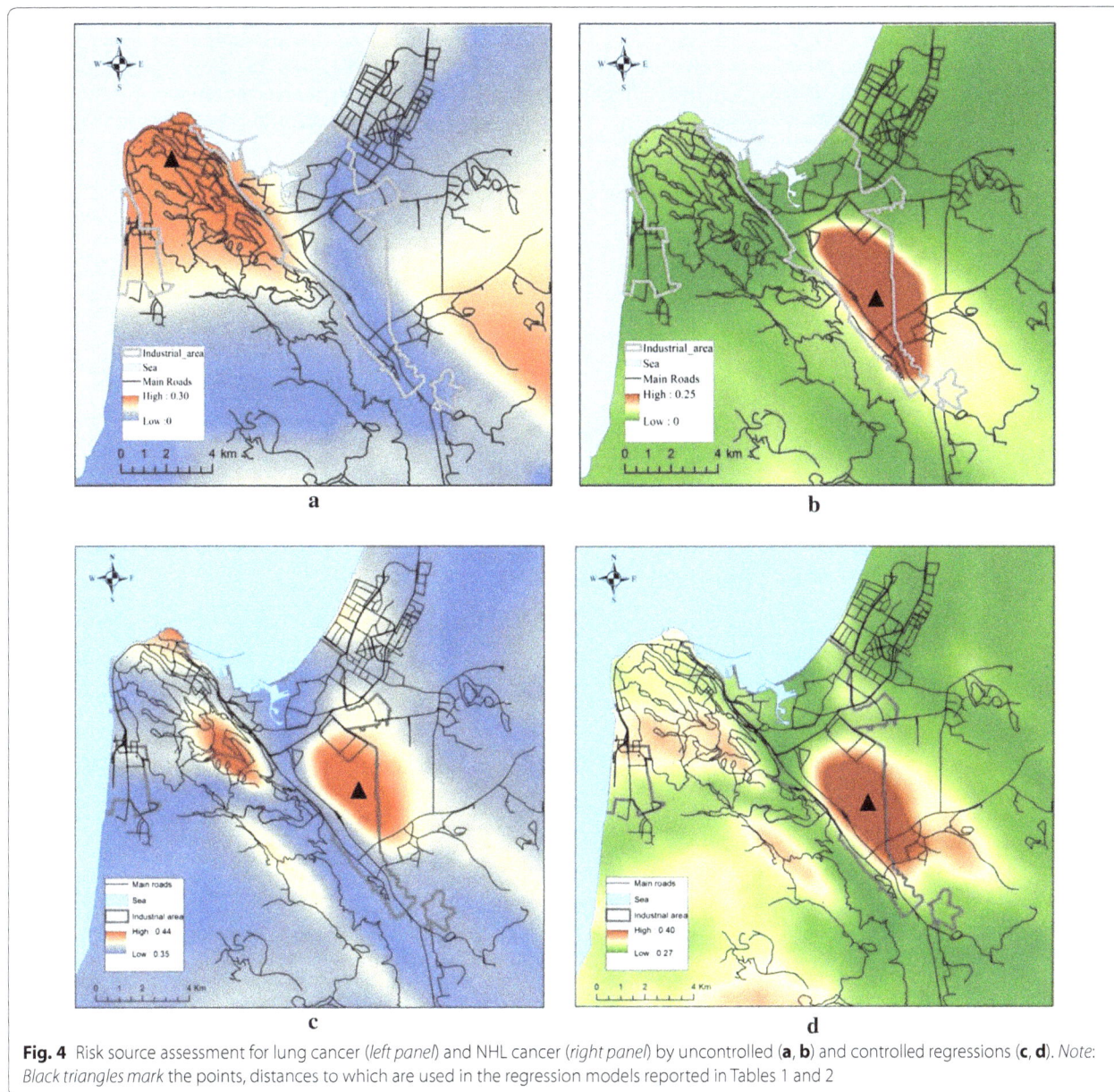

Fig. 4 Risk source assessment for lung cancer (*left panel*) and NHL cancer (*right panel*) by uncontrolled (**a**, **b**) and controlled regressions (**c**, **d**). *Note: Black triangles mark* the points, distances to which are used in the regression models reported in Tables 1 and 2

combinations included the constant set of confounders and a number of vectors of wind-weighted distances between alternative potential health risk sources and morbidity observations.

In several theoretical examples we designed, the proposed approach helped to identify correctly the predefined locations of health hazards, while in a real-world case study, the main health hazard were identified as a spot in the industrial zone, which hosts petrochemical facilities, and a major transportation hub in the central business district of the city. According to previous studies (see *inter alia*, [11, 38, 67]), petrochemical industries are known to be associated with evaluated cancer morbidity in surrounding residential areas. In a

separate study, [67] investigated morbidity near nuclear power plants and found it to be linked to childhood cancer.

The results of the present study also correspond to the findings of other studies which revealed geographic concentrations of cancer morbidity near heavy roads [30, 40, 41, 68], and in proximity to industrial areas [11, 38]. Thus, [69] identified the link between traffic-related pollution and respiratory morbidity, measured by lung function impairment.

Several limitations of our study need to be mentioned. First and foremost, the present study is an ecological analysis, in which explanatory variables are measured at the group level or as distance gradients,

Table 1 The association between double kernel density (DKD) of lung and NHL morbidity rates (cases per 100,000 residents) and distance to the revealed exposure sources (Method—*bivariate* regression, distance variables—linear and quadratic wind-adjusted distance terms)[c]

Variables	Model 1 B^a and (t^b)	Model 2 B^a and (t^b)
A. Lung cancer		
(Constant)	13.935 (58.947*)	1.131 (7.965*)
Distance	−5.500E−0.40 (−19.350*)	0.002 (4.364*)
Distance^2	–	−1.115E−07 (−4.152*)
No. of reference points	1000	1000
R^2	0.286	0.301
$R^2_{adjusted}$	0.285	0.299
F	374.419*	133.819*
B. NHL cancer		
(Constant)	4.656 (17.237*)	−3.697 (−5.219*)
Distance	3.380E−04 (8.409*)	0.003 (13.916*)
Distance^2	–	−2.189E−07 (−12.791*)
No. of reference points	1000	1000
R^2	0.070	0.205
$R^2_{adjusted}$	0.069	0.204
F	70.714*	120.722*

Model 1: Bivariate linear model

Model 2: Bivariate quadratic model

* indicates a 0.01 two-tailed significance level

[a] Regression coefficient

[b] *t*-statistics in the parentheses

[c] The models reported in the table are estimated for the distances to the "best performing" source locations, marked by small triangles in Fig. 4, that is, source locations distances to which help to improve the models' fits most significantly (see text for explanations)

Table 2 The association between double kernel density (DKD) of lung and NHL morbidity cancer rates (cases per 100,000) and distance to the revealed exposure sources (Method—*multivariate* regression, distance variables—linear and quadratic wind-adjusted distance terms)[c]

Variables	Model 3[d] B^a and (t^b)	Model 4[d] B^a and (t^b)
A. Lung cancer		
(Constant)	6.661 (2.591*)	−12.629 (−3.959*)
Distance	−5.159E−04 (−7.470*)	0.003 (8.235*)
Distance^2	–	−2.620E−07 (−8.159*)
N of reference points	1000	1000
R^2	0.393	0.458
$R^2_{adjusted}$	0.386	0.450
ΔR^2	–	0.065
F change[e]	–	36.658*
B. NHL cancer		
(Constant)	9.119 (5.231*)	−9.144 (−4.388*)
Distance	−2.862E−04 (−5.991*)	0.003 (13.359*)
Distance^2	–	−2.415E−07 (−12.791*)
N of reference points	1000	1000
R^2	0.242	0.369
$R^2_{adjusted}$	0.234	0.361
ΔR^2	–	0.127
F change[e]	–	92.855*

Model 3: Multivariate linear model

Model 4: Multivariate quadratic model

[a] Regression coefficient

[b] *t*-statistics in the parentheses

[c] The models reported in the table are estimated for the distances to the "best performing" source locations, marked by small triangles in Fig. 4, that is, source locations distances to which help to improve the models' fits most significantly (see text for explanations)

[d] The models are controlled for distance to the nearest main road (m), elevation above the sea level (m), percent of Jewish population in the SCA, SCA Socio-economic status, distance to the sea (m), manufacturing employment (% of total population of SCA), NO_x (ppb), $PM_{2.5}$ (ppb), total population over 65 (%), smoking rate in the SCA (%) and distance to the nearest main road (m)

[e] F-test of R^2-change compared to model without hazard source distances (i.e., Models 3A or 3B, respectively)

and not estimated for individuals. Therefore, we cannot attribute causality in the relationships we observed. However, the strength of population-level studies is that they represent large population groups and reflect varying levels of exposure. The purpose of such studies is not to prove the relationships but rather to generate hypotheses which can further be examined using individual level data [70].

Conclusions

This paper contributes to the existing body of literature by extending the traditional distance gradient method (DGM) to the identification of potential health hazards, which geographic location is a priori *unknown*. The results of the study demonstrate the utility of the proposed method for epidemiological studies which goal

is to identify potential sources of exposure to which the observed morbidity is related. We also consider it important that the proposed approach does not require extensive input information and can be used as a preliminary risk assessment tool, helping to identify potential environmental risk factors behind the observed population morbidity patterns.

The proposed approach can be used by researches worldwide in cases in which specific sources of locally elevated morbidity are unclear or cannot be identified by traditional methods. For instance, the proposed method

Table 3 The association between double kernel density (DKD) of lung and NHL morbidity rates (cases per 100,000 residents) and distance to the revealed exposure sources (Method—*multivariate* regression, distance variables—quadratic wind-adjusted distance terms; interaction terms added)[c]

Variables	Model 5 B^a and (t^b)	Model 6 B^a and (t^b)	Model 7 B^a and (t^b)
A. Lung cancer			
(Constant)	−15.663 (−7.937*)	−15.125 (−4.832*)	−15.791 (−4.948*)
Distance	0.004 (8.591*)	0.004 (9.314*)	0.004 (8.109*)
Distance^2	−2.689E−07 (−8.258*)	−2.945E−07 (−9.067*)	−2.715E−07 (−7.587*)
No. of reference points	1000	1000	1000
R^2	0.478	0.480	0.480
$R^2_{adjusted}$	0.470	0.471	0.472
F	56.308*	56.582*	56.790*
B. NHL cancer			
(Constant)	−9.890 (−4.709*)	−9.233 (−4.402*)	−10.001 (−4736*)
Distance	0.003 (13.563*)	0.003 (13.119*)	0.003 (12.436*)
Distance^2	−2.438E−07 (−12.930*)	−2.457 (−11.995*)	−2.486E−07 (−11.079*)
No. of reference points	1000	1000	1000
R^2	0.373	0.374	0.374
$R^2_{adjusted}$	0.364	0.364	0.364
F	39.311*	39.288*	36.704*

See comments to Table 2

Model 5: Multivariate quadratic model with the Side of Mountain Carmel vs. elevation above the sea level interaction term

Model 6: Multivariate quadratic model with the Side of Mountain Carmel vs. Distance to the identified hotspot interaction term

Model 7: Multivariate quadratic model with both interaction terms added

can be used in empirical studies in which available epidemiological data can help to map the existing morbidity patterns, and then to identify potential sources of exposure to which the observed morbidity patterns are related. However, future studies will be needed to extend the theoretical justification of the proposed approach, and to determine its applicability to other urban areas and to other health outcomes.

Abbreviations
CMB: chemical mass balance; DGM: distance gradient method; DKD: double Kernel density method; EBK: empirical Bayesian Kriging; GHMA: greater Haifa metropolitan area; KD: Kernel density; NHL: non-Hodgkin lymphoma cancer; PDF: probability density function; RTA: residence time analysis; SCA: small census area.

Authors' contributions
Ms. Svechkina carried out statistical analysis, performed mapping and drafted the manuscript. Dr. Zusman took part in statistical analysis, designed statistical scripts and assisted with mapping. Ms. Rybnikova helped with data assembling and processing. Prof. Portnov conceived of the study, assisted with the study design and implementation and helped to draft the manuscript. All authors read and approved the final manuscript.

Acknowledgements
The authors express their gratitude to the Israel Center of Disease Control for providing data on cancer morbidity.

Competing interests
The authors declare no conflict of interests, including personal or financial relationships pertinent to the study.

Funding
The present study was conducted as a part of the research project, entitled: "Epidemiological monitoring of the Haifa Bay Area: 2015–2020," funded by the Haifa Municipal Association for Environmental protection (Contract # 45783).

Appendix 1
See Table 4.

Table 4 Descriptive statistics of the variables used in the multivariate regressions

Variables	Minimum	Maximum	Mean	SD
DKD of NHL cancer cases (per 100,000)	0.00	18.54	6.78	2.49
DKD of Lung cancer cases (per 100,000)	0.00	27.22	10.08	4.04
Average distance to main industrial facilities (m)	755.57	9996.96	5402.55	2095.05
Distance to the nearest main road (m)	0.54	1217.84	163.71	182.13
Distance to the seashore (m)	2.38	14,302.92	4397.48	3872.51
Manufacturing employment (% of total population of the SCA)	0.00	29.30	14.68	6.20
Percent of Jewish population in the SCA	0.00	100.00	91.05	20.54
SCA socio-economic status (Index)	−1.62	2.88	0.44	1.08
NO_x in 2003 (IDW interpolation, ppb)	7.68	133.12	27.97	15.00
$PM_{2.5}$ in 2003 (IDW interpolation, ppb)	17.20	27.80	20.11	1.25
Total population over 65 (%)	0.00	0.39	0.17	0.06
Smoking rate in the SCA in 2003 (%)	15.07	41.78	18.87	3.49
Elevation above the sea level (m)	0.00	440.00	110.49	124.83

Appendix 2: Wind weighted transformation of distances

Adjustments for wind frequency and directions were implemented in a number of studies dealing with the measurements of directional concentrations of urban air pollutants (see *inter alia*, [48, 49, 71, 72]). The empirical literature reports several approaches to distance transformation, based on the seasonal analysis of data [48] or on the amount of precipitation, solar radiation, maximum and minimum temperatures [49] and average wind speed [71].

For the purpose of wind adjustment, we used the wind frequency rose of the study area, plotted at a one-degree angular resolution and showing the average annual distribution of wind frequencies for each one-degree angle. Since the probability of wind from point j to point i (w_{ji}) was assumed to be random, we used the probability density function (PDF) instead of a fixed distribution function. PDF describes the relative likelihood for the random variable, e.g., wind frequency to take on a given value (w_{ji}):

$$PDF_w\left(w_{ji}, \lambda_j\right) = \lambda_j \cdot e^{-\lambda_j \cdot W_{ji}}, \quad \forall W_{ji} \in (0, 1),$$

$$\lambda_j = \frac{1}{\overline{w_{ji}}}, \text{ for } \overline{w_j} = \frac{1}{n}\sum_{i=1}^{n} w_{ji}. \qquad (7)$$

where w_{ji} is annual wind frequency from point j to point i, $\overline{w_j}$ - average annual wind frequency from point j, n - is a number of i points, $\lambda_j > 0$ is the parameter of the distribution, also known as the *rate* parameter.

Next, distances between j and i ($dist_{ji}$) were adjusted for wind frequency and direction as follows:

$$\widetilde{dist_{ji}} = T\left(dist_{ji} | W_{ji}\right) = dist_{ji} \cdot PDF\left(W_{ji}, \lambda_j\right). \qquad (8)$$

According to this transformation, distances between point j and i with frequent winds are reduced, while distances between points with infrequent winds remain unchanged.

Appendix 3 Description of mathematical logic symbols used in the manuscript

∀—symbol indicates "for all", "for any", "for each";

→—symbol indicates domain and codomain of a function;

∈—symbol indicates affiliation to any set of elements.

References

1. Burkitt DP. Geography of a disease: purpose and possibilities from geographical medicine. In: Rothschild HR, editor. Biocultural aspects of disease. New York, NY: Academic Press; 1981. pp. 133–51.
2. Pope CA, Dockery DW. Health effects of fine particulate air pollution: lines that connect. J Air Waste Manag Assoc. 2006;56(6):709–42.
3. Kampa M, Castanas E. Human health effects of air pollution. Environ Pollut. 2008;151(2):362–7.
4. Chen X, Ye J. When the wind blows: spatial spillover effects of urban air pollution. Environment for Development Discussion: Paper Series 2015; EFD DP 15-15.
5. Cogliano V, Baan R, Straif K, Grosse Y, Lauby-Secretan B, El Ghissassi F, et al. Preventable exposures associated with human cancers. J Natl Cancer Inst. 2011;103(24):1827–39.
6. McKenzie LM, Witter RZ, Newman LS, Adgate JL. Human health risk assessment of air emissions from development of unconventional natural gas resources. Sci Total Environ. 2012;424(1):79–87.
7. Laumbach RJ, Howard MK. Respiratory health effects of air pollution: update on biomass smoke and traffic pollution. J Allergy Clin Immunol. 2012;129(1):3–11.
8. Tuna F, Buluc M. Analysis of PM10 pollutant in Istanbul by using Kriging and IDW methods: between 2003 and 2012. Int J Comput Inf Technol 2015;4(1):170–5.

9. Ramis R, Gomes-Barroso D, Tamayo I, Garcia-Perez J, Marales A, Romaguera EP, Lopez-Abente G. Spatial analysis of childhood cancer: a case control study. PLoS ONE. 2015;10(5):1–15.

10. Jacquez GM, Greiling DA. Geographic boundaries in breast, lung and colorectal cancers in relation to exposure to air toxics in Long Island, New York. Int J Health Geogr. 2003;2:4.

11. Zusman M, Dubnov J, Barchana M, Portnov BA. Residential proximity of petroleum storage tanks and associated cancer risks: double Kernel density approach vs. zonal estimates. Sci Total Environment. 2012;441:265–76.

12. Portnov BA, Reiser B, Karkabi K, Cohen-Kastel O, Dubnov J. High prevalence of childhood asthma in Northern Israel is linked to air pollution by particulate matter: evidence from GIS analysis and Bayesian model averaging. Int J Environ Health Res. 2012;22(3):249–69.

13. Hamra GB, Guha N, Cohen A, et al. Outdoor particulate matter exposure and lung cancer: a systematic review and meta-analysis. Environ Health Perspect. 2014;122(9):906–11.

14. Cooper JA, Watson JG. Receptor oriented methods of air particulate source apportionment. J Air Pollut Control Assoc. 1980;30(10):1116–24.

15. Stohl A. Trajectory statistics—a new method to establish source-receptor relationships of air pollutants and its application to the transport of particulate sulfate in Europe. Atmos Environ. 1996;30(4):579–87.

16. Lupu A, Maenhaunt W. Application and comparison of two statistical trajectory techniques for identification of source regions of atmospheric aerosol species. Atmos Environ. 2002;36:5607–18.

17. Pilz J, Spöck G. Why do we need and how should we implement Bayesian kriging methods. Stoch Env Res Risk Assess. 2008;22(5):621–32.

18. Zhu L, Huang X, Shi H, Cai X, Song Y. Transport pathways and potential sources of PM10 in Beijing. Atmos Environ. 2011;45:594–604.

19. Singh KP, Gupta S, Rai P. Identifying pollution sources and predicting urban air quality using ensemble learning methods. Atmos Environ. 2013;80:426–37.

20. Cesari R, Paradisi P, Allegrini P. A trajectory statistical method for the identification of sources associated with concentration peak events. Int J Environ Pollut. 2014;55:94–103.

21. Al-Harbi M. Assessment of air quality in two different urban localities. Int J Environ Res. 2014;8(1):15–26.

22. Belis CA, Pernigotti D, Karagulian F, Pirovano G, Larsen BR, Gerboles M, et al. A new methodology to assess the performance and uncertainty of source apportionment models in intercomparison exercises. Atmos Environ. 2015;119:35–44.

23. Salvador P, Artinano B, Alonso DG, Querol X, Alastuey A. Identification and characterisation of sources of PM10 in Madrid (Spain) by statistical methods. Atmos Environ. 2004;38:435–47.

24. Xie Y, Berkowitz CM. The use of positive matrix factorization with conditional probability functions in air quality studies: an application to hydrocarbon emissions in Houston, Texas. Atmos Environ. 2006;40:3070–91.

25. Wang C, Zhou X, Chen R, Duan X, Kuang X, Kan H. Estimation of the effects of ambient air pollution on life expectancy of urban residents in China. Atmos Environ. 2013;80:347–51.

26. Zhang ZY, Wong MS, Lee KH. Estimation of potential source regions of PM2.5 in Beijing using backward trajectories. Atmos Pollut. 2015;6:173–7.

27. Moore DA, Carpenter TE. Spatial analytical methods and geographic information systems: use in health research and epidemiology. Epidemiol Rev. 1999;20(2):143–61.

28. Rezaeian M, Dunn G, Leger S, Appleby L. Geographical epidemiology, spatial analysis geographical information system: a multidisciplinary glossary. J Epidemiol Community Health. 2007;61:98–102.

29. Gatrell AC, Bailey TC, Diggle PJ, Rowlingsont BS. Spatial point pattern analysis and its application in geographical epidemiology. Trans Inst Br Geogr. 1996;21(1):256–74.

30. Paz S, Linn S, Portnov BA, Lazimi A, Futerman B, Barchana M. Non-Hodgkin Lymphoma (NHL) linkage with residence near heavy roads—a case study from Haifa Bay, Israel. Health Place. 2009;15:636–41.

31. Hopke PK. Recent developments in receptor modelling. J Chemom. 2003;17:255–65.

32. Kim E, Hopke PK. Comparison between conditional probability function and nonparametric regression for fine particle source directions. Atmos Environ. 2004;38:4667–73.

33. Begum BA, Kimb E, Biswasa SK, Hopke PK. Investigation of sources of atmospheric aerosol at urban and semi-urban areas in Bangladesh. Atmos Environ. 2004;38:3025–38.

34. Sacks JD, Ito K, Wilson WE, Neas LM. Impact of covariate models on the assessment of the air pollution-mortality association in a single- and multipollutant context. Am J Epidemiol. 2012;176(7):622–34.

35. Banerjee T, Murari V, Kumar M, Raju MP. Source apportionment of airborne particulates through receptor modelling: Indian scenario. Atmospheric Research 2015; 164–87

36. Pirovano G, Colombi C, Balzarini A, Riva GM, Gianelle V, Lonati G. PM2.5 source apportionment in Lombardy (Italy): comparison of receptor and chemistry-transport modelling results. Atmos Environ. 2015;106:56–70.

37. Johnson S. The ghost map: the story of London's most terrifying epidemic—and how it changed science, cities and the modern world 2006; 195–196.

38. Sermage-Faure C, Laurier D, Goujon-Bellec S, Chartier M, Guyot-Goubin A, Rudant J, et al. Childhood leukaemia around French nuclear power plant. The Geocap study, 2002–2007. Int J Cancer. 2012;131(5):E769–80.

39. Yorifuji T, Kashima S. Air pollution: another cause of lung cancer. Lancet Oncol. 2013;14(9):788–9.

40. Su JG, Apte JS, Lipsitt J, Garcia-Gonzales DA, Beckerman BS, Nazelle A, Texcalac-Sangrador JL, Jerrett M. Populations potentially exposed to traffic-related air pollution in seven world cities. Environ Int. 2015;78:82–9.

41. Price K, Plante C, Goudreau S, Boldo EI, Perron S, Smargiassi A. Risk of childhood asthma prevalence attributable to residential proximity to major roads in Montreal, Canada. Can J Public Health. 2012;103(2):113–8.

42. Kim HH, Lee CS, Jeon JM, Yu SD, Lee CW, Park JH, Shin DC, Lim YW. Analysis of the association between air pollution and allergic diseases exposure from nearby sources of ambient air pollution within elementary school zones in four Korean cities. Environ Sci Pollut Res. 2013;20(7):4831–46.

43. Houston D, Ong P, Wu J, Winer A. Proximity of licensed child care facilities to near roadway vehicle pollution. Am J Public Health. 2006;96:1611–7.

44. Lumley T. Efficient execution of Stone's likelihood ratio tests for disease clustering. Comput Stat Data Anal. 1995;20(5):499–510.

45. Tango TA. Class of tests for detecting 'general' and 'focused' clustering of rare diseases. Stat Med. 1995;14(21–22):2323–34.

46. Bithell JF. The choice of test for detecting raised disease risk near a point source. Stat Med. 1995;14:2309–22.

47. Gatrel A. GIS and health. London; Philadelphia, PA: Taylor & Francis; 1998.

48. Dore AJ, Vieno M, Fournier N, Weston KJ, Sutton MA. Development of a new wind-rose for the British Isles using radiosonde data, and application to an atmospheric transport model. Q J R Meteorol Soc. 2006;132:2769–84.

49. Chen X, Ye J. When the wind blows: spatial spillover effects of urban air pollution. environment for development discussion: paper series 2015; EFD DP 15–15.

50. Bailey D, Plenys T, Solomon GM, Campbell TR, Feuer GR, Masters J et al. Harboring pollution: strategies to clean up US ports. Natural Resources Defence Council 2004.

51. Anand P, Kunnumakkara AB, Sundaram C, Harikumar KB, Tharakan ST, Lai OS, et al. Cancer is a preventable disease that requires major lifestyle changes. Pharm Res. 2008;25(9):2097–116.

52. Chen H, Goldberg MS, Villeneuve PJ. A systematic review of the relation between long-term exposure to ambient air pollution and chronic diseases. Rev Environ Health. 2008;23(4):243–97.

53. Krivoruchko K. Empirical Bayesian Kriging implemented in ArcGIS Geostatistical Analyst. http://www.esri.com (2016). Accessed 10 Feb 2016.

54. ESRI: ArcGIS desktop help 10.2. 2015. http://webhelp.esri.com. Accessed 20 Jan 2015.

55. Ministry of Health (MH): Israel National Cancer Registry. 2012. http://www.health.gov.il. Accessed 10 Feb 2016.

56. Rushton G, Armstrong MP, Gittler J, Greene BR, Pavlik CE, West MM, et al. Geocoding in cancer research: a review. Am J Prev Med. 2006;30(2):16–24.

57. Makimoto Y, Yamamoto S, Takano H et al. Imaging findings of radiation-induced sarcoma of the head and neck. BJR 2014;80(958):790.

58. Israel Ministry of Environmental Protection (IMEP). Map of the air monitoring stations. 2016. http://www.sviva.gov.il. Accessed 21 Feb 2016.

59. Nyberg F, Gustavsson P, Järup L, Bellander T, Berglind N, Jakobsson R, et al. Urban air pollution and lung cancer in Stockholm. Epidemiology. 2000;11(5):487–95.

60. Howard J. Minimum latency and types or categories of cancer. World Trade Center Health Program 2012; 17.

61. Norman RE, Ryan A, Grant K, Sitas F, Scott JG. Environmental contributions to childhood cancers. J Environ Immunol Toxicol. 2014;2(2):86–98.

62. IBM: SPSS Statistics desktop help 22. http://www.ibm.com. Accessed 1 Feb 2016.

63. Burnham KP, Anderson DR. Model selection and multimodel inference: a practical information-theoretic approach. Berlin: Springer; 2002.

64. Baltagi BH. A companion to theoretical econometrics. Malden: Blackwell Publishing Ltd; 2003.

65. Adams RJ, Piantadosi C, Ettridge K, Miller C, Wilson C, Tucker G, Hill C. Functional health literacy mediates the relationship between socio-economic status, perceptions and lifestyle behaviors related to cancer risk in an Australian population. Patient Educ Couns. 2013;91(2):206–12.

66. Quaglia A, Lillini R, Mamo C, Ivaldi E, Vercelli M. Socio-economic inequalities: a review of methodological issues and the relationships with cancer survival. Crit Rev Oncol/Hematol. 2013;85(3):266–77.

67. Spix C, Schmiedel S, Kaatsch P, Schulze-Rath R, Blettner M. Case-control study on childhood cancer in the vicinity of nuclear power plants in Germany 1980–2003. Eur J Cancer. 2008;44(2):275–84.

68. Amram O, Abernethy R, Brauer M, Davies H, Allen RW. Proximity of public elementary schools to major roads in Canadian urban areas. Int J Health Geogr. 2011;10:68–78.

69. Nuvolone D, Maggiore R, Maio S, Fresco R, Baldacci S, Carrozzi L, et al. Geographical information system and environmental epidemiology: a cross-sectional spatial analysis of the effects of traffic-related air pollution on population respiratory health. Environ Health. 2011;10:12.

70. Lindenmayer DB, Likens GE, Andersen A, Bowman DC, Bull M, Burnus E, et al. Value of long-term ecological studies. Austral Ecol. 2012;37(7):745–57.

71. Xu X, Akhtar US. Identification of potential regional sources of atmospheric total gaseous mercury in Windsor, Ontario, Canada using hybrid

72. receptor modeling. Atmos Chem Phys. 2010;10:7073–83.

72. Zoë L, Fleming ZL, Monks PS, Manning AJ. Review: untangling the influence of air-mass history in interpreting observed atmospheric composition. Atmos Res. 2012;104–105:1–39.

73. Israel Central Bureau of Statistics (ICBS). Statistical abstract of Israel: population, by population group, religion, sex and age. 2016. http://www.cbs.gov.il/. Accessed 21 Nov 2015.

74. Israel Central Bureau of Statistics (ICBS): Statistical abstract of Israel 2015: population, by district, sub district and religion. 2016. http://www.cbs.gov.il/. Accessed 1 Feb 2016.

75. Bithell JF. An application of density estimation to geographical epidemiology. Stat Med. 1990;9:691–701.

76. Shi X. Selection of bandwidth type and adjustment side in kernel density estimation over inhomogeneous backgrounds. Int J Geogr Inf Sci. 2010;24(5):643–60.

77. Portnov BA, Zusman M. Spatial data analysis using kernel density tools. In: Wang J, editor. Encyclopedia of business analytics and optimization. Hershey: Business Science Reference; 2014. p. 2252–64.

78. Kloog I, Haim A, Portnov BA. Using kernel density function as an urban analysis tool: investigating the association between nightlight exposure and the incidence of breast cancer in Haifa, Israel. Comput Environ Urban Syst. 2009;33:55–63.

79. Portnov BA, Dubnov J, Barchana M. Studying the association between air pollution and lung cancer incidence in a large metropolitan area using a kernel density function. Socio-Econ Plan Sci. 2009;43(3):141–50.

80. Zusman M, Broitman D, Portnov BA. Application of the double kernel density approach to the multivariate analysis of attributeless event point dataset. Lett Spatial Resour Sci 2015; 1–20.

81. Silverman BW. Density estimation for statistics and data analysis. London, New York: Chapman and Hall; 1986.

82. Lambe M, Blomqvist P, Bellocco R. Seasonal variation in the diagnosis of cancer: a study based on national cancer registration in Sweden. Br J Cancer. 2003;88(9):1358–60.

Spatially explicit assessment of heat health risk by using multi-sensor remote sensing images and socioeconomic data in Yangtze River Delta, China

Qian Chen[1], Mingjun Ding[2], Xuchao Yang[1]* ⓘ, Kejia Hu[1] and Jiaguo Qi[1,3]

Abstract

Background: The increase in the frequency and intensity of extreme heat events, which are potentially associated with climate change in the near future, highlights the importance of heat health risk assessment, a significant reference for heat-related death reduction and intervention. However, a spatiotemporal mismatch exists between gridded heat hazard and human exposure in risk assessment, which hinders the identification of high-risk areas at finer scales.

Methods: A human settlement index integrated by nighttime light images, enhanced vegetation index, and digital elevation model data was utilized to assess the human exposure at high spatial resolution. Heat hazard and vulnerability index were generated by land surface temperature and demographic and socioeconomic census data, respectively. Spatially explicit assessment of heat health risk and its driving factors was conducted in the Yangtze River Delta (YRD), east China at 250 m pixel level.

Results: High-risk areas were mainly distributed in the urbanized areas of YRD, which were mostly driven by high human exposure and heat hazard index. In some less-urbanized cities and suburban and rural areas of mega-cities, the heat health risks are in second priority. The risks in some less-developed areas were high despite the low human exposure index because of high heat hazard and vulnerability index.

Conclusions: This study illustrated a methodology for identifying high-risk areas by combining freely available multi-source data. Highly urbanized areas were considered hotspots of high heat health risks, which were largely driven by the increasing urban heat island effects and population density in urban areas. Repercussions of overheating were weakened due to the low social vulnerability in some central areas benefitting from the low proportion of sensitive population or the high level of socioeconomic development. By contrast, high social vulnerability intensifies heat health risks in some less-urbanized cities and suburban areas of mega-cities.

Keywords: Spatial risk assessment, Heat health risk, Remote sensing, GIS, Yangtze River Delta

*Correspondence: yangxuchao@zju.edu.cn
[1] Institute of Island and Coastal Ecosystems, Ocean College, Zhejiang University, Zhoushan 316021, China
Full list of author information is available at the end of the article

Background

Climate change, with global warming as the main feature, has become the biggest challenge for human health [1, 2]. Extreme heat events (EHEs), as one of the most serious meteorological disasters, are projected to increase in frequency, intensity, and duration in the background of future climate warming [3]. Exposure to high ambient temperature not only is the leading cause of weather-related morbidity (e.g., cardiovascular, cerebrovascular, and respiratory diseases) [4] but may also lead to human deaths in extreme cases. For example, two devastating heat wave in Europe in 2003 and Russia in 2010 led to a death toll of 70,000 and 55,000, respectively [5, 6]. The health implications of extreme heat events highlight the significance of studies on risk assessment and identification of high-risk population. Climate change adaptation is also increasingly linked to natural hazard risk management [7, 8].

There are ongoing observational studies that show a significant increase in the incidence and mortality of urban residents during EHEs [9, 10], which are associated with the urban heat island (UHI) whose effects are aggravated during heat waves [4, 11, 12]. Dousset et al. [13] analyzed mortality in Paris during EHEs in the summer of 2003; results showed that mortality is related to the distribution of high nighttime temperatures generally driven by the enhanced UHI effects at night. Urban residents are therefore particularly vulnerable to severe and sustained heat stress [14, 15]. Spatially explicit identification of high-risk hotspots will ensure appropriate development of targeted prevention and mitigation of EHEs in a warmer future world considering the projected augmentation in urban population and frequency of EHEs.

An increasing number of studies utilized the risk conceptual framework proposed by Crichton [8, 16] to fully understand heat-related risk patterns. However, there usually exist two deficiencies in previous heat health risk assessment, which related to heat hazard and human exposure respectively. For heat-related health risk, hazards refer to the possibility of EHEs occurring in a specific space where people live or engage in anthropogenic activities, characterizing the closeness of humans to EHEs [17, 18]. For a large study area, available air temperature data are commonly from the sparse government-operated stations. Those existing data are constrained by their spatial locations and are therefore inadequate for capturing the temperature gradient within a specific area. Previous studies on the association between ambient temperature and mortality also pointed out that the use of temperature data from sparse weather stations led to underestimation of the temperature effects [19]. In addition to coarse heat hazard information obtained from meteorological station [20, 21], satellite-derived

land surface temperature (LST) data were increasingly used to measure heat risk because they offer spatially-detailed heat-related information [22–25]. Moreover, it is noteworthy that although the synergies between UHI and heat waves have received increasing attention because of their potential health and environmental impacts [11, 26], most studies on spatial heat hazard assessment only considered the daytime temperature but ignored the UHI-related nighttime temperature [23, 27], which may result in significant underestimation of heat health risk in urban areas.

For human exposure analysis, demographic data is a fundamental component of disaster risk models. Detailed population information is required to assess casualties, determine shelter needs, and properly implement evacuation plans in pre-disaster and post-disaster phases [28, 29]. The absence of population data is a major obstacle to decision-making and disaster relief in parts of the developing world due to the lack of data collection or the unavailability of useful accompanying geographical data [30]. Population density maps on the basis of census data lack sufficient spatial details of the geographically-heterogeneous population distribution within the border of the census units, leading to a spatial mismatch with spatially explicit hazard data in risk assessment [17]. Emerging geospatial technologies, such as remote sensing and geographical information systems (GIS) techniques, are powerful tools for estimating population density at a finer scale. The GIS-based integration of multi-source remote sensing images can serve as a proxy for spatially explicit assessment of human exposure [24]. Therefore, the widely available datasets and the flexibility of GIS techniques make it possible to develop an effective and low-cost method for identifying the high exposure hotspots at finer scales, even for developing countries.

Currently, most studies on heat health risk assessment have been conducted in developed countries and mainly focused on cities. It is noteworthy that the spatial distribution of heat risk in developing countries is generally less well known [15, 31]. Furthermore, existing studies have been mainly implemented at the administrative unit level while few attempts focus on the specializing of heat-related health risk at a raster level. In this study, we aim to assess heat-related health risk at regional scale and explore its driving factors at a high spatial resolution. Herein, we took the Yangtze River Delta (YRD) in east China as a case study. A composite heat risk index aggregating three risk elements (heat hazard, human exposure, and vulnerability) was generated to improve the spatial delineation of heat health risk by comprehensive utilization of multi-source data. The spatially explicit heat health risk map and its driving factors were explored at the 250 m pixel level across the YRD, which can provide scientific foundation for effective resource targeting and beneficial program interventions with the least field-collection efforts.

Methods

Study area

The YRD lies along the eastern coast of China, including Shanghai, Hangzhou, Ningbo, Jiaxing, Shaoxing, Zhoushan, Huzhou, Taizhou, Nanjing, Suzhou, Yangzhou, Changzhou, Nantong, Wuxi, Zhenjiang, and Taizhou cities that are highly prosperous and populous (Fig. 1). The region is bounded by 116.78°E to 124.21°E and 26.99°N to 34.64°N and spread around 112,642 km². The YRD is located in the subtropical monsoon climate zone with a humid monsoon climate. Its annual average temperature ranges from 18 to 23 °C, and the average annual rainfall is approximately 1500 mm. During summer the YRD is frequently threatened by EHEs due to the long-lasting impact of the west Pacific subtropical high [32]. In July and August, there are usually a total of 20–30 hot days (daily maximum temperature ≥ 35 °C), with more than 40 hot days in some specific years. For example, in the summer of 2013, air temperature observations and the number of hot days in many cities of the YRD broke the historical records of the last 50 years [33]. The numbers of hot days were 47, 53, and 37 for

Shanghai, Hangzhou, and Nanjing, respectively. In addition, the YRD has experienced unprecedented economic development and urban expansion in the past 4 decades [34], which has resulted in the intensified UHI effect and a large increase in the heat-related health risk [35, 36].

Data collection and pre-processing

Satellite data

1. Temperature data. LST data based on moderate-resolution imaging spectroradiometer (MODIS) on board the National Aeronautics and Space Administration (NASA) EOS Terra and Aqua satellites are distributed as the MOD11A1 (daytime) and MYD11A1 (nighttime) products [37]. The MODIS LST images include daytime and nighttime measurements with spatial resolution of 1 km. In this study, we chose LST data from an exceptional hot day of August 7, 2013, with maximum air temperature exceeding 40 °C in many cities of YRD. Two clear sky LST images acquired at 10:30 a.m. and 1:30 a.m. were used. The MODIS reprojection tool was used for the mosaicking, reprojection, and resampling of original images, and the new LST images were generated with Albers conical equal area projection at the resolution of 250 m.

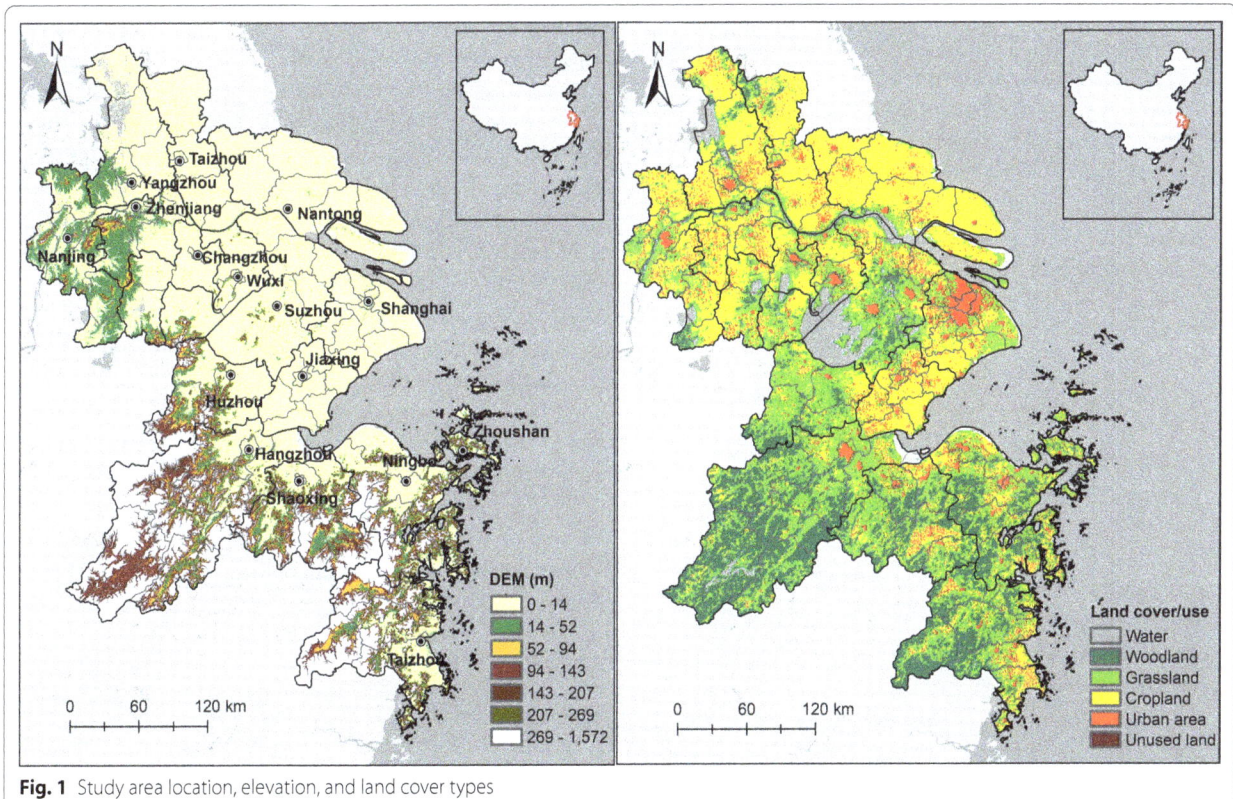

Fig. 1 Study area location, elevation, and land cover types

2. Vegetation Index data. The MODIS enhanced vegetation index (EVI) dataset (MOD13Q1) in 2013 was freely downloaded from the NASA website at a resolution of 250 m [37]. In comparison with the normalized differential vegetation index, EVI was produced by further minimization of the atmospheric effects and background spectral signals and was more sensitive to high biomass regions. To further eliminate cloud contamination and other noises, maximum value composite method was employed on the multitemporal MODIS EVI dataset to generate a new EVI composite (EVI_{max}), as expressed in Eq. (1):

$$EVI_{max} = MAX(EVI_1, EVI_2, \ldots, EVI_{23}), \qquad (1)$$

where $EVI_1, EVI_2, \ldots, EVI_{23}$ are the original 16 d EVI images in the study area in 2013. Then, the MODIS reprojection tool was utilized for data mosaicking. The new EVI_{max} image was re-projected into the Albers conical equal area projection.

3. Nighttime light data. The Defense Meteorological Satellite Program's Operational Linescan System (DMSP/OLS) images can monitor the lights associated with nighttime human activities. Since 1992, the National Geophysical Data Center annually releases global stable DMSP/OLS nighttime light composites that eliminated the cloud, accidental fire, and other noises with a spatial resolution of 30 arc-second [38]. The digital number (DN) values of DMSP/OLS data ranging from 0 to 63 and high DN values in the images generally indicate highly concentrated human activities or settlements. In this study, the original DMSP/OLS data for the year 2012 were projected and resampled to a new raster with Albers conical equal area projection at a resolution of 250 m.

4. Digital elevation model (DEM) data. The elevation data used in this study were downloaded from the website of ERSDAC of Japan [39], comprised the ASTER GDEM (Advanced Spaceborne Thermal Emission and Reflection Radiometer Global Digital Elevation Model) Version 2 with a spatial resolution of 30 m. The original DEM data were re-projected into Albers conical equal area projection and resampled to a new image at a spatial resolution of 250 m to match other datasets.

Census data

Census-aged population data at the county level of the study area were derived from China's Sixth National Census in 2010. Other demographic and socioeconomic statistical data were obtained from the statistical yearbooks of Shanghai, Zhejiang, and Jiangsu provinces and from some local bureaus of statistics for the year 2013.

Heat health risk assessment framework

The characteristics of natural disasters and their impact depend not only on the frequency or intensity but also on the human exposure and vulnerability [40]. We utilized a spatial heat health risk assessment framework based on the Crichton's risk triangle [16], which described risk as a function of hazard, human exposure, and vulnerability. For EHEs, heat hazard increased with enhanced temperature and presented a spatial gradient. This enhancement in temperature and resulting heat hazard index was measured using the satellite measured LST data across the YRD. A human settlement index integrated by multisource data was used to obtain the gridded human exposure index, matching the hazard layer at the spatial scale. For heat vulnerability assessment, multiple demographic and socioeconomic indicators have been reported to associate with hot weather mortality in previous studies [41–43]. Based on literature review [44–47] and data availability, six indicators were chosen to construct a heat vulnerability index. We selected significant components through principal component analysis (PCA) and derived their spatial distribution. The normalized heat hazard index, human exposure index, and heat vulnerability index were multiplied by equal weights to develop a final heat risk index layer given that standard conclusion on the determination of weightings among each indicator in the current risk assessment did not exist [20, 41].

Hazard

Although the remote-sensed LST that describes the radiometric surface temperature cannot directly represent air temperature, many studies have shown the strong correlation between these two disparate data, particularly at night [48, 49]. Satellite thermal data are therefore increasingly employed to estimate heat hazard [22–24, 27]. The MODIS LST data were selected in this case for their increased spatial coverage, daily measurement, and thermal accuracy, which make it possible to capture complex intra-urban gradient of surface temperature across the study area. Two clear sky LST images for daytime and nighttime during an exceptional heat wave were utilized for heat hazard analysis, considering the quality of LST image and cloud contamination in the study area [50]. Very few no-data pixels were replaced by the mean value of the surrounding 3×3 pixel. Then, two LST images were simply added and normalized to obtain the heat hazard index in the study area ranging from 0 to 1 using the ArcGIS software.

Exposure

The DMSP/OLS image was widely used as a valuable covariate for population density estimation across the world [51, 52]. However, the application of this method is limited by the spatial resolution, overglow, and saturation effects [53, 54]. By combining the vegetation indices (e.g. NDVI) and DMSP/OLS data, the saturation effect in DMSP/OLS data can be greatly reduced [55, 56]. By further incorporating elevation information, Yang et al. [57] proposed an elevation-adjusted human settlement index (EAHSI) at 250 m resolution that can reduce errors in the population estimation among areas with complex terrain. On the basis of the method proposed by Yang et al., an EAHSI at 250 m resolution was obtained in this study by combining DMSP/OLS night light images, EVI, and DEM data using the following formula:

$$EAHSI = \frac{(1 - EVI_{max}) + OLS_{nor}}{1 - OLS_{nor} + EVI_{max} + OLS_{nor} \times EVI_{max}} \times e^{-0.003DEM},$$

(2)

where

$$OLS_{nor} = (OLS - OLS_{min})/(OLS_{max} - OLS_{min}).$$

(3)

The OLS_{nor} is the normalized value of DMSP/OLS DN image, while OLS_{max} and OLS_{min} are the maximum and minimum DN values across the study area, respectively. Correlation analysis between census population and EAHSI in the next section suggested a highly linear relationship (Fig. 4). Then, EAHSI was normalized to generate a heat exposure index ranging from 0 to 1 to characterize the human exposure of EHEs.

Vulnerability

Many studies suggested that the elderly are more sensitive to EHEs because of their relatively special physiological characteristics and low tolerance to high temperatures [45]. More pressingly, elderly who live alone experience difficulty in obtaining quick and effective aid under emergency conditions [58], exposing them to the considerable threat of EHEs [59]. Meanwhile, individual or regional socioeconomic status plays a role in reducing the vulnerability of related populations. Higher socioeconomic status implies lower heat-related mortality [47]. Air conditioners are considered powerful tools to alleviate the hazardous effects of high temperature [46, 58]. The occupant's educational background and knowledge of environmental risks affect the individual's cognitive ability and avoidance behavior to EHEs [20, 60], while the regional economic level and accessibility to medical resources and facilities generally determine human adaptability to EHEs [15].

Based on the review of existing literature and the data availability in the study area, six vulnerability variables were obtained at county level, including age (≥ 65), the

elderly who live alone (≥ 60), illiteracy or semi-illiteracy rates of population aged ≥ 15, total beds of health institutions, number of air-conditioning units per 100 households, and per capita GDP. PCA is the primary statistical procedure for constructing social vulnerability index following the methodology by Cutter et al. [61]. PCA could provide information about the spatial structure of the data [62], which enables a few independent components to capture the multi-dimensionality of social vulnerability on the basis of underlying relationships between variables [63]. In this study, PCA was performed to a set of census variables with SPSS software, and the groups of variables with similar spatial patterns were identified as principal components. Once the principal components were produced, the heat vulnerability index was created by summing all the principal components using equal weighting according to their positive (+) or negative (−) effect on vulnerability. Finally, the heat vulnerability index was re-normalized to [0, 1] and mapped at the county level.

Results

Heat hazard

As shown in Fig. 2, strong and heterogeneous UHI effects for both daytime and nighttime were apparent in the YRD under heat wave conditions. During daytime, the LST varied from 27 to 48 °C, which depicted obvious spatial temperature gradient (Fig. 2a). The daytime hotspots were mainly distributed in the Z-shaped urban agglomeration in YRD, including Changzhou, Wuxi, Suzhou, Shanghai, Hangzhou, Shaoxing, and Ningbo (Fig. 2a). The LST was generally above 40 °C and reached a maximum of 45 °C in the downtowns of Hangzhou and Ningbo. Low daytime temperatures were observed in northern YRD and areas covered by forest and water bodies (such as Taihu Lake with LST ≤ 30 °C). During nighttime, the LST presented weaker temperature gradient across the YRD (Fig. 2b). Nighttime warming centers also concentrated in highly urbanized areas (≥ 30 °C) and expanded to neighboring area, demonstrating a considerable UHI effect at night. The lowest nighttime temperatures were observed in coastal areas and pixels covered by the flourish vegetation in the southern area. The heat hazard index by combining the daytime and nighttime LSTs indicated that the highly-affected areas during EHEs in the YRD are generally concentrated in urban areas, resulting from the coupling effect of the UHI (Fig. 3).

Exposure

Figure 4 displays the scatter plot between the accumulated EAHSI and the total population at county level in 2013. The strong linear correlation, with R^2 equal to 0.87,

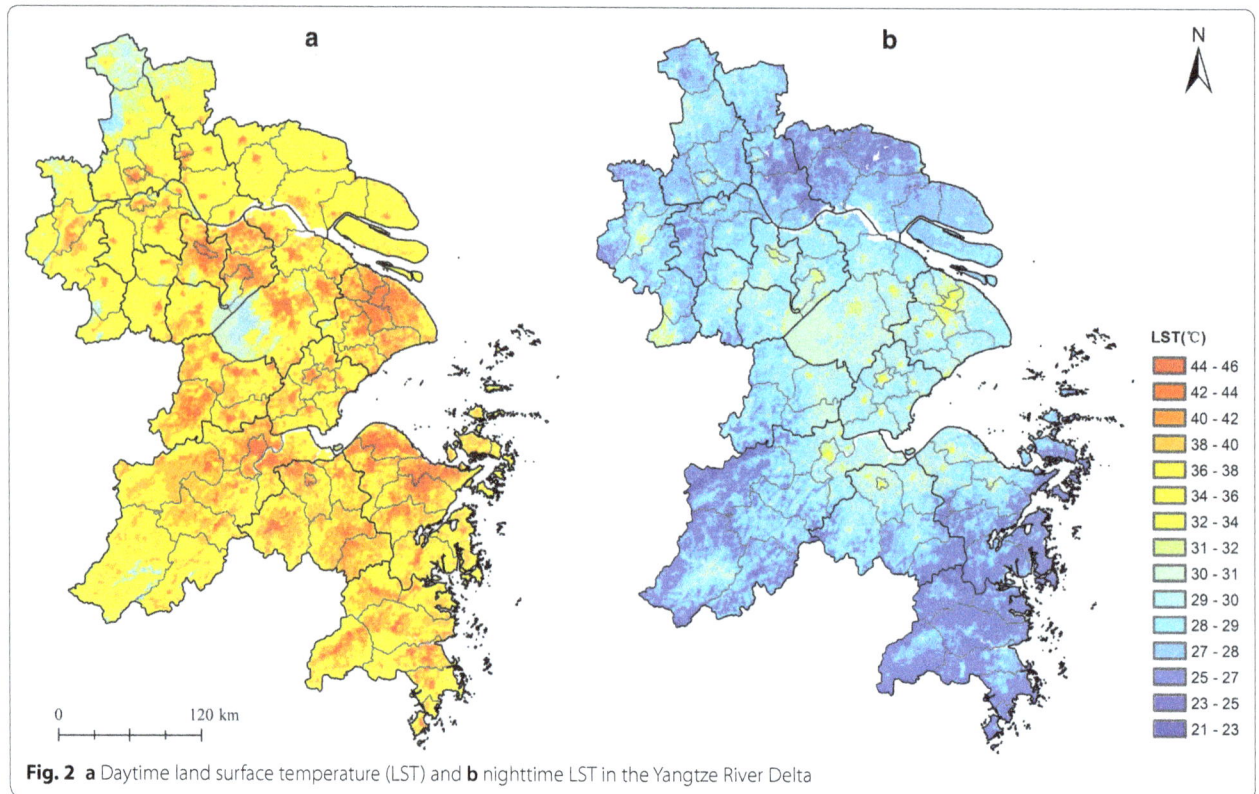

Fig. 2 **a** Daytime land surface temperature (LST) and **b** nighttime LST in the Yangtze River Delta

indicates that the EAHSI is a good proxy for the spatial delineation human exposure estimation in the YRD. The map of gridded human exposure index (Fig. 5) identifies a concentration of very high human exposure within the central areas of big cities, while moderate human exposure was found in some less-urbanized cities.

Vulnerability

As shown in Table 1, many of the six vulnerability variables were significantly correlated. Using the PCA method, the principal components with eigenvalues greater than 1.0 were used in the analysis (Table 2). These extracted factors were named based on their dominant loadings. The first factor, socioeconomic status, contributes 48.24% of the total variation among all the 6 variables. This factor is dominated by the variables that imply a high air conditioner ownership, per capita GDP and total beds of health institutions, low illiteracy rates of population (≥ 15 years), and low percentage of the elderly (≥ 60 years) living alone. Overall, the first factor identifies a group of study units with higher socioeconomic level, which contributes to a lower heat vulnerability. As depicted in Fig. 6a, areas with high socioeconomic status were mainly distributed in the most developed study units such as the downtown of Shanghai, Nanjing, Suzhou, Wuxi and Nantong. These cities were characterized by high economic conditions,

good medical service access, as well as a high percentage of educated population. The second factor, age, contributes 17.12% of the total variance. It identifies a group of units with a low percentage of population over 65 years old, which contributes to a lower heat vulnerability. Areas with a high percentage of elderly population were generally scattered throughout the northeast of the study area (Fig. 6b).

A composite heat vulnerability index based on the above two principle components was mapped in Fig. 6c. Very high heat vulnerability index values in the YRD were evident in the Rudong County of Nantong City, Chongming County of Shanghai, and mountainous areas in the southern YRD, which were mainly driven by the low economic and education level. In addition, vulnerability in some areas with relatively high economic level, such as the suburbs of Shanghai, were not significant but should not be ignored. Heat vulnerability in those areas was seemingly associated with a high percentage of elderly people, especially those living alone. Areas with low and very low heat vulnerability index values were generally scattered throughout the urbanized areas of Wuxi, Nanjing, Yangzhou, Hangzhou, Suzhou, Ningbo, and the downtown of Shanghai with generally high economic level, mature infrastructure, and low proportion of population sensitive to thermal risk (such as the elderly).

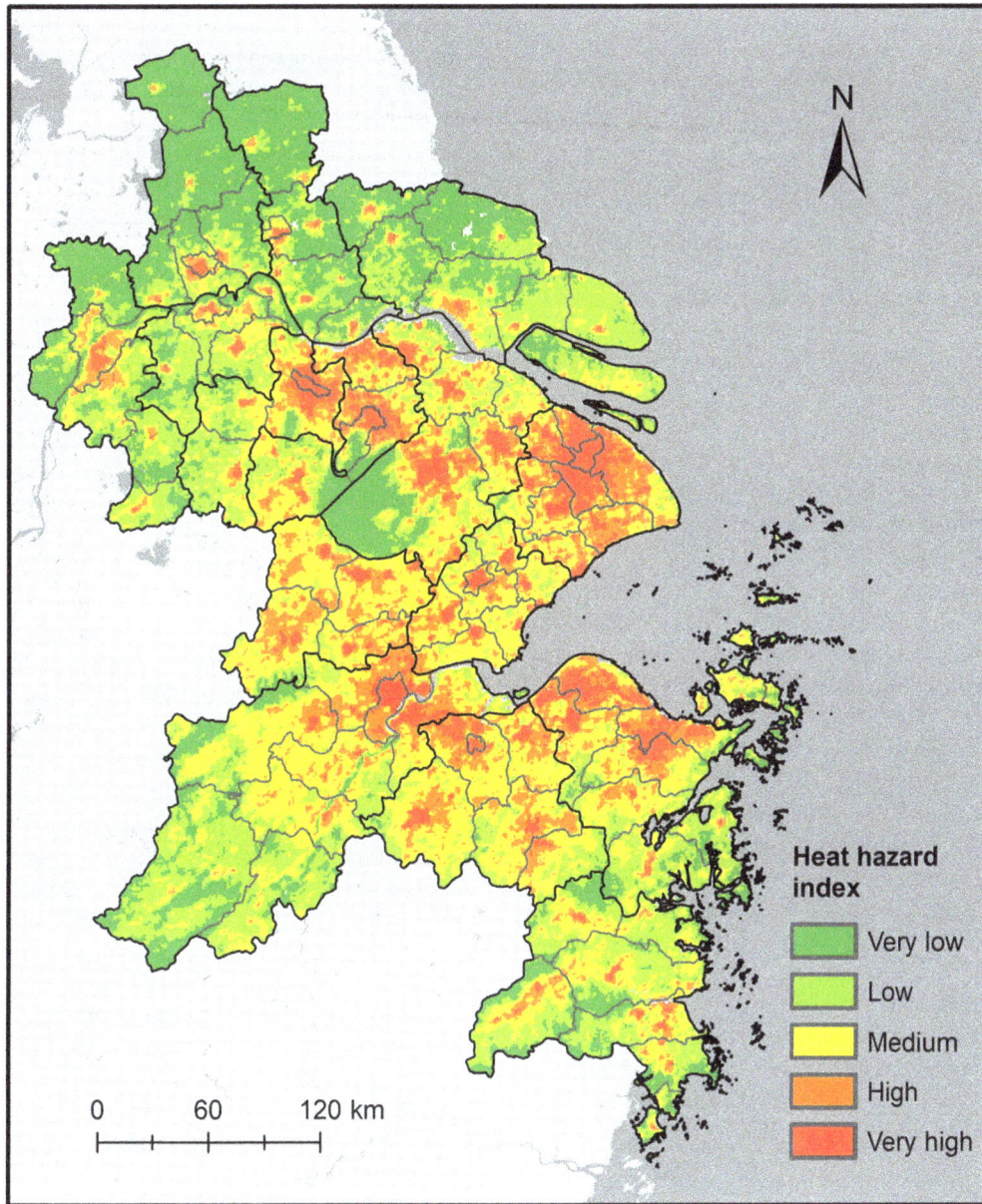

Fig. 3 Map of the heat hazard index of the Yangtze River Delta

Heat health risk

The spatial pattern of heat risk index in YRD was obtained by equally weighted aggregation of three risk elements (Fig. 7). The majority of the high-risk areas are grouped together in the central urbanized areas of Changzhou, Yangzhou, Taizhou (Jiangsu Province), Jiaxing, Taizhou (Zhejiang Province), Cixi and Yuyao City of Ningbo. Notably, the heat risk index values are high in the northern area of the YRD (such as Xinghua City and Baoying County), the eastern coastal areas of Jiangsu (such as Hai'an County), and the rural areas of the southwestern study area, and this can be explained by the distribution of vulnerability index.

Driving factors

In addition to identifying the high heat health risk areas, it is also important for decision makers to recognize risk factors which play a leading role in forming these high risk areas. Here, pixels with medium or higher risk grade were considered as potential high risk areas. The heat hazard, human exposure, and heat vulnerability index were also reclassified into two grades in the same

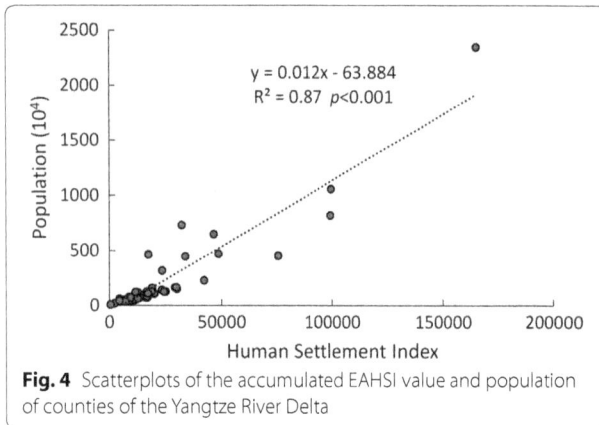

Fig. 4 Scatterplots of the accumulated EAHSI value and population of counties of the Yangtze River Delta

way. Then, the main driving factors that contributed to potential high heat risk areas in the YRD were identified (Fig. 8). For example, the legend "Hazard/vulnerability" in Fig. 8 means that both heat hazard and heat vulnerability grades were high whereas the heat exposure was low in the corresponding area. Heat hazard and heat vulnerability were therefore defined as the driving factors of high heat risk.

Risk areas driven by a single factor, which accounted for only 2.62% of the potential risk area, were less distributed, as depicted in Fig. 8. The heat risk patterns in 31.76% of the area were mostly driven by the distribution of heat hazard and human exposure, particularly in highly-urbanized areas of the YRD. However, in the suburbs encircling the city centers and in urban areas of some relatively small cities (e.g., suburbs of Shanghai), high vulnerability also contributes to the high risks. The heat health risks in some less-developed areas, with low human exposure index in the south and north sections of the YRD, remained high due to the assigned high heat hazard and heat vulnerability grades.

Discussion

Previous studies have pointed out the necessity for heat health risk assessment at a finer scale [21, 23]. Given the lack of attempts of spatially explicit assessment for heat health risk, especially in developing countries, this study developed a methodology built on previous risk assessment framework and aggregating the knowledge and technologies from GIS, remote sensing and epidemiological sciences. By fully considering heat hazard, human exposure, and multidimensional vulnerability and integrating multi-sensor remote sensing images and sociodemographic data, the GIS-based methodology has been designed to be transparent and to make use of readily freely available data. The resulting pixel-level heat health risk map and the identification of driving factors

can convey more information for understanding specific human risk during EHEs. It is particularly valuable in guiding local planners to develop more efficient mitigation and adaptation planning in developing countries with limited cost, time, and labour.

Previous studies pointed out that the daily minimum temperatures in the urban area were considerably higher than those in the rural area because of UHI effects [64, 65], thereby exacerbating the heat health risk on urban residents [27]. However, most spatial heat health risk studies only considered the daytime high temperature and generally omitted the impact of nighttime high temperature due to the nocturnal UHI effect. Here, cloud-free MODIS LST images were adopted to represent heat hazard during an exceptional heat wave. The nighttime LST data, which were restricted to only thermal infrared radiance from the ground, are considered a powerful proxy to more accurately represent the spatial distribution of UHI than the daytime LST [66]. Comprehensive analysis of the heat hazard in the YRD illustrated that both daytime and nighttime LSTs in urban areas were generally higher than those in rural areas. Therefore, urban residents were more likely to suffer from lasting heat stress at both day and night during EHEs, which agreed with similar work performed in other countries [13, 65, 67].

A better understanding of human exposure to EHEs required precise and spatially explicit estimation of population distribution [22, 24, 68]. In comparison with the previous studies based only on census population data, the present study conducted human exposure assessment at high spatial resolution by integrating multisource satellite images, thereby bridging the spatial mismatch with heat hazard layer. This represents a clear contribution that can lead to a better estimation of disaggregated exposure and risk at finer scales. The method for grid-based exposure assessment is characterized by the wide application of the readily available remote sensing data and flexibility of GIS technique.

It is now widely appreciated that spatial viabilities in demographic characteristics and socioeconomic status are key contributors to overall vulnerability to extreme weather events [41]. In this study, six heat vulnerability-related variables were represented by two principal components through PCA analysis to create the final heat vulnerability map. Our vulnerability map in YRD agree with the results by Chen et al. [69], which suggested that highly urbanized areas are generally much less vulnerable than rural areas. According to the PCA analysis, there exists inequity in the allocation of social resources like education opportunities and medical services between urban and rural areas. Areas with the high socioeconomic level are city districts. However, some of

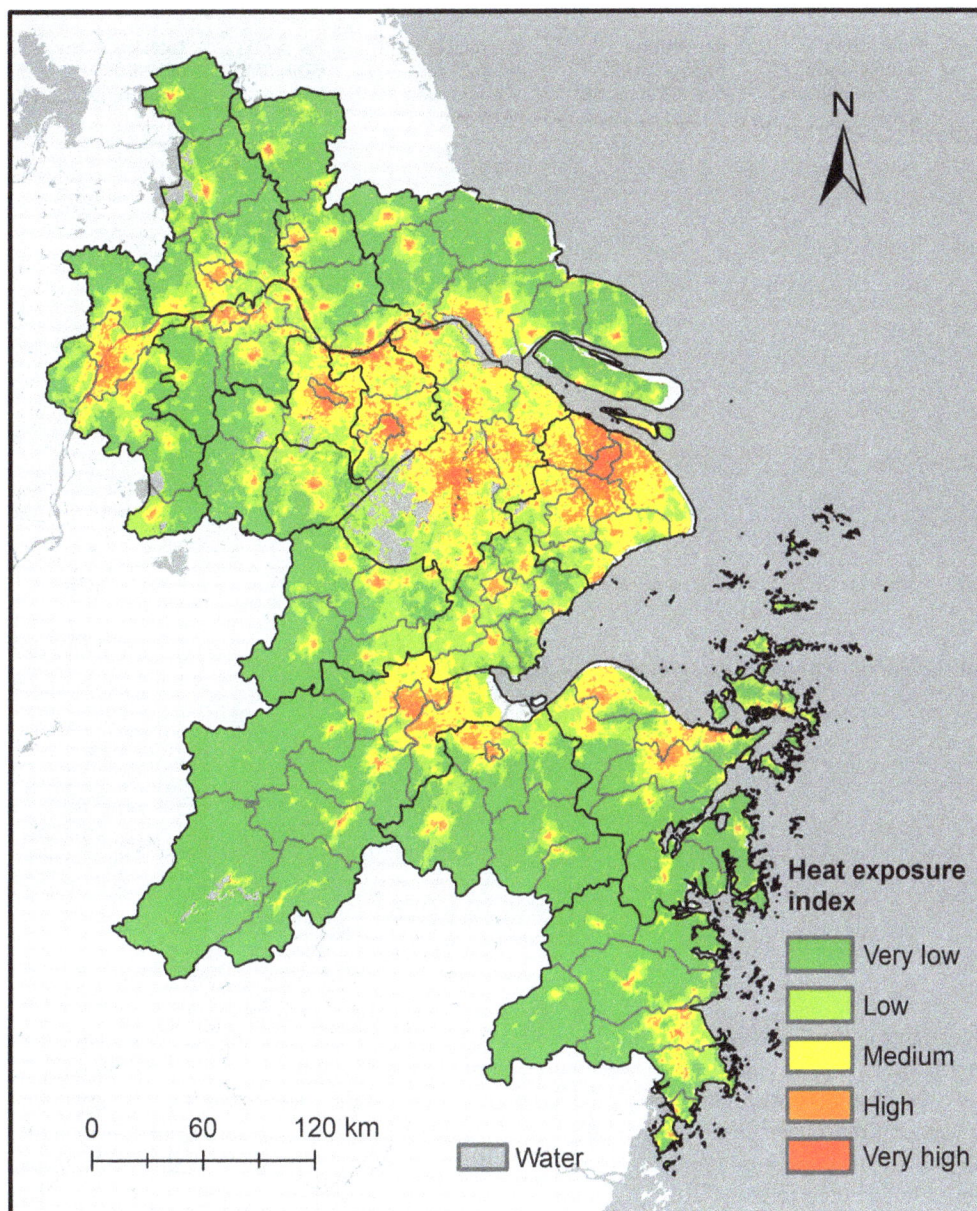

Fig. 5 Map of the heat exposure index of the Yangtze River Delta

these places exhibit other dimensions of vulnerability. For example, Nantong City of Jiangsu Province ranks high on socioeconomic status while have a relatively high percentage of elderly people. Therefore, by separating various dimensions of vulnerability, it is possible for decision makers to understand what contributes to vulnerability and decide tailored adaptation strategies.

However, there are still some limitations that should be pointed out in this study. Firstly, the verification of the results becomes a significant gap because health and

mortality records associated with previous EHEs in YRD are not available. Hospital data can be helpful in quantitative validation of heat health assessment, although the utility may be limited due to its restricted availability at temporal and spatial scales.

Secondly, we only considered the LST for the hazard analysis in this study, but the impact of EHEs on public health is in fact a function of temperature, humidity, wind speed, and other meteorological and environmental factors [15, 22]. Some studies demonstrated that the

Table 1 Spearman's correlation values for vulnerability variables (n = 76)

	Percentage of the elderly (≥ 60 years) living alone	Percentage of population over 65 years old	Illiteracy or semi-illiteracy rates of population (≥ 15 years)	Per capita GDP (RMB Yuan)	Total beds of health institutions	Air conditioners per 100 household
Percentage of the elderly (≥ 60 years) living alone	1.00					
Percentage of population over 65 years old	*0.07*	1.00				
Illiteracy or semi-illiteracy rates of population (≥ 15 years)	0.49	*0.20*	1.00			
Per capita GDP (RMB Yuan)	− 0.39	− 0.48	− 0.40	1.00		
Total beds of health institutions	*− 0.26*	*− 0.19*	− 0.37	0.38	1.00	
Air conditioners per 100 household	− 0.44	*− 0.28*	− 0.47	0.61	0.46	1.00

All values are statistically significant at $p < 0.001$ except for those in italics

Table 2 Principle component analysis result of social vulnerability

Components	Eigenvalue	Percentage variance explained	Variables	Loadings
(1) Socioeconomic status	2.667	48.24	Air conditioners per 100 household	0.818
			Per capita GDP (RMB Yuan)	0.801
			Illiteracy or semi-illiteracy rates of population (≥ 15 years)	− 0.715
			Percentage of the elderly (≥ 60 years) living alone	− 0.649
			Total beds of health institutions	0.641
(2) Age	1.018	17.12	Percentage of population over 65 years old	− 0.769

effects of air pollutants as confounders of the UHI would pose a serious threat to public health [15]; meanwhile, the "urban dry island" effect may potentially alleviate heat stress to a certain extent [70]. The synergies between temperature and the factors mentioned above should be further considered in future hazard analyses.

Thirdly, grid datasets for demographic and socioeconomic indicators are essential for vulnerability assessment but are not available at resolutions needed. In the current study, for the three risk elements, grid-based assessments on heat hazard and human exposure were conducted at a fine spatial resolution using multi-sensor remote sensing data. The spatial mismatch between exposure and hazard was therefore overcome. Still, the required grid-based datasets for other socio-economic vulnerability indicators at a finer resolution are not available for the study area. Therefore, the resulting vulnerability assessments were inevitably homogeneous within the border of the administrative units, and the spatial mismatch between vulnerability and other risk elements

still exist in the current study. Furthermore, some vulnerability variables could not be considered due to the data availability. For example, although people with pre-existing illness are quite vulnerable to high temperature because of their limited mobility and self-care ability [15, 27], this important variable was not considered in this study because these data are unfortunately unavailable at the county level due to privacy. Moreover, based on the epidemiological evidence that the elderly are the most vulnerable subgroup to extreme heat and data availability [71, 72], we therefore chose the percentage of the elderly who live alone as social isolation proxy in heat vulnerability assessment following recent studies [73, 74]. Other factors such as home relocation, friends, social support, social participation, and social networks are not included because these data are not available in China census databases.

Finally, although previous literature shows the disparate contribution of heat hazard, human exposure, and heat vulnerability to human health during EHES, there

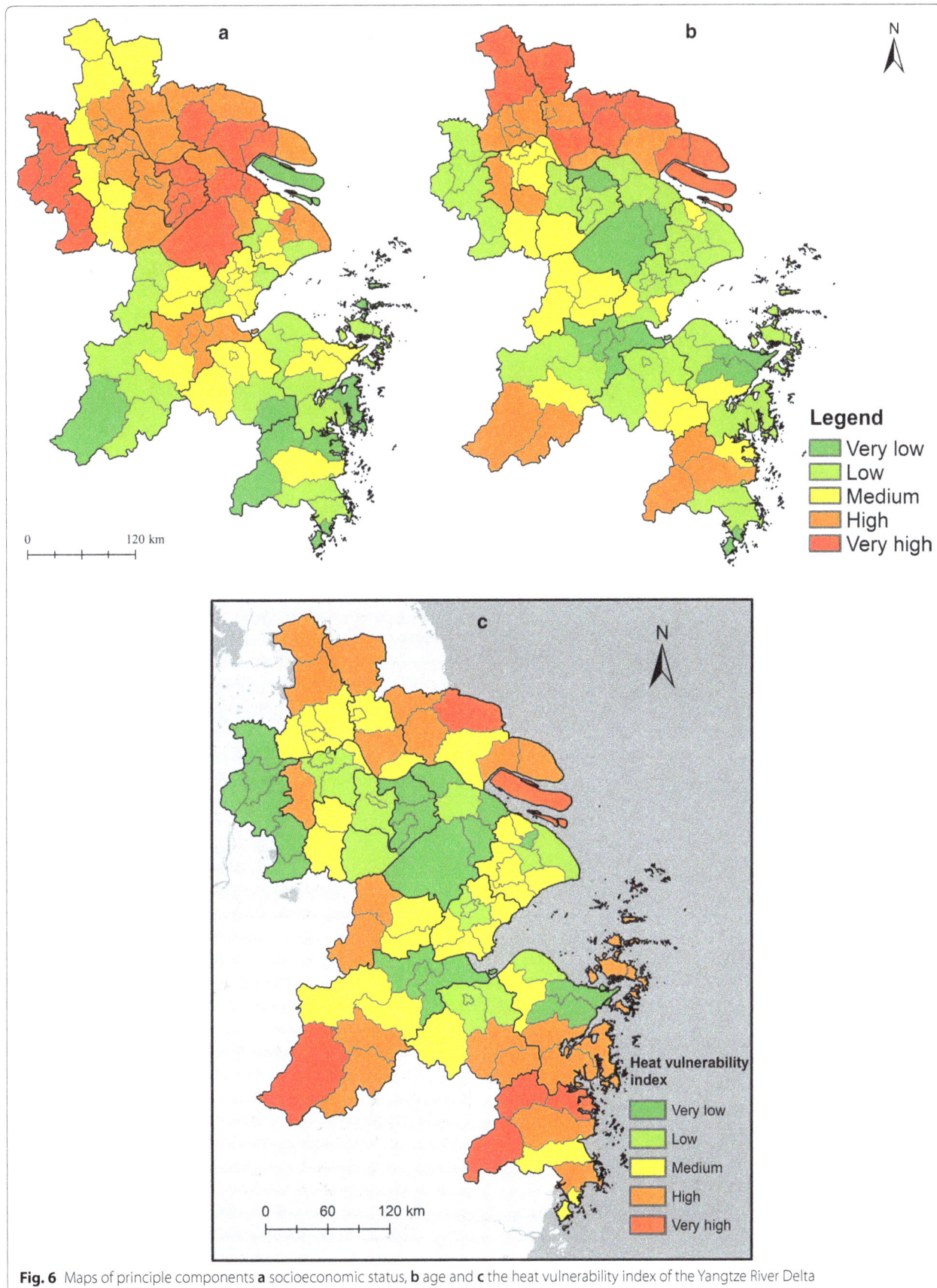

Fig. 6 Maps of principle components **a** socioeconomic status, **b** age and **c** the heat vulnerability index of the Yangtze River Delta

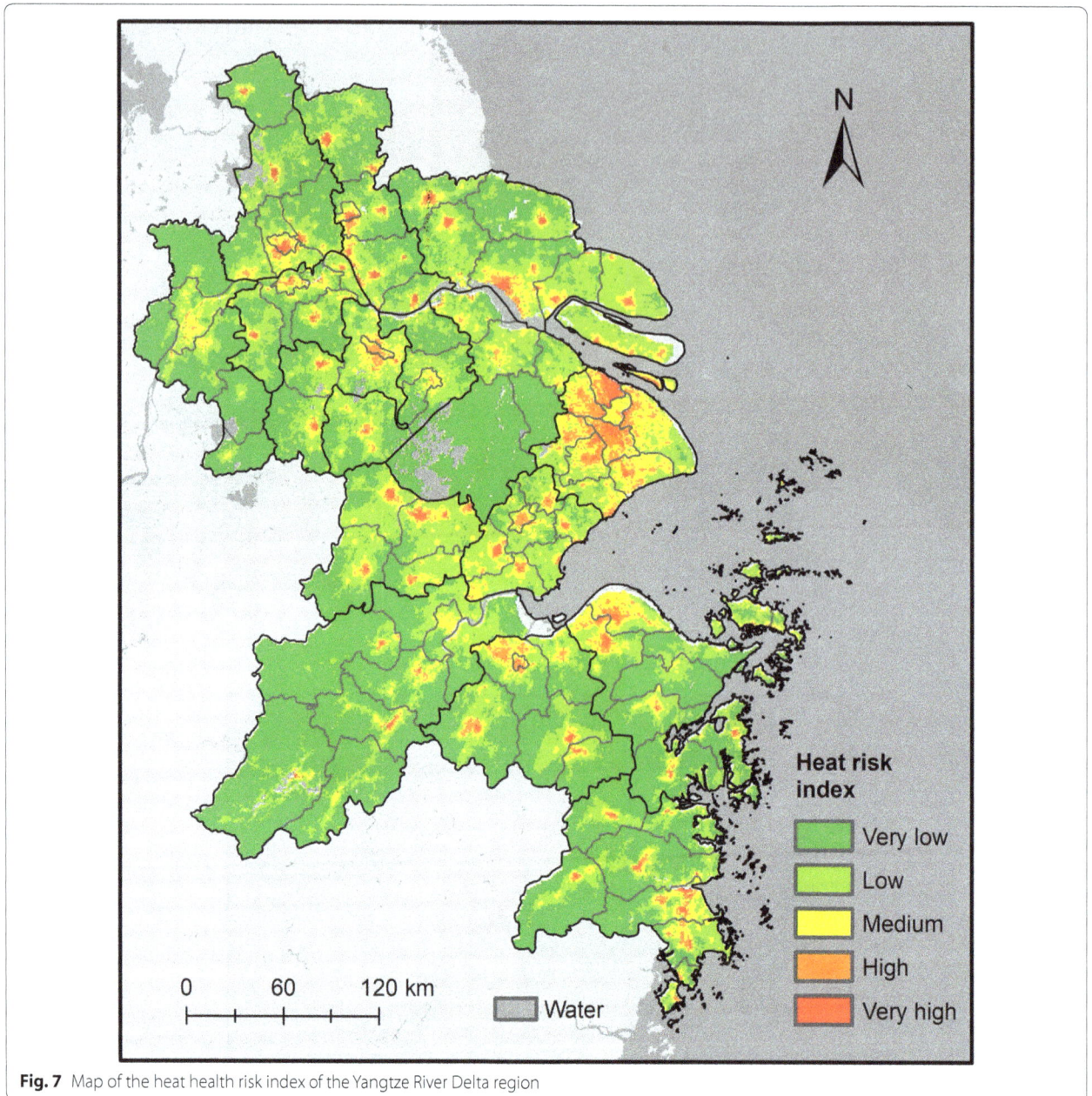

Fig. 7 Map of the heat health risk index of the Yangtze River Delta region

are no standard weights that are widely applied [20, 41]. The identification of weightings required further knowledge about the relationships between all three elements in the specific location. Therefore, three risk elements among our heat risk index were weighted equally. Previous studies have used equal weighting with success for various factors to estimate heat health risk [21, 23, 27, 75]. Moreover, weightings can be easily modified according to new available knowledge and specific local authority requirements [23].

Conclusion

This study presents a methodology for spatial heat risk assessment by combining freely available multi-source data, which allows for greater replicability in many other countries, especially in developing countries. Spatially, areas with higher heat hazard and human exposure are mainly concentrated in highly urbanized areas, which largely resulted in high heat health risk in the urban areas. However, the health effects of overheating during EHEs could be weakened due to low social vulnerability (associated with a

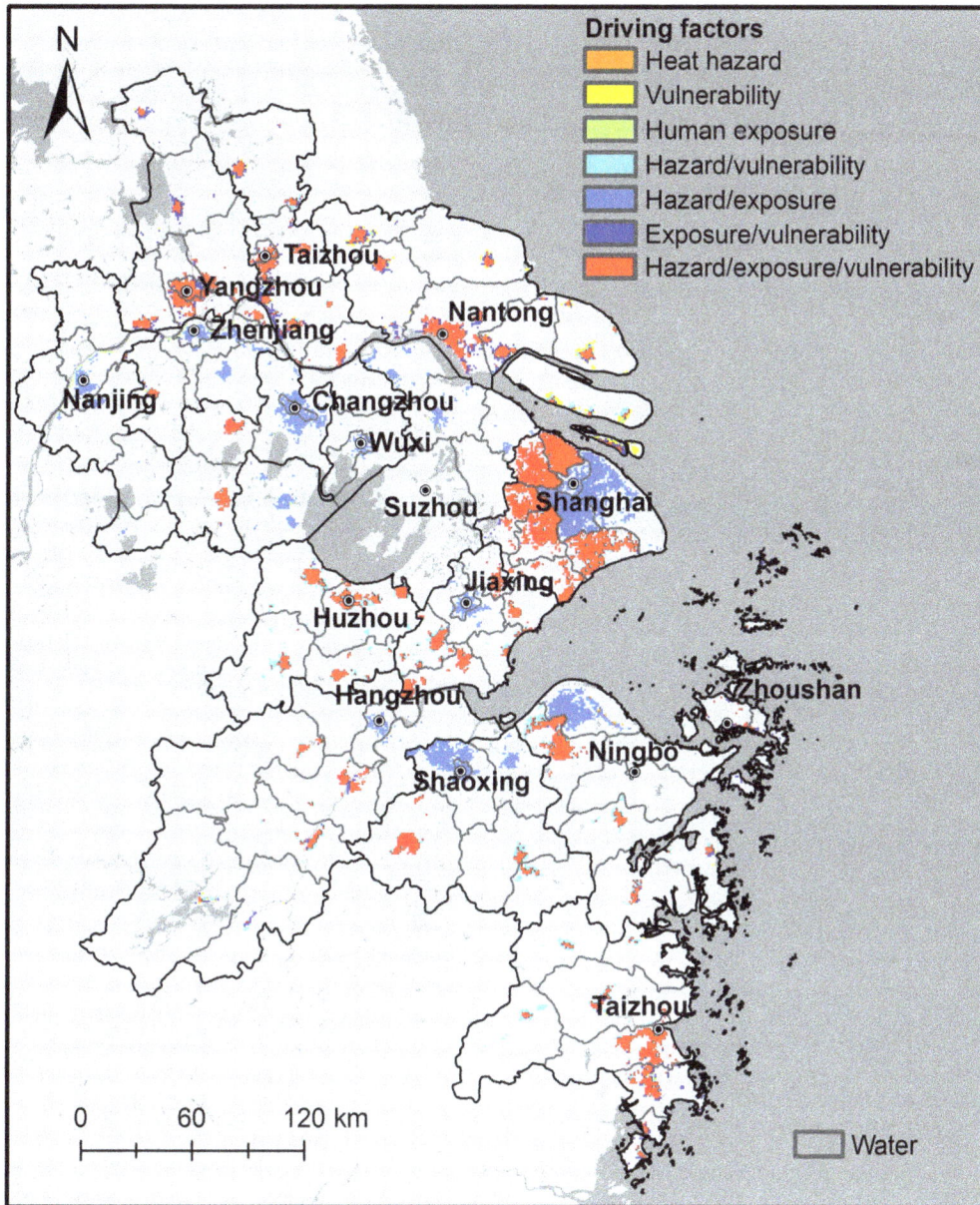

Fig. 8 Driving factors of heat health risks in the Yangtze River Delta region

low proportion of sensitive population or a high level of social and economic development) in some areas, especially Hangzhou, the central area of Shanghai, and Nanjing City. By contrast, high social vulnerability plays an important role in high heat health risk in some less-urbanized cities and in the suburban areas of mega-cities. Low-risk areas are generally found in high-altitude areas. The resultant heat health risk map is potentially applicable to decision makers when

considering tailored adaptation strategies and emergency planning of heat risk.

Abbreviations

EHEs: extreme heat events; EVI: enhanced vegetation index; DEM: digital elevation model; LST: land surface temperature; YRD: the Yangtze River Delta region; UHI: urban heat island; GIS: geographical information system; DN: digital number; MODIS: moderate-resolution imaging spectroradiometer; EAHSI: elevation-adjusted human settlement index; PCA: principal component analysis.

Authors' contributions

QC carried out the risk analysis and drafted the manuscript, XY conceived of the study and participated in its design, MD, KH and JQ offered advice throughout the research and feedback on the manuscript. All authors read and approved the final manuscript.

Author details

[1] Institute of Island and Coastal Ecosystems, Ocean College, Zhejiang University, Zhoushan 316021, China. [2] Key Lab of Poyang Lake Wetland and Watershed Research of Ministry of Education, School of Geography and Environment, Jiangxi Normal University, Nanchang 330022, China. [3] Center for Global Change and Earth Observations, Michigan State University, East Lansing, MI 48823, USA.

Acknowledgements

This study was funded by the National Natural Science Foundation of China (Grants 41671035 and 41371068). The authors acknowledge the two anonymous reviewers and Editor for their constructive comments and suggestions.

Competing interests

The authors declare that they have no competing interests.

Funding

This study was funded by the National Natural Science Foundation of China (Grant 41671035).

References

1. WHO. The world health report 2008: primary health care-now more than ever. Geneva: World Health Organization; 2008.
2. Kan H. Climate change and human health in China. Environ Health Perspect. 2011;119(2):A60–1.
3. Meehl GA, Tebaldi C. More intense, more frequent, and longer lasting heat waves in the 21st century. Science. 2004;305(5686):994–7.
4. Ward K, Lauf S, Kleinschmit B, Endlicher W. Heat waves and urban heat islands in Europe: a review of relevant drivers. Sci Total Environ. 2016;569:527–39.
5. Robine J-M, Cheung SLK, Le Roy S, Van Oyen H, Griffiths C, Michel J-P, Herrmann FR. Death toll exceeded 70,000 in Europe during the summer of 2003. C R Biol. 2008;331(2):171–8.
6. Barriopedro D, Fischer EM, Luterbacher J, Trigo RM, García-Herrera R. The hot summer of 2010: redrawing the temperature record map of Europe. Science. 2011;332(6026):220–4.
7. Stone B Jr, Vargo J, Liu P, Habeeb D, DeLucia A, Trail M, Hu Y, Russell A. Avoided heat-related mortality through climate adaptation strategies in three US cities. PLoS ONE. 2014;9(6):e100852.
8. Field C, Barros V, Stocker T, Qin D, Dokken D, Ebi K, Mastrandrea M, Mach K, Plattner G, Allen S. A special report of working groups I and II of the intergovernmental panel on climate change. Managing the risks of extreme events and disasters to advance climate change adaptation 2012.
9. Fouillet A, Rey G, Laurent F, Pavillon G, Bellec S, Guihenneuc-Jouyaux C, Clavel J, Jougla E, Hemon D. Excess mortality related to the August 2003 heat wave in France. Int Arch Occup Environ Health. 2006;80(1):16–24.
10. Tan J, Zheng Y, Song G, Kalkstein L, Kalkstein A, Tang X. Heat wave impacts on mortality in Shanghai, 1998 and 2003. Int J Biometeorol. 2007;51(3):193–200.
11. Li D, Bou-Zeid E. Synergistic interactions between urban heat islands and heat waves: the impact in cities is larger than the sum of its parts. J Appl Meteorol Climatol. 2013;52(9):2051–64.
12. Founda D, Santamouris M. Synergies between urban heat island and heat waves in Athens (Greece), during an extremely hot summer (2012). Sci Rep. 2017;7(1):10973.
13. Dousset B, Gourmelon F, Laaidi K, Zeghnoun A, Giraudet E, Bretin P, Mauri E, Vandentorren S. Satellite monitoring of summer heat waves in the Paris metropolitan area. Int J Climatol. 2011;31(2):313–23.
14. Smargiassi A, Goldberg MS, Plante C, Fournier M, Baudouin Y, Kosatsky T. Variation of daily warm season mortality as a function of micro-urban heat islands. J Epidemiol Commun Health. 2009;63(8):659–64.
15. Romero-Lankao P, Qin H, Dickinson K. Urban vulnerability to temperature-related hazards: a meta-analysis and meta-knowledge approach. Glob Environ Change. 2012;22(3):670–83.
16. Crichton D. The risk triangle. In: Ingleton J, editor. Natural disaster management. London: Tudor Rose; 1999. p. 102–3.
17. Chen KP, McAneney J, Blong R, Leigh R, Hunter L, Magill C. Defining area at risk and its effect in catastrophe loss estimation: a dasymetric mapping approach. Appl Geogr. 2004;24(2):97–117.
18. Heaton MJ, Sain SR, Greasby TA, Uejio CK, Hayden MH, Monaghan AJ, Boehnert J, Sampson K, Banerjee D, Nepal V, et al. Characterizing urban vulnerability to heat stress using a spatially varying coefficient model. Spat Spat Temp Epidemiol. 2014;8:23–33.
19. Lee M, Shi L, Zanobetti A, Schwartz JD. Study on the association between ambient temperature and mortality using spatially resolved exposure data. Environ Res. 2016;151:610–7.
20. Johnson DP, Stanforth A, Lulla V, Luber G. Developing an applied extreme heat vulnerability index utilizing socioeconomic and environmental data. Appl Geogr. 2012;35(1):23–31.
21. Aubrecht C, Ozceylan D. Identification of heat risk patterns in the U.S. National Capital Region by integrating heat stress and related vulnerability. Environ Int. 2013;56:65–77.
22. Johnson DP, Wilson JS, Luber GC. Socioeconomic indicators of heat-related health risk supplemented with remotely sensed data. Int J Health Geogr. 2009;8(1):57.
23. Buscail C, Upegui E, Viel JF. Mapping heatwave health risk at the community level for public health action. Int J Health Geogr. 2012;11(1):38.
24. Johnson D, Lulla V, Stanforth A, Webber J. Remote sensing of heat-related health risks: the trend toward coupling socioeconomic and remotely sensed data. Geogr Compass. 2011;5(10):767–80.
25. Weber S, Sadoff N, Zell E, de Sherbinin A. Policy-relevant indicators for mapping the vulnerability of urban populations to extreme heat events: a case study of Philadelphia. Appl Geogr. 2015;63:231–43.
26. Dan L, Ting S, Maofeng L, Long Y, Linlin W, Zhiqiu G. Contrasting responses of urban and rural surface energy budgets to heat waves explain synergies between urban heat islands and heat waves. Environ Res Lett. 2015;10(5):054009.
27. Tomlinson CJ, Chapman L, Thornes JE, Baker CJ. Including the urban heat island in spatial heat health risk assessment strategies: a case study for Birmingham, UK. Int J Health Geogr. 2011;10(1):42.
28. Aubrecht C, Özceylan D, Steinnocher K, Freire S. Multi-level geospatial modeling of human exposure patterns and vulnerability indicators. Nat Hazards. 2013;68(1):147–63.
29. Tenerelli P, Gallego JF, Ehrlich D. Population density modelling in support of disaster risk assessment. Int J Disaster Risk Reduct. 2015;13:334–41.
30. Council NR. Tools and methods for estimating population at risk from natural disasters and complex humanitarian crises. Washington: National Academy of Science; 2007.
31. Zhu Q, Liu T, Lin H, Xiao J, Luo Y, Zeng W, Zeng S, Wei Y, Chu C, Baum S, et al. The spatial distribution of health vulnerability to heat waves in Guangdong Province, China. Glob Health Action. 2014;7(1):25051.

32. Gong DY, Pan YZ, Wang JA. Changes in extreme daily mean temperatures in summer in eastern China during 1955–2000. Theor Appl Climatol. 2004;77(1–2):25–37.

33. Zhou B, Rybski D, Kropp JP. On the statistics of urban heat island intensity. Geophys Res Lett. 2013;40(20):5486–91.

34. Wang Z, Fang C, Zhang X. Spatial expansion and potential of construction land use in the Yangtze River Delta. J Geogr Sci. 2015;25(7):851–64.

35. Yang XC, Leung LR, Zhao NZ, Zhao C, Qian Y, Hu KJ, Liu XP, Chen BD. Contribution of urbanization to the increase of extreme heat events in an urban agglomeration in east China. Geophys Res Lett. 2017;44(13):6940–50.

36. Yang XC, Hou YL, Chen BD. Observed surface warming induced by urbanization in east China. J Geophys Res Atmos. 2011. https://doi.org/10.1029/2010JD015452.

37. LAADS DAAC. https://ladsweb.modaps.eosdis.nasa.gov/. Accessed 3 Mar 2018.

38. NGDC. http://ngdc.noaa.gov/eog/download.html. Accessed 3 Mar 2018.

39. ASTER GDEM. http://www.gdem.aster.ersdac.or.jp/search.jsp. Accessed 3 Mar 2018.

40. Field CB. Managing the risks of extreme events and disasters to advance climate change adaptation: special report of the intergovernmental panel on climate change. Cambridge: Cambridge University Press; 2012.

41. Reid C, O'Neill M, Gronlund C, Brines S, Brown D, Diez-Roux A, Schwartz J. Mapping community determinants of heat vulnerability. Environ Health Perspect. 2009;117(11):1730–6.

42. Reid CE, Mann JK, Alfasso R, English PB, King GC, Lincoln RA, Margolis HG, Rubado DJ, Sabato JE, West NL, et al. Evaluation of a heat vulnerability index on abnormally hot days: an environmental public health tracking study. Environ Health Perspect. 2012;120(5):715–20.

43. Harlan SL, Declet-Barreto JH, Stefanov WL, Petitti DB. Neighborhood effects on heat deaths: social and environmental predictors of vulnerability in Maricopa County, Arizona. Environ Health Perspect. 2013;121(2):197–204.

44. Filleul L, Cassadou S, Medina S, Fabres P, Lefranc A, Eilstein D, Le Tertre A, Pascal L, Chardon B, Blanchard M, et al. The relation between temperature, ozone, and mortality in nine french cities during the heat wave of 2003. Environ Health Perspect. 2006;114(9):1344–7.

45. Yu WW, Vaneckova P, Mengersen K, Pan XC, Tong SL. Is the association between temperature and mortality modified by age, gender and socioeconomic status? Sci Total Environ. 2010;408(17):3513–8.

46. Naughton M, Henderson A, Mirabelli M. Heat-related mortality during a 1999 heat wave in Chicago. Am J Prev Med. 2002;22(4):221–7.

47. Chan EYY, Goggins WB, Kim JJ, Griffiths SM. A study of intracity variation of temperature-related mortality and socioeconomic status among the Chinese population in Hong Kong. J Epidemiol Community Health. 2012;66(4):322–7.

48. Sohrabinia M, Zawar-Reza P, Rack W. Spatio-temporal analysis of the relationship between LST from MODIS and air temperature in New Zealand. Theor Appl Climatol. 2015;119(3–4):567–83.

49. Vancutsem C, Ceccato P, Dinku T, Connor SJ. Evaluation of MODIS land surface temperature data to estimate air temperature in different ecosystems over Africa. Remote Sens Environ. 2010;114(2):449–65.

50. Wang J, Yan Z, Quan X-W, Feng J. Urban warming in the 2013 summer heat wave in eastern China. Clim Dyn. 2017;48(9–10):3015–33.

51. Chowdhury PKR, Maithani S, Dadhwal VK. Estimation of urban population in Indo-Gangetic Plains using night-time OLS data. Int J Remote Sens. 2012;33(8):2498–515.

52. Bennett MM, Smith LC. Advances in using multitemporal night-time lights satellite imagery to detect, estimate, and monitor socioeconomic dynamics. Remote Sens Environ. 2017;192:176–97.

53. Letu H, Hara M, Yagi H, Naoki K, Tana G, Nishio F, Shuhei O. Estimating energy consumption from night-time DMPS/OLS imagery after correcting for saturation effects. Int J Remote Sens. 2010;31(16):4443–58.

54. Townsend AC, Bruce DA. The use of night-time lights satellite imagery as a measure of Australia's regional electricity consumption and population distribution. Int J Remote Sens. 2010;31(16):4459–80.

55. Roy Chowdhury PK, Maithani S. Monitoring growth of built-up areas in indo-gangetic plain using multi-sensor remote sensing data. J Indian Soc Remote Sens. 2010;38(2):291–300.

56. Lu D, Tian H, Zhou G, Ge H. Regional mapping of human settlements in southeastern China with multisensor remotely sensed data. Remote Sens Environ. 2008;112(9):3668–79.

57. Yang XC, Yue WZ, Gao DW. Spatial improvement of human population distribution based on multi-sensor remote-sensing data: an input for exposure assessment. Int J Remote Sens. 2013;34(15):5569–83.

58. Semenza J, Rubin C, Falter K, Selanikio J, Flanders W, Howe H, Wilhelm J. Heat-related deaths during the July 1995 heat wave in Chicago. N Engl J Med. 1996;335(2):84–90.

59. Kenny GP, Yardley J, Brown C, Sigal RJ, Jay O. Heat stress in older individuals and patients with common chronic diseases. Can Med Assoc J. 2010;182(10):1053–60.

60. Pisello AL, Rosso F, Castaldo VL, Piselli C, Fabiani C, Cotana F. The role of building occupants' education in their resilience to climate-change related events. Energy Build. 2017;154(Supplement C):217–31.

61. Cutter SL, Boruff BJ, Shirley WL. Social vulnerability to environmental hazards. Soc Sci Q. 2003;84(2):242–61.

62. Johnston RJ. Multivariate statistical analysis in geography; a primer on the general linear model. London: Longman; 1980.

63. Abdi H, Williams LJ. Principal component analysis. Wiley Interdiscip Rev Comput Stat. 2010;2(4):433–59.

64. Tan J, Zheng Y, Tang X, Guo C, Li L, Song G, Zhen X, Yuan D, Kalkstein AJ, Li F. The urban heat island and its impact on heat waves and human health in Shanghai. Int J Biometeorol. 2010;54(1):75–84.

65. Antics A, Pascal M, Laaidi K, Wagner V, Corso M, Declercq C, Beaudeau P. A simple indicator to rapidly assess the short-term impact of heat waves on mortality within the French heat warning system. Int J Biometeorol. 2013;57(1):75–81.

66. Nichol J. Remote sensing of urban heat islands by day and night. Photogramm Eng Remote Sens. 2005;71(5):613–21.

67. Hu K, Yang X, Zhong J, Fei F, Qi J. Spatially explicit mapping of heat health risk utilizing environmental and socioeconomic data. Environ Sci Technol. 2017;51(3):1498–507.

68. Golden JS, Hartz D, Brazel A, Luber G, Phelan P. A biometeorology study of climate and heat-related morbidity in Phoenix from 2001 to 2006. Int J Biometeorol. 2008;52(6):471–80.

69. Chen W, Cutter SL, Emrich CT, Shi P. Measuring social vulnerability to natural hazards in the Yangtze River Delta region, China. Int J Disaster Risk Sci. 2014;4(4):169–81.

70. Wang J, Feng JM, Yan ZW, Hu YH, Jia GS. Nested high-resolution modeling of the impact of urbanization on regional climate in three vast urban agglomerations in China. J Geophys Res Atmos. 2012. https://doi.org/10.1029/2012JD018226.

71. Benmarhnia T, Deguen S, Kaufman JS, Smargiassi A. Vulnerability to heat-related mortality: a systematic review, meta-analysis, and meta-regression analysis. Epidemiology. 2015;26(6):781–93.

72. Kovats RS, Hajat S. Heat stress and public health: a critical review. Annu Rev Public Health. 2008;29:41–55.

73. Gronlund CJ, Berrocal VJ, White-Newsome JL, Conlon KC, O'Neill MS. Vulnerability to extreme heat by socio-demographic characteristics and area green space among the elderly in Michigan, 1990–2007. Environ Res. 2015;136:449–61.

74. Nayak SG, Shrestha S, Kinney PL, Ross Z, Sheridan SC, Pantea CI, Hsu WH, Muscatiello N, Hwang SA. Development of a heat vulnerability index for New York State. Public Health. 2017. https://doi.org/10.1016/j.puhe.2017.09.006.

75. Dong W, Liu Z, Zhang L, Tang Q, Liao H, Xe Li. Assessing heat health risk for sustainability in Beijing's urban heat island. Sustainability. 2014;6(10):7334.

The role of the built environment in explaining educational inequalities in walking and cycling among adults in the Netherlands

Daniël C. van Wijk[1,2], Joost Oude Groeniger[2], Frank J. van Lenthe[2] and Carlijn B. M. Kamphuis[1*]

Abstract

Background: This study examined whether characteristics of the residential built environment (i.e. population density, level of mixed land use, connectivity, accessibility of facilities, accessibility of green) contributed to educational inequalities in walking and cycling among adults.

Methods: Data from participants (32–82 years) of the 2011 survey of the Dutch population-based GLOBE study were used (N = 2375). Highest attained educational level (independent variable) and walking for transport, cycling for transport, walking in leisure time and cycling in leisure time (dependent variables) were self-reported in the survey. GIS-systems were used to obtain spatial data on residential built environment characteristics. A four-step mediation-based analysis with log-linear regression models was used to examine to contribution of the residential built environment to educational inequalities in walking and cycling.

Results: As compared to the lowest educational group, the highest educational group was more likely to cycle for transport (RR 1.13, 95% CI 1.04–1.23), walk in leisure time (RR 1.12, 95% CI 1.04–1.21), and cycle in leisure time (RR 1.12, 95% CI 1.03–1.22). Objective built environment characteristics were related to these outcomes, but contributed minimally to educational inequalities in walking and cycling. On the other hand, compared to the lowest educational group, the highest educational group was less likely to walk for transport (RR 0.91, 95% CI 0.82–1.01), which could partly be attributed to differences in the built environment.

Conclusion: This study found that objective built environment characteristics contributed minimally to educational inequalities in walking and cycling in the Netherlands.

Keywords: Walking, Cycling, Built environment, Neighborhood, Health inequalities, GIS

Background

The twenty-first century is going to be an urban one. It is estimated that 54% of the world's population was living in urban areas by the year of 2014, and this figure will rise steadily over the following decades [1]. While urban areas are now believed to be of great importance in sustaining economic growth, it is less clear-cut what the consequences of this urban growth will be for population health. Living in an urban area may have positive as well as negative health consequences (e.g., urban areas offer better accessibility to various health-promoting resources, but in most cases have worse air quality), resulting in the use of the concepts of an 'urban health advantage' and an 'urban health penalty' simultaneously [2].

One of the key aspects of a healthy lifestyle is enough physical activity; 30 min of moderate-intensity activity a day is widely believed to have great health benefits [3, 4]. One way to promote physical activity is by facilitating the use of active travel modes (i.e. walking and cycling), either for transport-related or for recreational purposes. Increasing walking and cycling levels seems an attractive option, because walking and cycling are accessible

*Correspondence: c.b.m.kamphuis@uu.nl
[1] Department of Human Geography and Spatial Planning, Faculty of Geosciences, Utrecht University, Heidelberglaan 2, 3584 CS Utrecht, The Netherlands
Full list of author information is available at the end of the article

options to (almost) everyone and can be easily integrated into an individuals' daily activity program.

It is becoming increasingly clear that spatial planning has an important role to play in the promotion of a healthy urban lifestyle. While personal factors are critical in determining individual health, the built environment has the potential to exacerbate or mitigate health outcomes for large populations groups [5]. Various studies suggest a relationship exists between the built environment and the amounts of walking and cycling [6]. The built environment can thus play a vital role in promoting a healthy, physically active, urban lifestyle.

An important theme in health policy is the reduction of health inequalities [7]. Unhealthy lifestyles tend to be present more in lower socioeconomic groups, resulting in poorer health and higher mortality rates [8]. This general relationship is, however, less obvious in the case of physical activity, where the direction of socioeconomic inequalities seems to differ considerably by domain. A high socioeconomic position is related to higher levels of leisure-time physical activity [9], but socioeconomic inequalities in active transport do not show a consistent pattern [10]. Although the built environment is often presumed to be an explanatory factor of socioeconomic inequalities in walking and cycling, little research has yet investigated this issue. Because place of residence is strongly patterned by socioeconomic position, the neighborhood could be an important contributor to socioeconomic inequalities in health [11, 12]. Yet, pathways may be less straightforward: exposure to more facilities for example may increase walking for transport purposes, but decrease walking in leisure time. Moreover, if and to what extent higher and lower socioeconomic groups are differentially exposed to built environmental characteristics requires further investigation.

The Netherlands offer an interesting study setting for this issue, because Dutch cities are generally characterized by a relatively dense urban context, which is more conducive to walking and cycling [13].

Therefore the overall aim of this study is to examine to what extent objective built environment characteristics contribute to socioeconomic inequalities in walking and cycling—both transport-related and in leisure time—in the Netherlands. More specifically, we investigate (1) to what extent educational inequalities in walking and cycling exist in the Netherlands, (2) to what extent higher and lower educational groups reside in neighborhoods with different objective built environment characteristics, i.e. density, level of mixed use, connectivity, accessibility of facilities and accessibility of green, (3) the associations of these built environment characteristics with walking and cycling, and (4) to what extent these built environment characteristics contribute to the explanation

of educational inequalities in walking and cycling in the Netherlands. Figure 1 schematically represents the relationships between the different factors that are examined in this study.

Methods
Study population
This study uses survey data from the GLOBE cohort study, collected among adults living in the Dutch region of Eindhoven and surroundings in the year 2011. The GLOBE study is a cohort study that started in 1991. The city of Eindhoven and its surrounding villages was chosen as study location, because its composition was reasonably representative for the Netherlands in terms of age, sex, and educational level. Follow-up data collections were conducted in 1997, 2004, 2011 and 2014 (for more information on the GLOBE study, see [14]). This study uses data from the GLOBE survey of 2011 (N = 2888; mean age 60.69 (SD = 13.27); range 32–91 years). The 2011 survey was chosen because this survey contains the most detailed information on various sorts of walking and cycling activities. Respondents who had missing data for educational level, sex, age, employment status, or built environment variables (N = 513; some neighborhoods had missing data on accessibility of green variables due to neighborhood reorganizations since 2008) were excluded from the analysis, reducing the sample to N = 2375, residing in N = 209 neighborhoods (the neighborhood is defined in section "Built environment characteristics of the neighborhood").

Walking and cycling
Walking and cycling activity was measured using the SQUASH questionnaire [15]. Respondents were asked how many days per week they walked and cycled (1) in leisure time, (2) to shops and other facilities, and (3) to work or school. Walking to shops and other facilities and walking to work or school were grouped together to compose a 'walking for transport' variable. The same was done for cycling to shops and other facilities and cycling to work or school. For each of the outcome variables, a high share of the respondents indicated to walk '0 days per week'. Therefore, each outcome was dichotomized in either walking/cycling at least once per week versus no weekly walking/cycling. Thus, four dichotomous variables were created: walking for transport (yes/no) cycling for transport (yes/no), walking in leisure time (yes/no), and cycling in leisure time (yes/no).

Educational level
Educational level was used as indicator of socioeconomic position. A study by Winkleby et al. [16, see also 17] showed that education was the best socioeconomic

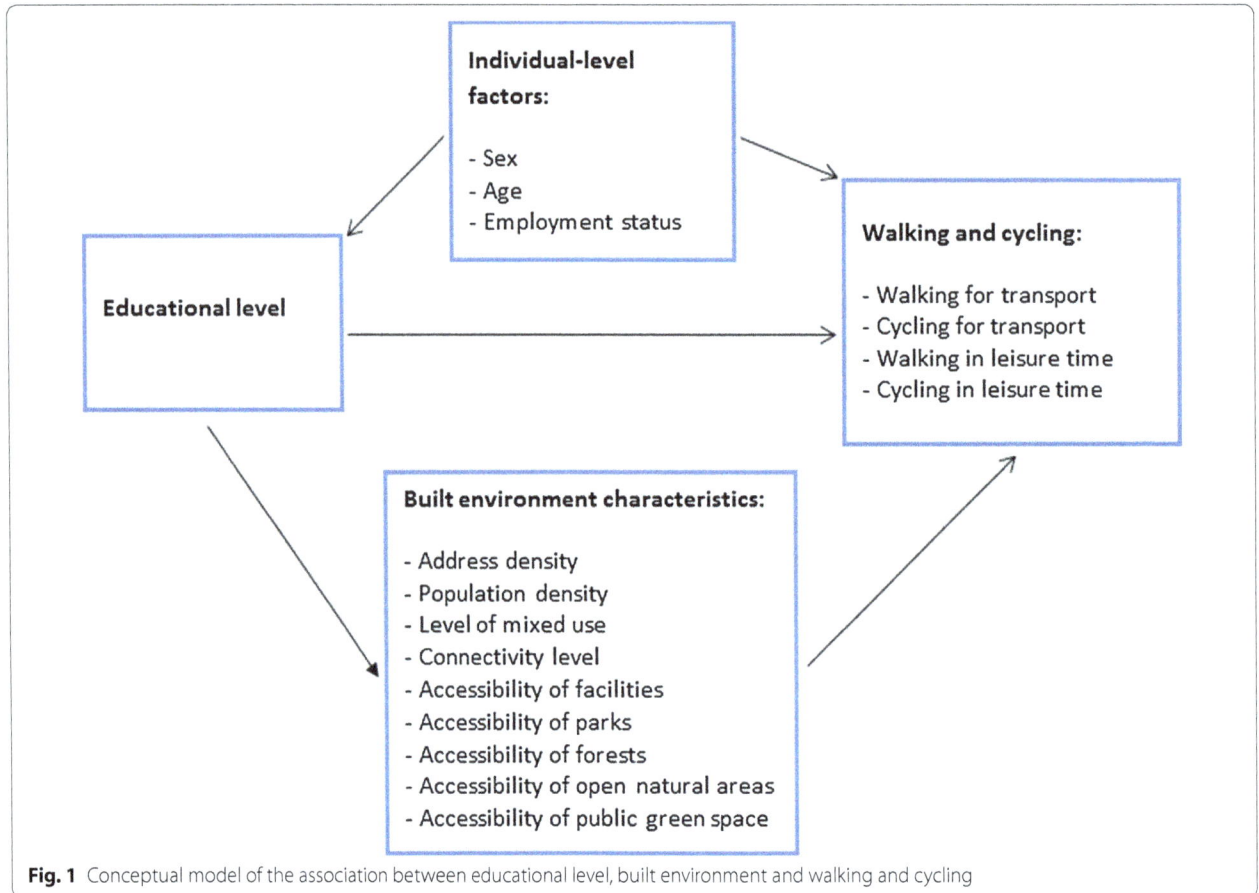

Fig. 1 Conceptual model of the association between educational level, built environment and walking and cycling

predictor of good health. Also, in the 2011 GLOBE survey, educational level was characterized by high response rates (i.e. higher than income). In the 2011 survey, information of respondents' educational level was acquired through questions on highest education completed (with options ranging from no education to university education). This information was grouped into three categories, based on a categorization used by Statistics Netherlands [18]. The 'low' educational group comprised respondents with no education and respondents who completed only primary education or lower secondary education (ISCED 0–2). The 'middle' educational group comprised respondents who completed either 'middle-level applied education' or higher secondary education (ISCED 3–4). The 'high' educational group comprised respondents who completed higher vocational education or university education (ISCED 5–7).

Built environment characteristics of the neighborhood

The spatial level on which the built environment data for this study were collected was the neighborhood level, which is the smallest geographical unit used in the Netherlands for statistical purposes. In 2013, neighborhoods

included in this study had an average population of 2558 (range 25–10,355) and an average size of 179 hectares (range 13–4243) [19]. The neighborhood level was deemed appropriate because it was expected to be of sufficient size to be of significant importance for people's daily walking and cycling activities, yet small enough for local variation in exposures and outcomes to exist. Also, Statistics Netherlands frequently uses the neighborhood level to collect spatial data, which were used in this study.

In general, built environment aspects that seem to be of significant importance for walking and cycling are population density, street connectivity, accessibility of facilities, a mixed land use, greenery, aesthetics, the presence of recreational facilities such as parks and the availability of walking and cycling paths [6, 20]. However, due to data availability not all aspects could be included in this study. Also, characteristics can be operationalized in different ways, sometimes yielding different results (see, for example, [21]). Table 1 gives an overview of the built environment variables that were used in this study, and their sources. The variables used in the study partly measured the same characteristics, and some are expected to be highly correlated (e.g., a neighborhood with high levels of

Table 1 Description and source of all built environment variables used in the study

Variable	Description	Mean (SD)	Range	Data source
Address density	Degree of concentration by number of addresses within a 1 km radius on January 1, 2013	1533 (779.6)	16–3684	Statistics Netherlands [19]
Population density	Number of residents per km^2 in a neighborhood on January 1, 2013	3999.3 (1904.7)	8–11,151	Statistics Netherlands [19]
Level of mixed use	Degree of mixed use of a neighborhood, measured by an entropy measure containing the categories 'residential' and 'other' in 2013	0.517 (0.203)	0.069–1	Kadaster [41]
Connectivity	Number of intersections per km^2 in a neighborhood in November 2012	140.2 (51.5)	2–303	Kadaster [42]
Accessibility of facilities	Number of facilities within a 1 km radius in 2013. The following facilities were used to calculate this variable (weights between brackets): big supermarkets (10), other daily provisions (5), cafes (1), cafeteria (1), restaurants (1), nurseries (1), out-of-school care (1) and schools (5)	68.9 (61.8)	0–424	Statistics Netherlands [19]
Accessibility of parks	Accessibility measure based on the mean distance to a park for all residents of a neighborhood in 2008	0.613 (0.544)	0.1–4.6	Statistics Netherlands [30]
Accessibility of forests	Accessibility measure based on the mean distance to a forest for all residents of a neighborhood in 2008	1.078 (0.512)	0.2–2.7	Statistics Netherlands [30]
Accessibility of open natural areas	Accessibility measure based on the mean distance to an open natural area for all residents of a neighborhood in 2008	3.197 (1.442)	0.5–6.3	Statistics Netherlands [30]
Accessibility of public green space	Accessibility measure based on the mean distance to public green space (i.e. one of the above) for all residents of a neighborhood in 2008	0.441 (0.196)	0.1–1.2	Statistics Netherlands [30]

mixed use is expected to be more accessible). The combination of various factors might, however, provide additional explanatory power [22]. Below the calculations of all variables are described. Because of their distributional characteristics (i.e. highly skewed with some extreme outliers), for the analyses, the values of all built environment variables have been grouped into tertiles (low, medium, high).

Address density was derived from Statistics Netherlands [19] and comprised the mean number of addresses per km^2 within a 1 km radius of each address within the neighborhood. For the calculation of this variable, first, the address density for each address (x–y- coordinate) in the neighborhood was calculated. Then the mean address density of the neighborhood was calculated by dividing the sum of all address densities in the neighborhood by the total number of addresses in the neighborhood [23].

Population density was calculated by Statistics Netherlands [19] as the number of residents of a neighborhood divided by the total land area of the neighborhood. A first difference between population density and address density is that address density contains all sorts of human activity (e.g. shops, offices), whereas population density only contains residential activity. A second

difference is the geographic area of measurement: while the population density variable comprised the density of the neighborhood area, the address density variable includes all addresses in a 1 km radius. This difference in calculation may yield substantial differences in outcomes. For example, a densely populated neighborhood located at the edge of a city will be characterized by high levels of population density, but low levels of address density.

The *level of mixed use* was based on the distribution of land use in an area. It was calculated using an entropy equation to form a measure that ranges from 0 to 1, with 0 representing complete homogeneity of land use and 1 representing an even distribution of all types of land use [24, 25]. In the present study, the level of mixed use was not calculated using proportions of land area. Instead, the type of land use was derived from individual addresses. The variable can therefore be seen as the degree of mixing of different address types. Because of the high proportion of addresses in the study area that were characterized as residential, the entropy measure is based solely on two categories: 'residential' and 'other' (e.g. retail, industry). It was calculated using the following equation (adapted from [26]):

$$-1 \frac{\frac{proportion\,'residential'}{total\ number\ of\ addresses} \times \ln\left(\frac{proportion\,'residential'}{total\ number\ of\ addresses}\right) + \frac{proportion\,'other'}{total\ number\ of\ addresses} \times \ln\left(\frac{proportion\,'other'}{total\ number\ of\ addresses}\right)}{\ln\,(2)}$$

The level of *connectivity* was calculated as the sum of intersections with at least three converging roads or pathways in a neighborhood, divided by the size of the neighborhood to control for differences in neighborhood size. For the purpose of this study, intersections that were primarily used by cars (e.g. highways, provincial roads) were excluded. This measure has been used previously [22, 25, 27], where it was shown to be a significant predictor of walking and cycling.

The *accessibility of facilities* was based on data derived from Statistics Netherlands [19] containing the mean number of various facility types within a road distance of 1 km. This was calculated using the number of facilities within a road distance of 1 km from every address in the neighborhood, divided by the total number of addresses [23]. Weights were assigned by the authors based on their expected frequency of visits (see Table 1). This variable can be seen as an elaboration of the 'cumulative opportunities' measure distinguished by Handy and Niemeier [28], which emphasizes the number of potential opportunities within a given travel distance (see also [29]).

The four accessibility of green variables (i.e. *accessibility of parks*, *accessibility of forests*, *accessibility of open natural areas*, and *accessibility of public green space*) were derived from Statistics Netherlands [30] and were calculated using data on the mean distance of all residents of a neighborhood to the closest park. For reasons of interpretation, after categorization this figure was 'swapped' (i.e. the lowest scores were turned into the highest and vice versa) to turn 'distance' into 'accessibility'. The *accessibility of public green space* variable is a combination of the other three accessibility of green variables, based on the mean distance of all residents of a neighborhood to the closest green space.

Statistical analysis

We applied a four-step mediation-based analysis approach, largely similar to previous studies [25]. In all steps, the models were adjusted for potential confounders, i.e. age, sex and employment status (the categorization used, and the distribution of respondents across these control variables, are shown in Table 2). In the first step, walking and cycling for different purposes (the dependent variables) were separately regressed on educational level (the independent variable). Second, educational level was separately correlated with each built environment variable. Third, each walking and cycling variable was separately regressed on each of the built environment variables, adjusted for educational level. Fourth, all built environment variables that were significant in the third analysis were added to the regression of the different walking and cycling variables on educational level. Comparison between the first and fourth analysis showed the contribution of the built environment variables to educational differences in walking and cycling levels [25].

The second step in the analysis (correlation between educational level and built environment variables) was conducted using crosstabs and Kendall's Tau-b (conducted in SPSS 22). All other analyses were conducted using multilevel log-linear analysis (conducted in Stata 14). Although in all analyses the variance at the neighborhood level was very small, multilevel models were nevertheless used to account for the clustering of individuals within neighborhoods. Log-linear regression instead of logistic regression was used because the distribution of respondents across the dependent variables was characterized by relatively high numbers of respondents in the 'no walking/cycling' groups (i.e. more than 10%), raising the problem of 'non-collapsibility' of odds ratios in a logistic regression mediation analysis. Log-linear analysis—which uses risk ratios instead of odds ratios—was used to tackle this problem [31].

All statistical analyses were weighted to be representative for the population of Eindhoven and surroundings aged 25–75 in the year 2004.

Results

A description of demographic characteristics and an initial examination of the distribution of walking and cycling variables among the three educational groups can be found in Table 2. This table shows that respondents in the low educational category were more frequently female (65.4%), older than 60 (64.8%), and not working (70.7%) than respondents in the higher educational categories (48.2, 33.8, and 32.7%, respectively, for the high educational category). Also, walking and cycling were in all cases practiced by more than half of the respondents.

In addition, maps of the various built environment variables and of the spatial distribution of respondents by educational level can be found in the Additional file 1: Appendix. These maps show that most built environment variables (both density variables, connectivity, accessibility of facilities and accessibility of parks) had higher levels in the Eindhoven city center and other urban centers in the area (those of Best and Helmond), while a few built environment variables (level of mixed use, accessibility of forests and accessibility of open natural areas) showed higher values in more suburban and rural areas. A correlation analysis between built environment variables (see Additional file 1: Appendix) showed that none of the paired variables showed problematically high correlation outcomes [the highest correlations were found between accessibility of parks and accessibility of public green ($\tau_B = 0.65$) and between population density and connectivity ($\tau_B = 0.63$)], so each variable can be assumed to contain unique characteristics.

Table 2 Distribution of respondents across variables in different educational groups (N = 2375)

Sex	Low education		Middle education		High education		Total	
	N	%	N	%	N	%	N	%
Female	674	65.4	277	54./	363	48.2	1314	56.3
Male	354	34.6	283	45.3	424	51.8	1061	43.7
Age								
30–39	22	3.5	70	15.0	114	18.1	206	11.9
40–49	68	9.9	138	29.1	165	24.0	371	20.2
50–59	140	21.7	113	24.0	172	24.3	425	23.3
60–69	331	36.2	137	21.3	175	21.1	643	26.7
70–79	405	24.6	84	8.6	144	10.8	633	15.2
80–89	62	4.0	18	2.1	17	1.7	97	2.7
Employment status								
Full-time	97	15.4	151	32.0	258	38.0	506	28.1
Part-time	93	13.8	147	30.8	192	29.3	432	24.0
Not working	838	70.7	262	37.2	337	32.7	1437	47.8
Walking for transport								
No	368	38.2	197	37.2	321	41.8	886	39.2
Yes	660	61.8	363	62.8	466	58.2	1489	60.8
Cycling for transport								
No	445	36.7	188	33.2	219	27.1	852	32.3
Yes	583	63.3	372	66.8	568	72.9	1523	67.7
Walking in leisure time								
No	352	31.6	124	21.7	173	22.6	649	25.6
Yes	676	68.4	436	78.3	614	77.4	1726	74.4
Cycling in leisure time								
No	419	35.9	167	29.6	206	26.2	792	30.7
Yes	609	64.1	393	70.4	581	73.8	1583	69.3

Frequencies are not weighted, percentages are

Educational level and walking and cycling

The highest educational group was more likely to cycle for transport (RR 1.13, 95% CI 1.04–1.23) walk in leisure time (RR 1.12, 95% CI 1.04–1.21) and cycle in leisure time (RR 1.12, 95% CI 1.03–1.22) than its low-educated counterpart. Respondents in the group with the highest education were less likely to walk for transport (RR 0.91, 95% CI 0.82–1.01) than their lower-educated counterparts, but this association was not significant (see Table 3).

Educational level and built environment

There was a weak but significant inverse association between educational level and address density ($\tau_B = -0.065$), educational level and population density ($\tau_B = -0.037$), educational level and level of mixed use ($\tau_B = -0.080$), educational level and accessibility of facilities ($\tau_B = -0.059$), and a positive association between educational level and accessibility of forests ($\tau_B = 0.036$). No significant association was found between educational level and connectivity, accessibility of parks, accessibility of open natural areas, and accessibility of public green space.

Table 3 Associations between educational level and walking and cycling for transport and in leisure time (N = 2375)

Educational level	RR (95% CI)	Sig.
Walking for transport		
Low	1.00	0.152
Middle	0.98 (0.86–1.10)	
High	0.91 (0.82–1.01)	
Cycling for transport		
Low	1.00	0.009
Middle	1.02 (0.93–1.12)	
High	1.13 (1.04–1.23)	
Walking in leisure time		
Low	1.00	0.006
Middle	1.12 (1.04–1.21)	
High	1.12 (1.04–1.21)	
Cycling in leisure time		
Low	1.00	0.021
Middle	1.07 (0.98–1.16)	
High	1.12 (1.03–1.22)	

All analyses were adjusted for variations in sex, age and employment status

Built environment and walking and cycling

Residents of neighborhoods with higher levels of address density, population density, connectivity and accessibility of facilities were more likely to walk for transport than residents of neighborhoods with the lowest scores, all significant at the 5% level. For example, residents of neighborhoods with the highest level of address density were 1.33 times more likely to walk for transport than residents of neighborhoods with the lowest scores (RR 1.33, 95% CI 1.21–1.47; see Table 4 for more results). Walking for transport was less prevalent among residents of neighborhoods that were close to a forest [RR 0.87, 95% CI 0.78–0.96 (high category)]. No significant impact on walking for transport was found for the other accessibility of green variables and for the level of mixed use variable. Residents of neighborhoods with higher levels

Table 4 Associations between walking and cycling and built environment (N = 2375)

	Walking for transport		Cycling for transport		Walking in leisure time		Cycling in leisure time	
	RR (95% CI)	Sig.	RR (95% CI)	Sig.	RR (95% CI)	Sig.	RR (95% CI)	Sig.
Address density								
1 (low)	1.00	0.000	1.00	0.293	1.00	0.005	1.00	0.004
2	1.04 (0.93–1.16)		0.96 (0.86–1.06)		0.90 (0.85–0.96)		0.90 (0.83–0.98)	
3 (high)	1.33 (1.21–1.47)		0.92 (0.84–1.02)		0.99 (0.94–1.04)		0.89 (0.82–0.96)	
Population density								
1 (low)	1.00	0.001	1.00	0.049	1.00	0.781	1.00	0.048
2	1.07 (0.97–1.19)		0.96 (0.86–1.06)		0.99 (0.93–1.05)		0.96 (0.89–1.04)	
3 (high)	1.22 (1.10–1.35)		0.89 (0.81–0.98)		1.01 (0.94–1.08)		0.91 (0.84–0.98)	
Level of mixed use								
1 (low)	1.00	0.159	1.00	0.549	1.00	0.821	1.00	0.740
2	1.10 (1.00–1.21)		1.04 (0.96–1.13)		1.02 (0.95–1.08)		1.03 (0.95–1.12)	
3 (high)	1.05 (0.94–1.18)		1.00 (0.89–1.12)		1.02 (0.95–1.09)		1.02 (0.94–1.11)	
Connectivity								
1 (low)	1.00	0.027	1.00	0.505	1.00	0.966	1.00	0.284
2	1.10 (0.997–1.22)		0.95 (0.86–1.06)		1.00 (0.94–1.07)		1.00 (0.92–1.08)	
3 (high)	1.14 (1.03–1.26)		0.94 (0.86–1.04)		1.01 (0.94–1.07)		0.94 (0.87–1.02)	
Accessibility of facilities								
1 (low)	1.00	0.000	1.00	0.890	1.00	0.037	1.00	0.959
2	1.09 (0.98–1.21)		1.02 (0.93–1.12)		0.96 (0.90–1.03)		1.01 (0.93–1.10)	
3 (high)	1.26 (1.13–1.41)		1.01 (0.91–1.12)		1.04 (0.99–1.11)		1.00 (0.92–1.08)	
Accessibility of parks								
1 (low)	1.00	0.354	1.00	0.530	1.00	0.632	1.00	0.538
2	1.03 (0.94–1.14)		1.00 (0.91–1.11)		1.01 (0.96–1.07)		0.99 (0.91–1.07)	
3 (high)	0.95 (0.86–1.06)		0.96 (0.86–1.07)		0.98 (0.91–1.05)		0.96 (0.88–1.04)	
Accessibility of forests								
1 (low)	1.00	0.015	1.00	0.218	1.00	0.758	1.00	0.592
2	0.89 (0.80–0.99)		1.08 (0.98–1.19)		0.98 (0.92–1.05)		1.03 (0.95–1.12)	
3 (high)	0.87 (0.78–0.96)		1.07 (0.98–1.17)		0.98 (0.91–1.04)		1.04 (0.96–1.13)	
Accessibility of open natural areas								
1 (low)	1.00	0.605	1.00	0.603	1.00	0.378	1.00	0.088
2	0.95 (0.85–1.06)		1.05 (0.96–1.15)		1.01 (0.95–1.08)		1.08 (1.01–1.17)	
3 (high)	0.96 (0.88–1.06)		1.02 (0.93–1.13)		0.96 (0.90–1.03)		1.02 (0.94–1.11)	
Accessibility of public green space								
1 (low)	1.00	0.379	1.00	0.539	1.00	0.292	1.00	0.040
2	0.95 (0.86–1.04)		0.95 (0.87–1.04)		0.99 (0.94–1.04)		0.93 (0.87–1.00)	
3 (high)	0.92 (0.79–1.06)		0.97 (0.84–1.11)		0.92 (0.83–1.02)		0.89 (0.80–0.99)	

All built environment variables were analyzed separately from each other

All analyses were adjusted for variations in sex, age, employment status and educational level of population density were less likely to cycle for transport [RR 0.89, 95% CI 0.81–0.98 (high category)].

Residents of neighborhoods with higher levels of address density were less likely to walk in leisure time [RR 0.90, 95% CI 0.85–0.96 (middle); RR 0.99, 95% CI 0.94–1.04 (high)]. Next to this, a significant association was found between accessibility of facilities and walking in leisure time, which was negative for the middle group but positive for the high one [RR 0.96, 95% CI 0.90–1.03 (middle); RR 1.04, 95% CI 0.99–1.11 (high). Also, when compared to their counterparts of neighborhoods in the lowest density category, residents of neighborhoods with higher levels of address density (RR 0.90, 95% CI 0.83–0.98 (middle); RR 0.89, 95% CI 0.82–0.96 (high)] and population density (RR 0.96, 95% CI 0.89–1.04 (middle); RR 0.91, 95% CI 0.84–0.98 (high)] were less likely to cycle in leisure time. Lastly, residents of neighborhoods that were close to public green space were less likely to cycle in leisure time [RR 0.93, 95% CI 0.87–1.00 (middle); RR 0.89, 95% CI 0.80–0.99 (high); see Table 4].

Educational level, objective built environment, and walking and cycling

The negative association between educational level and walking for transport attenuated after adjustment for built environment variables [RR 1.01, 95% CI 0.90–1.13, ΔRR +0.03 (middle educational group), RR 0.94, 95% CI 0.85–1.04, ΔRR +0.03 (high)]. Adjustment for built environment variables had only minimal effect on the associations between educational level and cycling for transport [RR 1.01, 95% CI 0.93–1.11, ΔRR −0.01 (middle), RR 1.12, 95% CI 1.03–1.22, ΔRR −0.01 (high)] and educational level and cycling in leisure time [RR 1.05, 95% CI 0.97–1.14, ΔRR −0.01 (middle), RR 1.11, 95% CI 1.02–1.20, ΔRR −0.01 (high)], and no effect was found for the association between educational level and walking in leisure time. After adjustment for built environment variables, middle and high educational groups were still significantly more likely to cycle for transport and to walk and cycle in leisure time than their counterparts in the low educational group (see Table 5).

Discussion

Lower educational groups were less likely to cycle for transport and to walk and cycle in leisure time, but only minimal effects of mediating built environment variables were found. On the other hand, lower educational groups were more likely to walk for transport, which could partly be attributed to differences in the built environment. These results suggest that neighborhood density, level of mixed use, connectivity, accessibility of facilities and accessibility of green only make a small contribution to

Table 5 Associations between educational level and walking and cycling adjusted for significant built environment variables

Educational level	RR (95% CI)	Sig.	ΔRR
Walking for transport[a]			
Low	1.00	0.262	
Middle	1.01 (0.90–1.13)		+0.03
High	0.94 (0.85–1.04)		+0.03
Cycling for transport[b]			
Low	1.00	0.014	
Middle	1.01 (0.93–1.11)		−0.01
High	1.12 (1.03–1.22)		−0.01
Walking in leisure time[c]			
Low	1.00	0.004	
Middle	1.12 (1.04–1.21)		0.00
High	1.12 (1.04–1.21)		0.00
Cycling in leisure time[d]			
Low	1.00	0.039	
Middle	1.05 (0.97–1.14)		−0.01
High	1.11 (1.02–1.20)		−0.01

The changes in risk ratios (ΔRR) compare the risk ratios after adjustment for built environment variables to the risk ratios before adjustment for built environment variables (see Table 3)

[a] Adjusted for variations in sex, age, employment status, address density, population density, connectivity, accessibility of facilities and accessibility of forests

[b] Adjusted for variations in sex, age, employment status and population density

[c] Adjusted for variations in sex, age, employment status, address density and accessibility of facilities

[d] Adjusted for variations in sex, age, employment status, address density, population density and accessibility of public green space

educational inequalities in walking and cycling behavior in the Netherlands.

Explaining educational inequalities in walking and cycling

Walking for transport was the only outcome that respondents with higher educational levels were less likely to perform. This study showed that this relationship attenuated after adjustment for built environment variables, indicating that respondents with a low educational level were more likely to walk for transport partly because their residential built environment was more conducive to this activity type. This is consistent with previous findings by Turrell et al. [25], who found that higher levels of walking for transport among residents of poorer neighborhoods in Australia could partly be explained by the higher connectivity, density and land use mix levels in those neighborhoods. It is also consistent with findings of a review of American studies, which found that low-income populations disproportionately resided in areas with higher population density and a more compact urban form ([32]; this review did not examine the impact of this relationship on walking and cycling out-comes). On the other hand, it diverges from findings by Cerin et al. [33], who found that the built environment contributed to higher levels of walking for transport among higher educational groups in Australia. One possible explanation of these divergent findings concerns the different type of built environment variables used in the studies: unlike the present study, Cerin et al. included 'micro' variables (which are smaller in scale and generally changeable more rapidly and with less cost; see [34] for a description of micro and macro built environment characteristics) like aesthetics, traffic load, physical barriers to walking, and the presence of separate footpaths.

Cycling for transport, walking in leisure time and cycling in leisure time were all significantly more prevalent among respondents with higher educational levels. Adjustment for built environment variables had no or only minimal effect on these educational inequalities. This lack of effect of objective built environment characteristics differs from findings by previous studies, which found objective built environment variables to be a significant contributor to socioeconomic inequalities in walking in leisure time [35], cycling in leisure time [36], and overall physical activity [37, 38]. However, the abovementioned studies again focused mostly on 'micro' built environment variables like aesthetics [36], the accessibility of physical activity-facilities (including parks, but also sport centers and youth clubs [37, 38]), and the presence of walking paths [35], whereas the present study used 'macro' characteristics such as density, land use pattern and overall accessibility measures. One possible explanation of these differences could be that 'micro' characteristics are more likely to be improved in the wealthier, better-organized neighborhoods of higher-educated residents (e.g. it is easier to remove graffiti or design a new bicycle path than to change the density of a neighborhood, and such small changes may take place more often in neighborhoods with high-educated residents). Next to this, the divergent results could be explained by the relatively small educational differences in built environment characteristics (see section "Educational level and built environment"). Although significant effects were found, the small size of these effects suggests that built environment characteristics were quite equally distributed among educational groups. This, together with the compact nature of the Dutch urban environment, might make walking and cycling-promoting resources almost equally accessible to all residents of urban areas.

Previous Dutch studies found that socioeconomic inequalities in recreational walking and cycling could partly be attributed to less favorable built environment characteristics in more disadvantaged neighborhoods [39, 40], which seems in contrast with our results. There are two possible explanations for these differences. Firstly, the divergent findings could be explained by the nature of the neighborhood variables included in the analyses. Where the present study used objective built environment variables, the two studies above used perceptions of either participants [40] or municipal professionals [39]. Also, other neighborhood characteristics than built environment characteristics were applied in those previous Dutch studies (e.g. safety, general attractiveness). Secondly, differences in findings could be explained by differences in the operationalization of socioeconomic position. Where one study [39] used the neighborhood socioeconomic environment and the other [40] used both educational attainment and income, this study used only educational level as an indicator of SEP, and as discussed above, only small educational differences in built environment characteristics were found.

This study showed that the residential patterning of different educational groups can also have positive effects on the accessibility of resources that influence health for groups with lower educational levels. This was the case for walking for transport, the variable that was most strongly correlated to built environment characteristics. Although effects were small due to the small magnitude of differences in built environment characteristics, respondents in lower educational groups had better access to built environment characteristics that positively influenced walking for transport. The health benefits for lower educational groups resulting from their higher levels of walking for transport may partly offset the negative effects of other less healthy behaviors (e.g. the negative effects of less cycling for transport and less recreational walking and cycling; [25]).

Built environment and walking and cycling

Consistent with previous studies [6, 20], a strong association was found between built environment variables within the walkability domain and walking for transport, with a higher chance of walking for transport among respondents of neighborhoods with high levels of address density, population density, connectivity and accessibility of facilities. Contrary to previous findings [6], the chances of walking in leisure time and cycling in leisure time were lower among respondents living in neighborhoods with higher scores on address density, indicating that an environment that is conducive to walking for transport may have adverse effects on recreational walking and cycling. The fact that this negative association was not found for other variables in the walkability domain (e.g. connectivity) shows that the inclusion of complementary variables can show different effects (i.e. using only a single 'walkability' variable would not give this detailed results).

Of all walking and cycling variables, walking for transport was most strongly related to the built environment, which is consistent with previous studies' findings [20]. For the other walking and cycling variables, relationships were less strong. This was especially the case for cycling for transport, where only one built environment variable was found to be significant: cycling for transport was less prevalent in areas with higher population density. One potential explanation is that in these neighborhoods, more facilities are within walking distance, thereby reducing the need to cycle for transport.

It may be that built environment variables not included in the present study could be more important for cycling for transport, walking in leisure time and cycling in leisure time levels (e.g. aesthetics, presence of walking paths), but it is also possible that these activity types are mainly affected by factors outside the built environment (this could still be neighborhood-level characteristics, such as safety or social features). Another explanation is that these activities may largely take place outside the residential neighborhood, and therefore do not show associations with neighborhood characteristics. Cycling in particular can easily reach beyond the residential neighborhood, enabling residents of lower density areas to reach facilities that are further away from their homes.

Study strengths
This study has combined survey data from the GLOBE study with objective built environment data from other sources, which has given unique insights into the role of objective built environment factors in explaining inequalities in walking and cycling in the Netherlands. Because this study has focused on the urban region of Eindhoven and its surroundings, the associations found concern an entire urban area, including more suburban and rural surroundings, instead of a single city (as studied in most previous research). This has increased both the variation of built environment characteristics investigated in the study and the possibility of generalizability of this study's results. Having said that, as compared to the situation in for example the US or Australia, the variation in our urban area might still be small. Another major strength of this study was that it included both walking and cycling, both for transport and in leisure time, whereas other studies have often focused on just one or two outcomes. This broad study design made it possible to compare educational level and built environment influences on different types of physical activity, revealing contrary mechanisms. Also, the incorporation of nine objective built environment variables made it possible to examine the effects of a broad array of different built environment types.

Study limitations
A number of methodological and analytical problems exist that need to be considered when interpreting this study's findings. First, the neighborhood area and its 1 km radius used as the spatial analysis units in this analysis may not be similar to the geographic area of residents' daily spatial movements. People do not take into account neighborhood boundaries in their daily activities, and their activity space may be much larger than just the neighborhood. This is expected to be of importance especially for cycling, where larger distances can be traversed more easily. Second, this study included a selection of built environment variables, while other built environment characteristics might also be important (e.g. aesthetics, presence of walking and cycling trails). Third, a gap of a few years existed between the dates of the various data used. Whereas the GLOBE data was collected in 2011, most built environment variables describe the situation in 2013, and the accessibility of green variables describe the situation in 2008. However, the built environment characteristics used are not expected to have changed much in just a few years. Fourth, the mediation analysis used in the study assumes that there is no misspecification of the causal order, no confounding between the exposure, mediators and outcomes, and no interaction between exposure and mediators [31]. Because the study used a cross-sectional research design, claims about causality cannot be made, but the causal order used in the study is in line with theoretical notions [11, 12]. The analyses were also adjusted for potential confounders (i.e. sex, age, employment status), but there may be other confounders which were not controlled for. The assumption of no interaction was met for walking for transport, cycling for transport and cycling in leisure time. For walking in leisure time an effect of exposure-mediator interaction was found between address density and educational level. Therefore, a stratified analysis of these variables was added in the Additional file 1: Appendix.

A final remark should be made about the possibility of generalization of this study's results. Like other studies that focused on the contribution of the built environment to socioeconomic inequalities in walking and cycling in the Netherlands [39, 40], this study focused on the city of Eindhoven and its surroundings. The specific spatial patterns that characterize this region should be taken into account when generalizing the results to other urban areas. One example is the spatial patterning of socioeconomic groups. Because the city of Eindhoven does not have a historical city center that tends to attract high socioeconomic groups to the extent that other Dutch cities do, higher-educated residents of Eindhoven might tend to live more in the suburban parts of the city, or even in the smaller urban centers. This pattern might make Eindhoven more comparable to American cities. However, because of other general differences (e.g. in overall density or in cycling behavior) findings should be generalized to other contexts with care. Such differences make comparative research in other cities very relevant.

Conclusion

Lower educational groups were less likely to cycle for transport, and to walk and cycle in leisure time. Some of the objective built environment characteristics of residential areas examined (i.e. address density, population density, accessibility of facilities and accessibility of public green space) were related to these outcomes. However, only minimal contributions of the built environment to educational inequalities in walking and cycling were found. This may indicate that factors that may explain educational inequalities in these activity types should be searched for outside the residential area, or in other environments than the built environment (e.g. the sociocultural environments). It could also be that smaller-scale ('micro') built environment characteristics of the neighborhood (e.g. aesthetics, presences of walking paths) offer a better explanation.

Despite this, the small effect that was found for walking for transport suggests that the spatial patterning of people by educational level can have a diminishing effect on health inequalities. Lower educational groups tend to live in more walkable neighborhoods, which partly explains their higher tendency to walk for transport. Policy makers that aim to reduce health inequalities should be aware of the positive impact of the residential environment of lower educational groups on walking for transport levels. Recent gentrification processes, in which lower educational groups are forced to relocate to the outskirts of the city, might pose a serious threat to this inequalities-reducing mechanism, and new neighborhoods should be designed to be walkable. Future research should shed more light on the causal mechanisms between socioeconomic position, walking and cycling, and the built environment. A specifically important research type is the comparative analysis of different cities, which might elucidate the role of various urban contexts in the relationships between physical activity and the built environment.

Authors' contributions
DCvW wrote the manuscript while being supervised by CBMK. DCvW and JOG conducted the analyses. FJvL guided the data collection process of the GLOBE study. JOG, FJvL and CBMK critically reviewed the manuscript. All authors read and approved the final manuscript.

Author details
[1] Department of Human Geography and Spatial Planning, Faculty of Geosciences, Utrecht University, Heidelberglaan 2, 3584 CS Utrecht, The Netherlands. [2] Department of Public Health, Erasmus University Medical Centre, Erasmus University Rotterdam, Wytemaweg 80, 3015 CN Rotterdam, The Netherlands.

Acknowledgements
None.

Competing interests
The authors declare that they have no competing interests.

Funding
The present project was financed by a grant from the Netherlands Organization for Health Research and Development (Healthy Food Program, Project No. 115100006).

References
1. United Nations. World urbanization prospects: The 2014 revision, highlights. New York: United Nations; 2014.
2. Vlahov D, Galea S, Freudenberg N. The urban health "advantage". J Urban Health Bull NY Acad Med. 2005;82:1–4.
3. Warburton DER, Nicol CW, Bredin SSD. Health benefits of physical activity: the evidence. CMAJ. 2006;174:801–9.
4. Haskell WL, Lee IM, Pate RR, Powell KE, Blair SN. Physical activity and public health: updated recommendation for adults from the American College of Sports Medicine and the American Heart Association. Circulation. 2007;116:1081–93.
5. Barton H. Land use planning and health and well-being. Land Use Policy. 2009;26(Suppl 1):S115–23.
6. Wang Y, Chau CK, Ng WY, Leung TM. A review on the effects of physical built environment attributes on enhancing walking and cycling activity levels within residential neighborhoods. Cities. 2016;50:1–15.
7. WHO. Closing the gap in a generation: health equity through action on the social determinants of health. Final Report of the Commission on Social Determinants of Health. Geneva: World Health Organization; 2008.
8. Savelkoul M. Overzicht sociaaleconomische gezondheidsverschillen [Overview of socioeconomic differences in health]. In: Volksgezondheid Toekomst Verkenning, Nationaal Kompas Volksgezondheid. Bilthoven: National Institute for Public Health and the Environment; 2014.
9. Beenackers MA, Kamphuis CBM, Giskes K, Brug J, Kunst AE, Burdorf A, van Lenthe FJ. Socioeconomic inequalities in occupational, leisure-time, and transport related physical activity among European adults: a systematic review. Int J Behav Nutr Phys Act. 2012;9:116.
10. Rind E, Shortt N, Mitchell R, Richardson EA, Pearce J. Are income-related differences in active travel associated with physical environmental characteristics? A multi-level ecological approach. Int J Behav Nutr Phys Act. 2015;12:73.
11. Diez Roux AV, Mair C. Neighborhoods and health. Ann NY Acad Sci. 2010;1186:125–45.

12. Gelormino E, Melis G, Marietta C, Costa G. From built environment to health inequalities: an explanatory framework based on evidence. Prev Med Rep. 2015;2:737–45.

13. de Vries SI, Hopman-Rock M, Bakker I, Hirasing RA, van Mechelen W. Built environmental correlates of walking and cycling in dutch urban children: results from the SPACE study. Int J Environ Res Public Health. 2010;7:2309–24.

14. van Lenthe FJ, Kamphuis CBM, Beenackers MA, Jansen T, Looman CWN, Nusselder WJ, Mackenbach JP. Cohort profile: understanding socioeconomic inequalities in health and health behaviours: the GLOBE study. Int J Epidemiol. 2014;43:721–30.

15. Wendel-Vos GCW, Schuit AJ, Saris WH, Kromhout D. Reproducibility and relative validity of the short questionnaire to assess health-enhancing physical activity. J Clin Epidemiol. 2003;56:1163–9.

16. Winkleby MA, Jatulis DE, Frank E, Fortmann SP. Socioeconomic status and health: how education, income, and occupation contribute to risk factors for cardiovascular disease. Am J Public Health. 1992;82:816–20.

17. Verweij A. Wat is sociaaleconomische status? [What is socioeconomic status?] In: Volksgezondheid Toekomst Verkenning, Nationaal Kompas Volksgezondheid. Bilthoven: National Institute for Public Health and the Environment; 2010.

18. Verweij A. Onderwijsdeelname: Indeling opleidingsniveau. In: Volksgezondheid Toekomst Verkenning, Nationaal Kompas Volksgezondheid. Bilthoven: National Institute for Public Health and the Environment; 2008.

19. Statistics Netherlands. Wijk- en Buurtkaart 2013 [District and neighborhood map 2013]. Den Haag/Heerlen: Statistics Netherlands; 2014.

20. McCormack GR, Shiell A. In search of causality: a systematic review of the relationship between the built environment and physical activity among adults. Int J Behav Nutr Phys Act. 2011;8:125.

21. Manaugh K, Kreider T. What is mixed use? Presenting an interaction method for measuring land use mix. J Transp Land Use. 2013;6:63–72.

22. Glazier RH, Creatore MI, Weyman JT, Fazli G, Matheson FI, Gozdyra P, Moineddin R, Shriqui VK, Booth GL. Density, destinations or both? A comparison of measures of walkability in relation to transportation behaviors, obesity and diabetes in Toronto, Canada. PLoS ONE. 2014;9:e85295.

23. Statistics Netherlands. Toelichting Wijk- en Buurtkaart 2012, 2013 en 2014: Respectievelijk Versie 3, 2 en 1 [Supplement district and neighborhood map 2012, 2013 and 2014: Version 3, 2 and 1 respectively]. Den Haag/ Heerlen: Statistics Netherlands; 2015.

24. Leslie E, Coffee N, Frank L, Owen N, Bauman A, Hugo G. Walkability of local communities: using geographic information systems to objectively assess relevant environmental attributes. Health Place. 2007;13:111–22.

25. Turrell G, Haynes M, Wilson LA, Giles-Corti B. Can the built environment reduce health inequalities? A study of neighbourhood socioeconomic disadvantage and walking for transport. Health Place. 2013;19:89–98.

26. Brown BB, Yamada I, Smith KR, Zick CD, Kowaleski-Jones L, Fan JX. Mixed land use and walkability: variations in land use measures and relationships with BMI, overweight, and obesity. Health Place. 2009;15:1130–41.

27. Witten K, Blakely T, Baheri N, Badland H, Ivory V, Pearce J, Mavoa S, Hinckson E, Schofield G. Neighborhood built environment and transport and leisure physical activity: findings using objective exposure and outcome measures in New Zealand. Environ Health Perspect. 2012;120:971–7.

28. Handy SL, Niemeier DA. Measuring accessibility: an exploration of issues and alternatives. Environ Plan A. 1997;29:1175–94.

29. Thornton LE, Pearce JR, Kavanagh AM. Using geographic information systems (GIS) to assess the role of the built environment in influencing obesity: a glossary. Int J Behav Nutr Phys Act. 2011;8:71.

30. Statistics Netherlands. Nabijheid voorzieningen; afstand locatie, wijk- en buurtcijfers 2006–2012 [Proximity of facilities; distance location, district and neighborhood figures 2006–2012]. Den Haag/Heerlen: Statistics Netherlands; 2014.

31. VanderWeele TJ. Explanations in causal inference: methods for mediation and interaction. Oxford: Oxford University Press; 2015.

32. Lovasi GS, Hutson MA, Guerra M, Neckerman KM. Built environments and obesity in disadvantaged populations. Epidemiol Rev. 2009;31:7–20.

33. Cerin E, Leslie E, Owen N. Explaining socio-economic status differences in walking for transport: an ecological analysis of individual, social and environmental factors. Soc Sci Med. 2009;68:1013–20.

34. Sallis JF, Slymen DJ, Conway TL, Frank LD, Saelens BE, Cain K, Chapman JE. Income disparities in perceived neighborhood built and social environment attributes. Health Place. 2011;17:1274–83.

35. Ball K, Timperio A, Salmon J, Giles-Corti B, Roberts R, Crawford D. Personal, social and environmental determinants of educational inequalities in walking: a multilevel study. J Epidemiol Community Health. 2007;61:108–14.

36. Kamphuis CBM, Giskes K, Kavanagh AM, Thornton LE, Thomas LR, van Lenthe FJ, Mackenbach JP, Turrell G. Area variation in recreational cycling in Melbourne: a compositional or contextual effect? J Epidemiol Community Health. 2008;62:890–8.

37. Estabrooks PA, Lee RE, Gyurcsik NC. Resources for physical activity participation: does availability and accessibility differ by neighborhood socioeconomic status? Ann Behav Med. 2003;25:100–4.

38. Gordon-Larsen P, Nelson MC, Page P, Popkin BM. Inequality in the built environment underlies key health disparities in physical activity and obesity. Pediatrics. 2006;117:417–24.

39. van Lenthe FJ, Brug J, Mackenbach JP. Neighbourhood inequalities in physical inactivity: the role of neighbourhood attractiveness, proximity to local facilities and safety in the Netherlands. Soc Sci Med. 2005;60:763–75.

40. Kamphuis CBM, van Lenthe FJ, Giskes K, Huisman M, Brug J, Mackenbach JP. Socioeconomic differences in lack of recreational walking among older adults: the role of neighbourhood and individual factors. Int J Behav Nutr Phys Act. 2009;6:1.

41. Kadaster. Basisregistratie Adressen en Gebouwen [Basic registration of addresses and buildings]. Apeldoorn: Kadaster; 2013.

42. Kadaster. Top10NL [Top10NL]. Apeldoorn: Kadaster; 2012.

Permissions

The contributors of this book come from diverse backgrounds, making this book a truly international effort. This book will bring forth new frontiers with its revolutionizing research information and detailed analysis of the nascent developments around the world.

We would like to thank all the contributing authors for lending their expertise to make the book truly unique. They have played a crucial role in the development of this book. Without their invaluable contributions this book wouldn't have been possible. They have made vital efforts to compile up to date information on the varied aspects of this subject to make this book a valuable addition to the collection of many professionals and students.

This book was conceptualized with the vision of imparting up-to-date information and advanced data in this field. To ensure the same, a matchless editorial board was set up. Every individual on the board went through rigorous rounds of assessment to prove their worth. After which they invested a large part of their time researching and compiling the most relevant data for our readers.

The editorial board has been involved in producing this book since its inception. They have spent rigorous hours researching and exploring the diverse topics which have resulted in the successful publishing of this book. They have passed on their knowledge of decades through this book. To expedite this challenging task, the publisher supported the team at every step. A small team of assistant editors was also appointed to further simplify the editing procedure and attain best results for the readers.

Apart from the editorial board, the designing team has also invested a significant amount of their time in understanding the subject and creating the most relevant covers. They scrutinized every image to scout for the most suitable representation of the subject and create an appropriate cover for the book.

The publishing team has been an ardent support to the editorial, designing and production team. Their endless efforts to recruit the best for this project, has resulted in the accomplishment of this book. They are a veteran in the field of academics and their pool of knowledge is as vast as their experience in printing. Their expertise and guidance has proved useful at every step. Their uncompromising quality standards have made this book an exceptional effort. Their encouragement from time to time has been an inspiration for everyone.

The publisher and the editorial board hope that this book will prove to be a valuable piece of knowledge for researchers, students, practitioners and scholars across the globe.

List of Contributors

Warren C. Jochem
Department of Geography and Environment, University of Southampton, University Road, Southampton SO17 1BJ, UK

Abdur Razzaque
Health Systems and Population Studies Division, icddr, b, 68, Shaheed Tajuddin Ahmed Sarani, Mohakhali, Dhaka 1212, Bangladesh

Elisabeth Dowling Root
Department of Geography, Division of Epidemiology, The Ohio State University, 1036 Derby Hall, 154 North Oval Mall, Columbus, OH 43212, USA

Tiina E. Laatikainen, Kamyar Hasanzadeh and Marketta Kyttä
Department of Built Environment, Aalto University, 00076 Aalto, Finland

Anna Roudot
Université Paris Ouest Nanterre La Défense, 200 Avenue de la République, 92000 Nanterre, France

Daouda Kassié
Université Paris Ouest Nanterre La Défense, 200 Avenue de la République, 92000 Nanterre, France
CIRAD, ASTRE, CIRAD TA C-22/E, Campus International de Baillarguet, 34398 Montpellier Cedex 5, France

Gérard Salem
Université Paris Ouest Nanterre La Défense, 200 Avenue de la République, 92000 Nanterre, France
CEPED, Institut de Recherche pour le Développement, 19 Rue Jacob, 75006 Paris, France

Nadine Dessay
ESPACE DEV, Institut de Recherche pour le Développement, Maison de la Télédetection, 500 rue Jean-François Breton, 34093 Montpellier Cedex 5, France

Jean-Luc Piermay
Université De Strasbourg, 4 Rue Blaise Pascal, 67081 Strasbourg, France

Florence Fournet
MIVEGEC, Institut de Recherche pour le Développement, 911, Avenue Agropolis, BP 64501, 34394 Montpellier Cedex 5, France
Institut de Recherche en Sciences de la Santé, 01 BP 545, Bobo-Dioulasso, Burkina Faso

Elizabeth A. Mack and Kevin Credit
Department of Geography, Environment and Spatial Sciences, Michigan State University, Geography Building, 673 Auditorium Rd, Room 202, East Lansing, MI 48824, USA

Daoqin Tong
School of Geographical Sciences and Urban Planning, Arizona State University, Tempe, AZ 85281, USA

C. El Khoury
Univ. Lyon, University Claude Bernard Lyon 1, HESPER EA 7425, 69008 Lyon, France
Emergency Department and RESCUe Network, Lucien Hussel Hospital, Vienne 38200, France

J. Freyssenge
Univ. Lyon, University Claude Bernard Lyon 1, HESPER EA 7425, 69008 Lyon, France
Emergency Department and RESCUe Network, Lucien Hussel Hospital, Vienne 38200, France
UMR 5600 Environnement Ville Société CNRS, University Jean Moulin Lyon 3, 18, rue Chevreul, 69007 Lyon, France

A. M. Schott
Univ. Lyon, University Claude Bernard Lyon 1, HESPER EA 7425, 69008 Lyon, France
Pôle IMER, Hospices Civils de Lyon, 69003 Lyon, France

L. Derex
Univ. Lyon, University Claude Bernard Lyon 1, HESPER EA 7425, 69008 Lyon, France
Department of Stroke Medicine, Hospices Civils de Lyon, 69003 Lyon, France

K. Tazarourte
Univ. Lyon, University Claude Bernard Lyon 1, HESPER EA 7425, 69008 Lyon, France

Emergency Department, Hospices Civils de Lyon, 69003 Lyon, France

F. Renard
UMR 5600 Environnement Ville Société CNRS, University Jean Moulin Lyon 3, 18, rue Chevreul, 69007 Lyon, France

N. Nighoghossian
Department of Stroke Medicine, Hospices Civils de Lyon, 69003 Lyon, France
Department of Neuroradiology, Hospices Civils de Lyon, 69003 Lyon, France
CREATIS, CNRS-UMR5220 INSERM-U1044, Lyon 69008, France
INSA-Lyon, Lyon 69008, France

Dörthe Brüggmann
Department of Obstetrics and Gynecology, Keck School of Medicine of USC, Los Angeles, CA, USA

Katharina Pulch, Doris Klingelhöfer and David A. Groneberg
Department of Female Health and Preventive Medicine, Institute of Occupational Medicine, Social Medicine and Environmental Medicine, Goethe-University, Theodor-Stern Kai 7, 60590 Frankfurt, Germany

Celeste Leigh Pearce
Department of Epidemiology, School of Public Health, University of Michigan, Ann Arbor, MI, USA.

Nick Warren Ruktanonchai, Corrine Warren Ruktanonchai, Jessica Rhona Floyd and Andrew J. Tatem
WorldPop Project, Geography and Environment, University of Southampton, Southampton SO17 1BJ, UK
Flowminder Foundation, Roslagsgatan 17, 11355 Stockholm, Sweden

Fei Gao and Nolwenn Le Meur
EHESP Rennes, Sorbonne Paris Cité, Paris, France
L'équipe REPERES, Recherche en Pharmaco-épidémiologie et recours aux soins, UPRES EA-7449, Rennes, France
Department of Quantitative Methods for Public Health, EHESP School of Public Health, Avenue du Professeur Léon Bernard, 35043 Rennes, France

Séverine Deguen
EHESP Rennes, Sorbonne Paris Cité, Paris, France

Department of Social Epidemiology, Sorbonne Universités, UPMC Univ Paris 06, INSERM, Institut Pierre Louis d'Epidémiologie et de Santé Publique (UMRS 1136), Paris, France

Wahida Kihal
LIVE UMR 7362 CNRS (Laboratoire Image Ville Environnement), University of Strasbourg, 6700 Strasbourg, France

Marc Souris
IRD, UMR_D 190 "Emergence des Pathologies Virales" (IRD French Institute of Research for Development, Aix-Marseille University, EHESP French School of Public Health), Marseille, France

Caglar Koylu
Department of Geographical and Sustainability Sciences, University of Iowa, Iowa City, USA

Rahmi Nurhan Celik and Selman Delil
Informatics Institute, Istanbul Technical University, Istanbul, Turkey

Diansheng Guo
Department of Geography, University of South Carolina, Columbia, USA

Christine B. Phillips, Jonathan M. Kurka and Marc A. Adams
School of Nutrition and Health Promotion, Arizona State University, Phoenix, AZ, USA

Jessa K. Engelberg, Carrie M. Geremia, Kelli L. Cain, James F. Sallis and Terry L. Conway
Department of Family and Preventive Medicine, University of California, San Diego, San Diego, CA, USA

Wenfei Zhu
School of Physical Education, Shaanxi Normal University, Xi'an, Shaanxi, China

Astrid Etman, Alex Burdorf and Frank J. Van Lenthe
Department of Public Health, Erasmus University Medical Centre, 3000 CA Rotterdam, The Netherlands

Carlijn B. M. Kamphuis
Department of Public Health, Erasmus University Medical Centre, 3000 CA Rotterdam, The Netherlands
Department of Human Geography and Spatial Planning, Utrecht University, Utrecht, The Netherlands

Frank H. Pierik
Department of Urban Environment and Safety, TNO, Utrecht, The Netherlands

Dominique Mathon and Philippe Apparicio
Environmental Equity Laboratory, INRS Centre Urbanisation Culture Société, 385, rue Sherbrooke Est, Montréal, Québec H2X 1E3, Canada

Ugo Lachapelle
Département d'études urbaines et touristiques, Université du Québec à Montréal, Case postale 8888, Succursale Centre-Ville, Montréal, Québec H3C 3P8, Canada

Gijs Klous and Dick J. J. Heederik
Julius Centre for Health Sciences and Primary Care, University Medical Centre Utrecht, Utrecht, The Netherlands
Institute for Risk Assessment Sciences (IRAS), Division Environmental Epidemiology and Veterinary Public Health (EEPI-VPH), Utrecht University, Yalelaan 2, 3584 CM Utrecht, The Netherlands

Mirjam E. E. Kretzschmar
Julius Centre for Health Sciences and Primary Care, University Medical Centre Utrecht, Utrecht, The Netherlands
National Institute for Public Health and the Environment (RIVM), Bilthoven, The Netherlands

Roel A. Coutinho
Julius Centre for Health Sciences and Primary Care, University Medical Centre Utrecht, Utrecht, The Netherlands
Faculty of Veterinary Medicine, Utrecht University, Utrecht, The Netherlands

Lidwien A. M. Smit and Anke Huss
Institute for Risk Assessment Sciences (IRAS), Division Environmental Epidemiology and Veterinary Public Health (EEPI-VPH), Utrecht University, Yalelaan 2, 3584 CM Utrecht, The Netherlands

Floor Borlée
Institute for Risk Assessment Sciences (IRAS), Division Environmental Epidemiology and Veterinary Public Health (EEPI-VPH), Utrecht University, Yalelaan 2, 3584 CM Utrecht, The Netherlands
Netherlands Institute for Health Services Research (NIVEL), Utrecht, The Netherlands

Alina Svechkina, Marina Zusman, Natalya Rybnikova and Boris A. Portnov
Department of Natural Resources and Environmental Management, Faculty of Management, University of Haifa, 3498838 Mount Carmel, Haifa, Israel

Qian Chen, Xuchao Yang and Kejia Hu
Institute of Island and Coastal Ecosystems, Ocean College, Zhejiang University, Zhoushan 316021, China

Jiaguo Qi
Institute of Island and Coastal Ecosystems, Ocean College, Zhejiang University, Zhoushan 316021, China
Center for Global Change and Earth Observations, Michigan State University, East Lansing, MI 48823, USA

Mingjun Ding
Key Lab of Poyang Lake Wetland and Watershed Research of Ministry of Education, School of Geography and Environment, Jiangxi Normal University, Nanchang 330022, China

Carlijn B. M. Kamphuis
Department of Human Geography and Spatial Planning, Faculty of Geosciences, Utrecht University, Heidelberglaan 2, 3584 CS Utrecht, The Netherlands

Daniël C. van Wijk
Department of Human Geography and Spatial Planning, Faculty of Geosciences, Utrecht University, Heidelberglaan 2, 3584 CS Utrecht, The Netherlands
Department of Public Health, Erasmus University Medical Centre, Erasmus University Rotterdam, Wytemaweg 80, 3015 CN Rotterdam, The Netherlands

Joost Oude Groeniger and Frank J. van Lenthe
Department of Public Health, Erasmus University Medical Centre, Erasmus University Rotterdam, Wytemaweg 80, 3015 CN Rotterdam, The Netherlands

Index

www.ingramcontent.com/pod-product-compliance
Lightning Source LLC
Chambersburg PA
CBHW061249190326
41458CB00011B/3621